D1316114

EARLY DIAGNOSIS
OF ALZHEIMER'S DISEASE

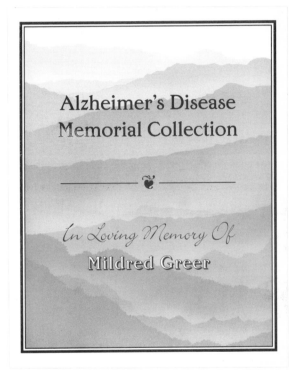

Alzheimer's Disease
Memorial Collection

In Loving Memory Of

Mildred Greer

CURRENT CLINICAL NEUROLOGY

Early Diagnosis of Alzheimer's Disease, edited by Leonard F. M. Scinto
and Kirk R. Daffner, *2000*
Sexual and Reproductive Neurorehabilitation, edited by Mindy Aisen, *1997*

EARLY DIAGNOSIS OF ALZHEIMER'S DISEASE

Edited by

LEONARD F. M. SCINTO, PhD
KIRK R. DAFFNER, MD

Department of Neurology
Brigham and Women's Hospital,
Harvard Medical School, Boston, MA

Foreword by

JOHN C. MORRIS, MD
Washington University School of Medicine
St. Louis, MO

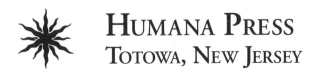

HUMANA PRESS
TOTOWA, NEW JERSEY

For additional copies, pricing for bulk purchases, and/or information about other Humana titles, contact Humana at the above address or at any of the following numbers: Tel.:973-256-1699; Fax: 973-256-8341; E-mail: humana@humanapr.com; or visit Humana on the Internet at: http://humanapress.com

This publication is printed on acid-free paper. ∞
ANSI Z39.48-1984 (American Standards Institute) Permanence of Paper for Printed Library Materials.

Cover illustration: Graph of theoretical progression of AD biomarkers superimposed over photomicrograph of AD tau pathology in the Edinger–Westphal nucleus. *Photomicrograph by Changiz Geula and Leonard F. M. Scinto.*

Due diligence has been taken by the publishers, editors, and authors of this book to assure the accuracy of the information published and to describe generally accepted practices. The contributors herein have carefully checked to ensure that the drug selections and dosages set forth in this text are accurate and in accord with the standards accepted at the time of publication. Notwithstanding, as new research, changes in government regulations, and knowledge from clinical experience relating to drug therapy and drug reactions constantly occurs, the reader is advised to check the product information provided by the manufacturer of each drug for any change in dosages or for additional warnings and contraindications. This is of utmost importance when the recommended drug herein is a new or infrequently used drug. It is the responsibility of the treating physician to determine dosages and treatment strategies for individual patients. Further it is the responsibility of the health care provider to ascertain the Food and Drug Administration status of each drug or device used in their clinical practice. The publisher, editors, and authors are not responsible for errors or omissions or for any consequences from the application of the information presented in this book and make no warranty, express or implied, with respect to the contents in this publication.

Printed in the United States of America. 10 9 8 7 6 5 4 3 2 1

Library of Congress Cataloging-in-Publication Data
Early diagnosis of Alzheimer's disease / edited by Leonard F. M. Scinto, Kirk R. Daffner.
        p.   cm. —(Current clinical neurology)
     Includes index.
     ISBN 0-89603-452-6 (alk. paper)
     1. Alzheimer's disease–Diagnosis. I. Scinto, Leonard F. M. II. Daffner, Kirk R. III. Series.
     [DNLM: 1. Alzheimer's Disease–diagnosis. 2. Alzheimer Disease–genetics. WT 155 E125 2000]
     RC523.E27   2000
     616.8'31075–dc21
     DNLM/DLC
     for Library of Congress   99-25252
                                                 CIP

In memory of Tom A. Sandson, MD *(1962–1999)*

FOREWORD

Dramatic increases in the life expectancy in the United States and other developed countries have resulted in unprecedented numbers and proportions of older adults in the population. This demographic evolution in turn has fueled growing interest in age-associated dementing illnesses, particularly Alzheimer's disease. The prevalence of Alzheimer's disease, by far the leading cause of dementia in the United States, doubles every 5 years after age 65 such that perhaps as many as one-half of all individuals age 85 years or older are demented.

Much has been learned about Alzheimer's disease since two milestone events occurred in 1984. First, uniform clinical diagnostic criteria were introduced by the Work Group convened by the National Institute on Neurological and Communicative Disorders and Stroke and the Alzheimer's Disease and Related Disorders Association (1) and provided the basis for the accurate recognition of the disorder. Second, Glenner and Wong isolated the beta amyloid peptide from meningeal vessels in Alzheimer's disease brain (2), thus ushering in an era of remarkable progress in deciphering the neurobiologic mechanisms underlying Alzheimer's disease and in developing drug therapies. The pace of scientific advance has been so rapid that it is easy to forget that only two decades ago the major issue regarding dementia was not therapy or biology, but simply whether it was possible to clinically differentiate Alzheimer's disease from other forms of "senile brain degeneration" and vascular dementia. Use of accurate clinical criteria with quantitative postmortem assessment, coincident with a reduction in vascular dementia owing to improved stroke prevention measures, now firmly establish Alzheimer's disease as the predominant cause of "senile" dementia.

There remain difficulties in dementia classification, however. In particular, it has not been possible to resolve whether aging and Alzheimer's disease are continuous or categorical processes because the clinical and pathological boundaries between the two conditions often are indistinct. The difficulty in distinguishing aging and Alzheimer's disease is underscored by the plethora of terms that have been introduced to characterize borderzone states in which the individual is neither clearly normal nor clearly demented: "benign senescent forgetfulness," "age-associated memory impairment," "pathological aging," "cognitive impairment, no dementia," and "mild cognitive impairment." At the same time, there is accumulating evidence to suggest that truly healthy brain aging can occur into the ninth and tenth decades of life and may be associated with less cognitive decline (3,4) and neuropathological changes (5) than usually are assumed. Such evidence indicates that more than minimal cognitive decline may not be "normal" for age and that much (perhaps most) of what presently is described as mild cognitive impairment (6) and similar states may represent incipient or very mild Alzheimer's disease.

It was not uncommon years ago to reserve the diagnosis of Alzheimer's disease for moderate-to-severe stages of dementia, a practice that reflected both uncertainty about distinguishing mild dementia from normal aging and the lack of incentive to make an "early" diagnosis when there was little to offer the patient. This attitude has been replaced by growing interest in diagnosing the disorder at earlier and earlier stages, stimulated by the advent of approved drugs for the symptomatic treatment of Alzheimer's disease (7) and the promise of newer agents that may halt dementia progression or even prevent the disease. Thus, therapeutic nihilism is being dispelled. Impetus for detection of early-stage Alzheimer's disease also comes from the realization that investigations of proposed causative mechanisms and putative biomarkers should not be limited to advanced disease, in which critical findings that distinguish disease from aging may be obscured.

This volume on the early diagnosis of Alzheimer's disease is both timely and compelling. It offers contributions from a superb group of experts who have helped define the relevant issues and led critical clinical and scientific advances in early-stage diagnosis. The first three chapters justify the importance of accurate diagnosis and describe the clinical and pathological phenotypes for early-stage Alzheimer's disease. Chapter 4 provides a masterful review of the molecular pathology of the disorder and proposes a schema for its initiating pathophysiologic events. Chapters 5 and 12 cogently discuss the current state of knowledge for the genetics of Alzheimer's disease as well as the important implications of genetic testing for early diagnosis and presymptomatic detection. The encouraging potential roles for structural and functional neuroimaging as tools for diagnosis and for monitoring response in therapeutic trials of antidementia agents are reviewed in Chapters 6 and 7. The clinical utility of cognitive testing in detecting and predicting early-stage Alzheimer's disease is cogently discussed in Chapter 8. Chapters 9 and 10 comprehensively review the promise and limitations of proposed biomarkers for Alzheimer's disease. Chapter 11 summarizes the status of currently approved therapies for Alzheimer's disease and convincingly argues that early-stage illness should be a target for intervention.

The editors are to be commended for the extraordinarily high quality of the contributing authors and the chapters and for focusing attention on the topic of early-stage Alzheimer's disease. As we move into the next century, I predict that the early diagnosis of Alzheimer's disease will become a dominant issue for clinicians, patients, and their families as new therapies are developed and new research discoveries occur. This volume not only serves as a testimonial to the value of early diagnosis, but provides clinicians and scientists with the basis to appreciate ongoing developments in this emerging and important field.

John C. Morris, MD

References

1. McKhann G, Drachman D, Folstein M, Katzman R, Price D, Stadlan EM. Clinical diagnosis of Alzheimer's disease: Report of the NINCDS-ADRDA Work Group under the auspices of Department of Health and Human Services Task Force on Alzheimer's disease. Neurology 1984;34:939–944.
2. Glenner GG, Wong CW. Alzheimer's disease: initial report of the purification and characterization of a novel cerebrovascular amyloid protein. Biochem Biophys Res Commun 1984;120:885–890.
3. Rubin EH, Storandt M, Miller JP, Kinscherf DA, Grant EA, Morris JC, et al. A prospective study of cognitive function and onset of dementia in cognitively healthy elders. Arch Neurol 1998;55:395–401.
4. Haan MN, Shemanski L, Jagust WJ, Manolio TA, Kuller L. The role of APOE ε4 in modulating effects of other risk factors for cognitive decline in elderly persons. JAMA 1999;282:40–46.
5. Price JL, Morris JC. Tangles and plaques in nondemented aging and preclinical Alzheimer's disease. Ann Neurol 1999;45:358–368.
6. Petersen RC, Smith GE, Waring SC, Ivnik RJ, Tangalos EG, Kokmen E. Mild cognitive impairment. Arch Neurol 1999;56:303–308.
7. Knopman D, Morris LC. An update on primary drug therapies for Alzheimer's disease. Arch Neurol 1997;54:1406–1409.

PREFACE

As the population ages, an increasing number of individuals are at risk for degenerative diseases such as Alzheimer's disease (AD). *Early Diagnosis of Alzheimer's Disease* has been written out of the conviction that without an understanding of the complex issues surrounding the search for early markers for Alzheimer's disease, the prospects for early diagnosis and, consequently, the development of new interventions for the disease will, at best, be delayed. In the past few years, we have seen a proliferation of research on methods to detect Alzheimer's disease early in its course. It is an excellent time to take stock of the progress of this rapidly expanding field.

The chapters in *Early Diagnosis of Alzheimer's Disease* review the most promising approaches in current research on early diagnostic markers for AD. These approaches include the elucidation of changes in the brain as seen in structural and functional neuroimaging, characteristic patterns of cognitive decline as documented by sensitive neuropsychological tests, various genetic markers, and a wide array of biological assays. We have placed these different approaches to early diagnosis within a broader context by also reviewing current clinical practice in diagnosing AD, major theories about its pathophysiology, and the therapeutic and ethical implications of early diagnosis. Each of the areas explored in *Early Diagnosis of Alzheimer's Disease* holds promise for contributing to the development of strategies for meeting the diagnostic and therapeutic challenge posed by AD.

Early Diagnosis of Alzheimer's Disease is addressed to a broad audience within the biomedical research and clinical communities. It should be of interest to clinicians who endeavor to care for an aging population, researchers working in the area of new therapeutic approaches to the disease, and policymakers who are concerned about the implications surrounding early diagnosis and the delivery of health care. Although the work gathered here provides a timely summary of different approaches for the early diagnosis of AD, we hope it will make a more lasting contribution in setting a framework for future research and critical thinking on the many issues surrounding early diagnosis. We are grateful to our fellow authors who have contributed their time and expertise to this work. Such a cooperative effort by many scholars from a variety of disciplines serves as a model for how important questions concerning diagnosis and therapy will need to be pursued to find adequate solutions to the puzzle of AD.

We thank the staff at Humana Press for their patience and care in the production of this volume. We appreciate the effort of Barbara Vericker during the planning and execution of this work. Her talents have added immeasurably to its successful completion.

Leonard F. M. Scinto, PhD
Kirk R. Daffner, MD

CONTENTS

CONTRIBUTORS

DAVID F. ANDREWS, PhD • *Department of Statistics, University of Toronto, Toronto, Ontario, Canada*

DEBORAH L. BLACKER, MD • *Department of Psychiatry, Massachusetts General Hospital, Harvard Medical School, Boston, MA*

KIRK R. DAFFNER, MD • *Brigham Memory Disorders Unit, Division of Cognitive and Behavioral Neurology, Brigham and Women's Hospital, Harvard Medical School, Boston, MA*

CHANGIZ GEULA, PhD • *Laboratory for Neurodegenerative and Aging Research, Beth Israel Deaconess Medical Center, Harvard Medical School, Boston, MA*

CLIFFORD R. JACK, JR., MD • *Department of Diagnostic Radiology, Mayo Clinic and Foundation, Rochester, MN*

KEITH A. JOHNSON, MD • *Department of Radiology, Brigham and Women's Hospital, Harvard Medical School, Boston, MA*

DAVID S. KNOPMAN, MD • *Department of Neurology, University of Minnesota, Minneapolis, MN*

KENNETH S. KOSIK, MD • *Center for Neurologic Diseases, Brigham and Women's Hospital, Harvard Medical School, Boston, MA*

MAIRE E. PERCY, PhD • *Departments of Physiology and Obstetrics & Gynecology, University of Toronto, Toronto, Ontario, Canada*

RONALD C. PETERSEN, PhD, MD • *Department of Neurology, Mayo Clinic and Foundation, Rochester, MN*

STEPHEN G. POST, PhD • *Center for Biomedical Ethics, Case Western Reserve University School of Medicine, Cleveland, OH*

HUNTINGTON POTTER, PhD • *Department of Biochemistry and Molecular Biology, University of South Florida College of Medicine, Tampa, FL*

KIMBERLY A. QUAID, PhD • *Department of Medical and Molecular Genetics, Indiana University School of Medicine, Indianapolis, IN*

DORENE M. RENTZ, PsyD • *Laboratory of Higher Cortical Functions, Brigham and Women's Hospital, Harvard Medical School, Boston, MA*

THOMAS A. SANDSON, MD • *Behavioral Neurology Unit, Beth Israel Deaconess Medical Center, Harvard Medical School, Boston, MA (Deceased)*

LEONARD F. M. SCINTO, PhD • *Laboratory of Higher Cortical Functions, Brigham and Women's Hospital, Harvard Medical School, Boston, MA*

DENNIS J. SELKOE, MD • *Center for Neurologic Diseases, Brigham and Women's Hospital, Harvard Medical School, Boston, MA*

REISA A. SPERLING, MD • *Brigham Memory Disorders Unit, Division of Cognitive and Behavioral Neurology, Brigham and Women's Hospital, Harvard Medical School, Boston, MA*

RUDOLPH E. TANZI, PhD • *Laboratory of Genetics and Aging Research, Masschusetts General Hospital–East, Harvard Medical School, Charlestown, MA*

SANDRA WEINTRAUB, PhD • *Center for Cognitive and Behavioral Neurology, Northwestern University Medical School, Chicago, IL*

1

Early Diagnosis of Alzheimer's Disease

An Introduction

Kirk R. Daffner and Leonard F.M. Scinto

Alzheimer's Disease: The Scope of the Problem

Alzheimer's disease (AD) is poised to become the scourge of the next century, bringing with it enormous social and personal costs. Depending on the methods of assessment used, estimates of the prevalence of dementia due to AD in Americans 65 and older range from 6% to 10% *(1–3)*. The prevalence of the disease doubles every 5 years after the age of 60 *(4–6)*. For the population 85 and older, estimates of the prevalence have been as high as 30–47% *(1–3)*. As many as 4 million Americans may suffer from a clinical dementia of the Alzheimer's type, with an annual cost of approximately $100 billion *(7)*. Based on current rates, and in the absence of effective prevention, it is estimated that in 50 years, there will be as many as 14 million cases of clinically diagnosed Alzheimer's disease in the United States alone. While AD is a major public health problem, it also has a very private face that causes tremendous suffering to families. For the elderly, it one of the most dreaded afflictions that threatens to rob them of their independence and dignity at the end of life.

Early Diagnosis: So What?

This book addresses issues surrounding early diagnosis in Alzheimer's disease. It is predicated on the belief that early, accurate diagnosis of AD is important and will become increasingly so in the future. At first glance, this proposition may seem foolish. Given the current absence of very effective therapies to reverse, arrest, or prevent the disease process, why should clinicians and scientists be concerned that diagnosis of this illness is accurate and occurs early in its course? Some might consider a book dedicated to

From: *Early Diagnosis of Alzheimer's Disease*
Edited by L. F. M. Scinto & K. R. Daffner © Humana Press, Inc., Totowa, NJ

"Early Treatment" to be much more relevant to current health-care concerns. Our position is simple. Early treatment is not feasible in the absence of early diagnosis. Interest in effective treatment demands attention to effective diagnosis. The development of clinical trials and the subsequent availability of therapies aimed at slowing the disease process early in its course will depend on our improved ability to identify patients in the earliest stages of the illness.

Alzheimer's disease is a progressive neurodegenerative disorder that leads to the death of brain cells that cannot be replaced once lost. Thus, the best hope for controlling the ravages of this disease that ultimately disrupt cognitive and behavioral functioning lies in early treatment aimed at stemming the pathological process. For treatment to have the greatest impact on the disease, we need to be able to recognize individuals in the earliest stages, before they manifest clinical symptoms such as significant memory impairment. Even "palliative" treatment, initiated during the period in which there is demonstrated cognitive impairment, but no major disruption of daily activities, may delay the progression of functional decline by several years and have a profound impact on the service needs of our aging population *(8).*

In the last few years, there has been a proliferation of reports on potential diagnostic markers or tests for AD *(9–59c).* Thus, it is a propitious time to carefully review the data on these varied approaches and help bring order to this growing field. In doing so, we hope to provide a framework for evaluating new techniques as they become available.

Even as we await the development of more effective treatments for AD, we should endeavor to ensure accurate diagnosis. This helps to guard against misdiagnosing dementias that are currently amenable to treatment, such as those due to depression, toxic-metabolic states, or normal pressure hydrocephalus. It is estimated that 10–15% of cases of dementia are due to a potentially reversible cause *(60,61).* Diagnostic accuracy also is important for families, who can better prepare for the future when they have been informed of the patient's prognosis. Pharmaceutical trials require accurate diagnosis to select appropriate subjects for study (see Chapters 8 and 11). The inappropriate inclusion of patients without underlying AD is likely to lead to incorrect conclusions about the efficacy of the therapy being evaluated. Most trials that have been conducted to date have studied patients in the moderate or mild-to-moderate stage of the illness. There is growing interest in testing medications in patients who are in the earliest clinical stages of the illness, when treatment can have a more profound impact on functional status and rate of decline. As new classes of medications are developed (e.g, aimed at slowing underlying disease progression), studies may be directed at individuals in the preclinical stages of the illness. Such future trials will depend on further advances in our ability to identify such individuals.

Clinical Versus Pathological Dimensions of AD

Rigorous study of a progressive neurological disease such as AD requires that we appreciate the distinction between its clinical and pathological dimensions. Clinically, AD most commonly manifests as an insidiously progressive decline in cognitive and functional status, with salient disruption of memory and other intellectual functions (see Chapter 2 for clinical definitions of AD). There are several different, but largely overlapping sets of criteria that specify the pattern of symptoms and signs required for a clinical diagnosis of AD (often designated as "probable Alzheimer's disease" or dementia of the Alzheimer's type) *(62–64)*. Pathologically, AD is characterized by the presence of plaques and tangles (more strictly by an excessive density of plaques and tangles). As with the clinical definition of the disorder, various consensus statements offer slightly different pathological criteria *(65–67)*. (This issue is detailed in Chapter 3.)

Demented patients who fit the clinical diagnostic criteria for probable AD have a high probability of having the underlying plaque and tangle pathology of AD. However, a small proportion of patients with symptoms and signs consistent with a clinical diagnosis of AD will turn out to have a different underlying pathology *(68–76)*. Likewise, a small proportion of demented individuals with underlying AD pathology will manifest clinical patterns that are atypical for dementia of the Alzheimer's type. Rather than exhibiting salient memory problems, these patients may present with relatively isolated disruption of language, visuospatial functions, or executive cognitive functions *(77–82)*.

A large body of evidence now points to the fact that the pathology of AD may represent an insidious process developing over as many as 15 to 20 years before there are any clinical manifestations *(83–89)*. While there is ongoing discussion over which pathological marker (i.e, tangle burden, plaque count, synaptic loss) is most closely linked to dementia severity *(90–95)*, there is no debate over the fact that overt clinical manifestations of the disease occur after the presence of significant neuropathological abnormality. In this regard, AD is similar to Parkinson's disease, in which 50–60% of the pigmented neurons in the substantia nigra pars compacta must be lost before the patient shows definite clinical signs *(96)*.

This distinction between the clinical and pathological dimensions of AD highlights some of the major challenges associated with early diagnosis and the search for biological markers of the disease. By the time a patient is recognized as clinically demented, considerable irreversible brain damage has already taken place. For example, in patients who have just begun to show the earliest clinical symptoms of dementia [i.e, with Clinical Dementia Rating (CDR) *(87,97)* score of 0.5 as defined below], 50% of the neurons in entorhinal cortex, a crucial anatomic component of memory processing, have already been lost *(98)*. Hence many individuals who are considered clinically "normal" will have definite neuropathological features of AD.

Some investigators might disagree with this perspective, arguing that since a large portion of "nondemented" elders have some degree of plaque and tangle pathology at autopsy, one should take the position that individuals who are not clinically symptomatic do not have the disease. The motive behind subordinating the pathological to the clinical dimension may be a desire to avoid distressing and stigmatizing elderly people who do not have any symptoms. Here, the pathological plane becomes subordinate to the clinical one in an effort not to call something a disease in the elderly before it manifests symptoms.* This viewpoint would be consistent with the position that aging individuals with progressive narrowing of the coronary arteries do not have a disease until they

---

*It is beyond the scope of this book to adequately address the debate over the relationship between so-called normal aging and AD (refs. *a–e*). Some of the pertinent issues are considered in the sections addressing AD pathology (Chapter 3) and early cognitive changes (Chapter 8). Two antithetical views have been posed: one emphasizing the continuity and the other the differences between normal aging and AD. On a pathological plane, some would argue that qualitatively, normal aging and AD are very similar. The differences are only quantitative, with AD reflecting greater plaque and tangle burden (ref. *f*). AD is seen as an inevitable consequence of the aging process, such that anyone who lived "long enough" would develop the disease. From this perspective, the "dividing line" between normal aging and AD is relatively arbitrary. If the more extreme version of this view turns out to be correct, it would pose a challenge to efforts to identify individuals in the presymptomatic stages of AD. Even on pathological grounds, there would be no way to distinguish such individuals from those undergoing the "normal" aging process. One way to deal with this perspective is to suggest that from a practical perspective, we could aim to develop diagnostic markers in the presymptomatic stage that indicate that "pathology" has surpassed some critical threshold, presumably because an individual was further along in the aging/AD process and closer to manifesting a dementia. Also, it is possible that, while plaques and tangles may be part of normal aging, AD involves a much faster rate of progression of this process, which could theoretically be determined by measuring plaque and tangle density at different points in time.

An alternative view is that AD is not inextricably linked to normal aging, but represents a specific disease process. Like many other illnesses, the incidence of AD increases with age. Some have argued that even the presence of diffuse amyloid plaques is not part of normal aging, but represents presymptomatic or unrecognized early AD (refs. *a,c,g*).

manifest symptoms of cardiac ischemia. As we gather more tools for identifying preclinical markers and more effective therapies for AD, we anticipate a shift toward a more pathology-oriented perspective because it favors early identification and secondary prevention.

The relationship between AD pathology and clinical symptoms is not necessarily a simple or linear one and is likely to be mediated by a range of factors, including the patient's education ("cerebral reserve") and concomitant medical illnesses *(99–104)*. There certainly are reports of individuals, who, in life, were viewed by their families and physicians as "normal," but at autopsy would have met established criteria for a pathological diagnosis of AD *(83–88,105–106)*. How then are we to understand the relationship between the clinical and pathological planes for aging individuals who are not currently demented? One way is to view AD neuropathology as the greatest risk factor for developing the clinical syndrome of probable AD. This view establishes a context in which early diagnosis and intervention are possible while conceding that some people developing AD pathology will die before they manifest clinical symptoms.

Stages of the Illness

Figure 1 schematically illustrates a proposed time line for the development of AD pathology and its impact on functional status. It posits progressive degenerative changes and a "threshold" degree of neuropathological damage beyond which an individual manifests the clinical syndrome of dementia. By definition, that threshold is marked by observable decline in functional status that interferes with a person's activities of daily living. Ideally, decline is judged on the basis of changes from a particular person's premorbid status. In practice, it is often more crudely assessed by noting a disruption of common activities such as maintaining a checkbook, household responsibilities and chores, and personal hygiene. However, the more the determination of functional decline is adjusted for the patient's baseline, the less the clinical diagnosis will be affected by her socioeconomic, cultural, and educational background.

For heuristic purposes, the "journey" between normal brain functioning and clinical dementia can be divided into different stages:

1. Presymptomatic
2. Preclinical
3. Very early, "questionable" dementia
4. Mild dementia
5. Moderate dementia
6. Severe dementia

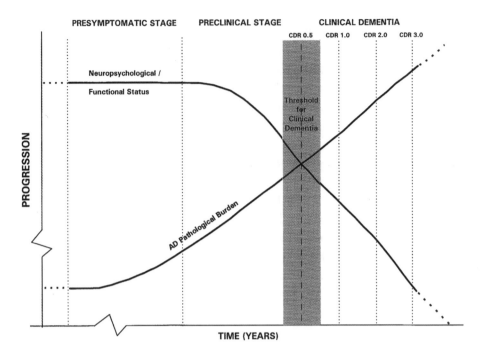

Fig. 1. Theoretical time line for Alzheimer's disease.

In the *presymptomatic* stage, there is an insidious pathological process in the brain, but there are no mental or behavioral symptoms, no impairment of everyday functioning, and no abnormalities on neuropsychological testing, even using tests sensitive to subtle decrements in performance. When baseline neuropsychological test data are available, results at the time of clinical evaluation would show no significant changes from the baseline. The existence of such a stage is supported by pathology series showing characteristic AD lesions in the absence of any observable or measurable clinical deficits on an antemortem evaluation *(83–88,105–106)*. The notion of a presymptomatic stage is further bolstered by evidence of such a period in patients with Down syndrome who, in middle age, invariably develop a clinical dementia marked by AD pathology at autopsy *(107–109)*. In this presymptomatic stage, some biological markers may be positive, permitting identification of candidates for intervention aimed at prevention of the disease.

In the *preclinical* stage, subtle deficits, especially in memory, are detectable by formal testing of cognitive performance. However, these deficits are not associated with any impairments in daily living. Such individuals would still rate a 0 classification on the CDR scale *(87,97)*. Deficits in this stage can be detected by employing a comprehensive and sensitive battery of neuropsychological tests (see Chapter 8 for a discussion of such batteries and preclinical AD).

As individuals approach the threshold for dementia, they may begin to exhibit subtle signs of functional and cognitive deterioration, suggestive of a clinical dementia. The Clinical Dementia Rating scale has designated this period with a score of 0.5. Such individuals exhibit mild forgetfulness, along with subtle impairment of judgment, home and community activities, or occupational functioning.* In one series by Morris and colleagues *(87)*, all 10 of the individuals at this stage were found at autopsy to meet pathological criteria for AD. Several research groups have demonstrated that elders who exhibit this kind of mild impairment in memory and daily functioning go on to develop a full-blown syndrome of dementia at a rate of 10% to 15% per year, which is approximately 5 to 7 times higher than for age-matched individuals who do not exhibit such impairment *(50,110)*.

By the time individuals reach a CDR stage of 1.0, there is no doubt that they have dementia, albeit of mild severity. Memory impairment interferes with everyday activities. There are growing difficulties handling complex problems and managing independence in household responsibilities and daily activities such as maintaining one's residence, handling finances, or reliably taking medication for concomitant medical illnesses.

Patients with dementia of moderate severity (CDR stage 2), exhibit significant memory loss, frequent disorientation, impairment of social judgment, and an increasing need for supervision in their daily living activities, including maintenance of personal hygiene and the cleanliness and safety of their residence. In the severe stages of the illness (CDR score of 3 and beyond), patients are totally dependent on others for personal care and everyday problem-solving. At the end of the disease, they lose the capacity to communicate, recognize caregivers, feed themselves, or walk without assistance.

According to this scheme for dementia staging, what is being "diagnosed" depends on whether we are considering the presypmtomatic or symptomatic stages of the illness. In the presymptomatic stages, what is being "diagnosed" is the underlying Alzheimer's pathological process, with the presumption that individuals with such markers are at high risk for developing a clinical dementia. In the symptomatic stages of the illness, what is being diagnosed is

---

*Individuals in this stage of the illness are likely to need more time when interacting with health care professionals in order to understand and carry out instructions. Currently, the system often fails to identify such individuals or provide them with the additional time they require.

the clinical syndrome of dementia and a specific brain disease that accounts for it. Most often, current clinical practice focuses on the latter goal, as reviewed in Chapter 2. Often, the major effort is on excluding ("ruling out") other potential causes of dementia rather than making a positive diagnosis of AD. Most of the new diagnostic strategies reviewed in this book have focused, at least initially, on patients in the mild to moderate stages of the illness. In the past few years, there has been growing research (using longitudinal studies) on at-risk individuals in early or preclinical stages of the disease.

Candidate Markers

Since the pathological process precedes the clinical manifestations of the disease, the earliest markers for the illness may not be found if the search for them begins with the first clinical symptoms. To aid diagnosis in the presymptomatic and preclinical stages, we need to find biological markers for the disease that are detectable well before even subtle clinical symptoms are apparent.

Many of the proposed markers for the AD process will be discussed throughout this book. Although, there are substantial differences in the existing approaches, in general, two major strategies have been employed. One strategy takes advantage of the characteristic anatomic distribution of the neuropathological changes of AD. The other strategy measures presumed byproducts of the underlying pathological process in, for example, cerebrospinal fluid (CSF), serum, urine, or skin.

Like any degenerative illness, AD does not afflict all neuroanatomical locations with equal severity. As is discussed in Chapter 3, there is a characteristic pattern of progression in the cortex that initially emphasizes limbic and posterior association regions and tends to spare primary sensorimotor areas *(21,94,98,111–121)*. This distribution differs substantially from other degenerative processes such as frontotemporal dementia, which has a predilection for frontal and anterior temporal lobes *(78,81,122–124)*. Many of the proposed diagnostic strategies take advantage of the relative anatomical selectivity of AD pathology, especially early in the course of the illness. The early involvement of limbic regions such as the entorhinal cortex and hippocampus is the basis for using morphometric MRI analysis of mesial temporal structures to distinguish patients with AD from normal controls, as discussed in Chapter 6. The early destruction of these regions essential to neuropsychological functions such as memory provides the anatomical basis for the pattern of neuropsychological deficits that mark the preclinical and early stages of the illness, as reviewed in Chapter 8. Functional imaging studies also take advantage of the predictable distribution of disrupted cortical metabolic or perfusion activity, which most often involves bilateral temporoparietal cortex, as reviewed in Chapter 7. Finally, the observations of exaggerated pupillary dilation to dilute tropicamide (a topical cholinergic antagonist) may be due to the early development of pathology in the Edinger-Westphal nucleus of the midbrain, a center for the regulation of pupillary response (see Chapter 10).

All strategies that take advantage of the distributional predilection of the AD pathological process suffer from the same potential limitations. The findings are not pathognomonic of AD. Other diseases that may affect similar areas of the brain could generate similar patterns and thus "false positive" results. Moreover, atypical cases of AD, with an unusual distribution of pathology, would likely yield false negative results. Although such problems might potentially diminish the utility of these diagnostic tools, we suspect that atypical presentations of AD and non-AD processes with overlapping anatomic distributional characteristics represent a relatively small percentage of cases. The impact of such cases on the diagnostic accuracy of these tests is an empirical question that will need to be addressed.

The second major strategy, measuring components or by-products of the pathological process of AD, relies on an understanding of the pathophysiology underlying AD. Chapter 4 presents one of the dominant theories about the pathogenesis of the illness. Additional information about the biology of the disease can be found in Chapter 5, addressing genetic factors, and Chapter 9 on peripheral markers. Despite major advances, many questions remain that have implications about "translating" our understanding of the biology of the illness into diagnostic strategies: Which products are directly linked to the pathologic process, and which represent nonspecific responses to ongoing cerebral injury? Which can be usefully measured without a brain biopsy? Which turn positive in the presymptomatic and preclinical phases? Some putative markers of AD, such as tau protein, are also found in other diseases. Thus, their specificity will depend in part on the distribution of the various dementing illnesses in a study population. Also, many assays currently require CSF. The need for a lumbar puncture is likely to limit their widespread application. Chapter 9 reviews a broad range of peripheral markers that have been proposed, including measurements of CSF tau, beta amyloid, neuronal thread protein, serum melanotransferin (P97), and mitochondrial DNA mutations. Recently, a consensus statement on criteria for evaluating potential biomarkers for the disease has been issued jointly by the Ronald and Nancy Reagan Research Institute of the Alzheimer's Association and the National Institute on Aging Working Group (*see* the Appendix, pp. 329–348, for the complete report).

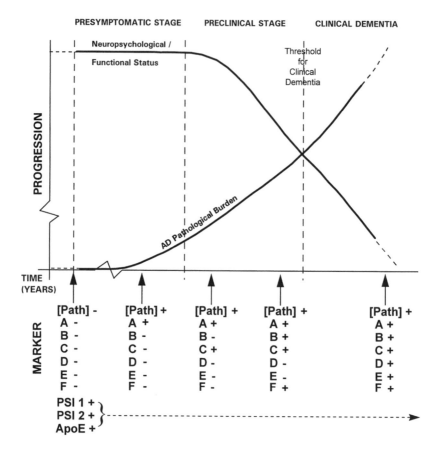

Fig. 2. Theoretical sequence of biological markers for Alzheimer's disease.

Biological markers must be capable of detecting some aspect of the pathological cascade of AD that leads to end-stage disease. Different markers will tap different components of this pathological cascade at different points in the pathological process. Some markers may be manifested at relatively early periods in the presymptomatic stage, while others may only become positive in response to the presence of pathology at later periods. The best markers are those most directly related to the pathologic process or that are uniquely a consequence of the pathology. Moreover, they would predict as early as possible the presence of a pathological process that leads to end-stage disease. Figure 2 illustrates the concept of biologic markers that "turn positive" in sequence. Since few data are available to order the currently proposed markers, the scheme is presented without naming specific markers.

It seems unlikely that any single marker will predict the development of clinical symptoms with 100% certainty. We suspect that in the future more researchers will take advantage of combining information from different techniques. For example, statistical techniques such as logistic regression and discrete-time survival analysis can be applied to data from longitudinal studies of at-risk elders, many, but not all, of whom subsequently become demented. These methods permit the development of models that reflect the relative predictive value of different biological markers. Once validated on a second sample, they can provide clinically useful estimates of the probability that individuals will develop dementia of the Alzheimer type. We can imagine setting a threshold probability level that would trigger the initiation of newly developed therapies. As we learn more about the relationship between specific indicators and the natural history of the disease, models assigning weights to different markers should have increasing clinical utility.

Distinguishing Between Diagnostic Tests and Risk Factors

When we consider diagnostic techniques, it is important to distinguish assays that mark the presence of a specific pathological process from tests that only assess the risk for the disease. This distinction is often blurred when genetic tests are considered. Chapter 5 is devoted to a review of genetic markers and AD. The presence of specific genetic abnormalities such as the presenilin mutations on chromosome 1 and 14, do signal that disease will follow with extremely high, if not 100%, certainty *(125,126)*. However, such findings are not diagnostic in the strict sense of the word. The presence of such mutations tell us that disease will inevitably develop, but they do not tell us if the disease process is currently active and ongoing, or exactly when it will begin. Other genetic markers such as an apolipoprotein ε4 allele do not signal the inevitable onset of disease. Rather, this genetic factor implies an increased risk for earlier onset of AD. Not all individuals who possess an ε4 allele will develop the disease. Several consensus statements have strongly argued against using ApoE status as a predictive or diagnostic test *(127–130)*.

Combining information about a patient's current cognitive status with her genetic inheritance may permit a more definitive set of inferences. For example, if a member of a family with an autosomal dominant form of AD secondary to a presenilin mutation exhibited cognitive impairment and early symptoms of dementia, it is extremely likely that the decline was due to underlying AD pathology. A similar argument has been made for late-onset dementias in patients with Apo ε4 alleles *(39,58)*. It has been proposed that the presence of an Apo ε4 allele in an older patient with the dementia syndrome raises the probability of AD from approximately 66% to over 90% *(39)*.

However, the pattern of clinical deficits characteristic of AD would also raise the probablity of having underlying AD pathology to 85–90% *(68–76)*. In such cases, the additional value of knowing Apo ε status in improving diagnostic accuracy is less clear. A large-scale multicenter study *(131)* suggested that ApoE genotyping in combination with clinical criteria for Alzheimer's disease can significantly improve the specificity of the diagnosis.

Assessing the Value of Candidate Tests: Epidemiological Considerations

Diagnostic tests are often judged on the basis of their sensitivity, specificity, and predictive value. Recall that sensitivity is defined as the probability that a test will be positive when the disease is present and specificity reflects the probability that a test will be negative if the disease is not present. Ideally, a test for AD would be both highly sensitive and specific. Most biological tests under consideration have a range of values. Establishing cutoff points for disease usually involves a tradeoff between sensitivity and specificity. The relationship between sensitivity and specificity can be characterized by a *receiver operator characteristic* (ROC) curve that plots the probability of having a true positive result against that of a false positive one for a range of cutoff scores (see Fig. 3). Generally, sensitivity is emphasized when failure to detect a disease has very deleterious consequences. Specificity is emphasized when a false-positive result leads to potential harm. In terms of tests for AD, the "ideal" set point of this balancing act will evolve over time as a reflection of changes in the risk:benefit ratio of treatments being developed. New tests that allow for improvement of both sensitivity and specificity (shifting the ROC curve) would be considered an advance over current diagnostic probes. Furthermore, tests also will need to be judged by how *early* they can sensitively detect the underlying AD pathologic process without generating a false-positive rate that is too high.*

Clinically, diagnostic tests are evaluated not by sensitivity and specificity, but rather their positive predictive value (PPV), that is, the probability that the disease is present if the test is positive and their negative predictive value, the probability that there is no disease if the test is negative. Such information is what clinicians and their patients are interested in knowing when a test has been ordered. The PPV is defined as the number of true positives divided by the sum of

---

*It is likely that diagnostic tests will have different ROC curves for each of the stages of AD that we have discussed. For example, the sensitivity of marker A for a given specificity (say 80%) may be 95% at CDR stage 2, 60% at CDR stage 0.5, and 30% for the preclinical stage. Conceivably, the most appropriate set point for a given ROC curve between sensitivity and specificity would be different for each stage.

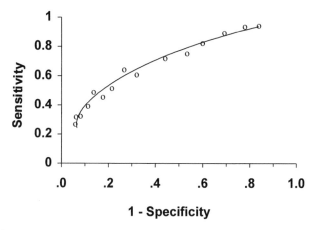

Fig. 3.   Example of a receiver operator characteristic (ROC) curve.

the true positives plus the false positives. Central to calculating the PPV is an estimate of the prevalence of the disease (prior probability) in the community being tested. According to the Bayes theorem, PPV can be calculated as follows:

$$PPV = (prevalence \times sensitivity) / [(prevalence \times sensitivity)$$
$$+ (1 - prevalence) \times (1 - specificity)].$$

Prior probability determines how much of an impact the false positive rate (i.e, $1 -$ specificity) has on the predictive value of the test. For example, even if a test were 99% sensitive and 99% specific, if the prior probability were only 1%, the PPV only would be 50%. By contrast, if the prior probability were 50%, the PPV would be 99%.

Thus, for Alzheimer's disease, if the estimated prevalence is relatively low, even a very sensitive and specific test would have limited predictive value. However, establishing true prevalence rates for AD is not as straightforward as it might first appear. The prevalence reported in the literature reflects an estimate of the number of clinically demented cases in a particular age range that are felt to be due to AD. Some reports have suggested that as many as 10% of Americans over the age of 65 and nearly 50% of elders over 85 suffer from a clinical dementia of the Alzheimer's type *(1)*. There are several limitations to using established prevalence estimates to evaluate the usefulness of newer diagnostic strategies. First, these numbers are based on current methods for diagnosing the disease. They identify individuals whose clinical state has declined to the point of being demented, but do not include individuals who are in the preclinical or presympotmatic stages of the illness. Currently, there is no definitive way to identify such individuals for an accurate estimate of the prevalence of AD pathology in the community. Several lines of evidence would suggest that the prevalence is quite high. For example, if 40–50% of individuals over 85 suffer from a clinical dementia of the Alzheimer's type and if the disease process begins 15–20 years before a person is clinically demented, then 40–50% of individuals in their early 70s may have developing AD pathology. While these particular numbers may represent the "worst-case scenario," the logic behind them needs to be taken seriously. Certainly, in evaluating tests for AD in the presymptomatic stages, we will need new ways of estimating prior probability of underlying pathology in order to assess the potential utility of the assays.

Review of the epidemiological aspects of early diagnosis of AD parallels discussions of screening tests in medicine that address ways of evaluating at-risk populations. However, the current approach to diagnosis in AD distinguishes it from other diseases for which screening tests are common. Most often, a positive result on a screening evaluation leads to "more definitive" tests (e.g, occult blood in the stool on a screening examination leads to colonoscopy and/or radiological studies; an abnormal screening digital prostate examination or positive PSA results in sonography and biopsy of the prostate). Unfortunately, short of brain biopsy, which is very rarely done, there is currently no "gold standard" marker for AD (see below) that could provide the next level of assessment. Thus, in AD the usual distinction between screening and diagnostic tests is blurred. Despite the absence of a definitive noninvasive marker for AD, one can still make use of test data. A positive test can help identify elders at greatest risk for becoming demented. Such information could result in following them with greater vigilance. Confirmatory evidence could come in the form of a convergence of other diagnostic markers or clinical signs that become positive over time. Depending on the risk:benefit profile of available therapies, the threshold for initiating treatment in such patients might be lowered. Unfortunately, there are also potential negative social consequences in identifying elders at increased risk for becoming demented. Such information could be used by insurance companies or other members of society to deprive them of potential benefits. These important issues are discussed in Chapter 12.

Assessing the Value of Candidate Tests: The Problem of No Gold Standard

As noted above, one of the greatest challenges facing the assessment of candidate early markers for AD, especially those in the presymptomatic phase of the illness, is the lack of an appropriate in vivo "gold standard" upon which to make a judgment. Consider, for example, two biological markers that are tested on a group of elderly individuals who currently are not clinically demented. If one of the markers is positive in a portion of these elders and the other is negative in all cases, how do we know which test is better. The former test either might have an unacceptably high false-positive rate, thus limiting the value of the test, or might usefully identify disease before other potential indicators turn positive. Markers of the illness that only turn positive after the onset of a clinical diagnosis of dementia ultimately will have limited value. However, they would enable the clinicians to "positively" confirm AD as the specific cause of dementia rather than only use a "rule-out" approach to the diagnosis of the illness.

Currently, cross-sectional designs are most commonly used to assess the accuracy of a proposed diagnostic marker. In one form of this research strategy, test results on a group of patients with a clinical diagnosis of AD are compared to test results on a group of matched, nondemented control subjects. In a related approach, test results of patients with probable AD are compared to test results of patients who carry a different clinical diagnosis such as multiinfarct dementia or Parkinson's disease. This assessment strategy makes the most sense if the proposed test is being used to delineate a clinical dementia of the Alzheimer's type from clinical dementia of another etiology. The utility of this kind of approach in the evaluation of markers of underlying AD pathology is much less clear.

Cross-sectional designs for evaluating the accuracy of a biological assay to identify underlying AD pathology are inherently flawed because of the difficulty of selecting an age appropriate sample of individuals who we can be certain are disease free (i.e., lack pathology). In such studies, purportedly "normal" control samples may have a significant prevalence of presymptomatic or preclinical disease. The use of patient control groups also can generate similar problems. For example, patients with the clinical diagnosis of a vascular dementia are commonly employed as a control group. Unfortunately, numerous reports have suggested that over 50% of patients with such a diagnosis will be found at autopsy to have AD pathology, with or without concomitant significant cerebrovascular disease *(132–135)*. Similarly, a significant number of patients with the clinical diagnosis of Parkinson's disease will have concomitant AD pathology, especially in individuals with cognitive decline *(136,137)*. Biological markers of AD pathology should be positive in such patients. However, if viewed on clinical grounds alone, such positive test results would be interpreted as indicating a lack of specificity.

Longitudinal studies are the most promising method for testing the accuracy of a biological marker to identify AD pathology early in its course. A clinically useful test for AD in presymptomatic individuals should accurately predict the eventual development of cognitive compromise and symptoms of dementia. Data from longitudinal studies also allow us to assess the temporal interval over which we may expect the development of clinical symptoms of dementia. Longitudinal studies of this kind present many formidable challenges. Until such studies are completed, we do not know how far in advance of clinical dementia the test may turn positive. Thus, it is difficult to establish the ideal duration of a longitudinal study. The need to follow large numbers of subjects over time is likely to be extraordinarily expensive and it is unclear if such endeavors will be funded.

Acquisition of pathological material may be very helpful in sorting out the accuracy of a diagnostic technique. Researchers are unlikely to obtain a sufficient number of brain biopsies on patients who have had a given diagnostic test to provide information about its accuracy. Autopsy series also are challenging and slow to yield results. However, autopsy series of patients on whom data for a particular biological marker exists can provide critical evidence. Results that favor the validity of a particular technique include the following: 1) positive test while the patient was alive, AD pathology on autopsy, and 2) negative test in life, no significant AD pathology at postmortem. An excessive number of positive tests in life without significant AD pathology at autopsy would strongly call into question the utility of the assay. However, a negative test during life and AD pathology at postmortem would be the more difficult to interpret, especially if there were a long delay (e.g, many years) between when the test was done and when the autopsy took place.

Assessing the Value of Candidate Tests: Administration and Cost

In addition to the predictive value of a test, its utility will be judged on practical criteria such as accessibility, ease of administration, and cost. At one extreme would be brain biopsy. Biopsy is almost never sought in elders who present with typical features of a dementia of the Alzheimer's type. Such an invasive, risky, and expensive procedure is an inappropriate tool for identifying elders in the preclinical stages of the illness. By contrast, an ideal test would not only be accurate, but also noninvasive, inexpensive, and easy to administer at a primary care provider's office. Unfortunately, we do not (yet) have such a test. Tests short of brain biopsy that demand invasive biological sampling or complex assay procedures, such as lumbar puncture or tissue culture are much less attractive option than tests without such requirements.

The cost of tests is an important consideration, given the large population at-risk for developing dementia. However, at this stage, we should not reject test candidates because of the cost. Technical advances or simply test volume may reduce cost, while effective early interventions would raise the benefit:cost ratio. If we had treatments that, when started early in the course of the illness, were effective in slowing the progression of the disease, the savings on support services and long-term care would easily outweigh the cost of even an expensive test. New diagnostic tests would also reduce cost by eliminating the necessity for part of the "standard" workup for individuals with cognitive impairments. Test results that accurately diagnose AD might obviate the need to routinely perform other expensive procedures like neuroimaging. On the other hand, one could argue for the importance of investigating abnormalities other than a degenerative process that may be contributing to the decline in a person's cognitive or functional status. Aging individuals are at risk for developing more that one disease that can disrupt central nervous system functioning and cognitive abilities *(104,138–139)*.

Early Diagnosis In Alzheimer's Disease: Summary

There is indeed a dual challenge that faces us in our efforts to conquer Alzheimer's disease. We need to develop early, definitive, and noninvasive diagnostic tests for the disease and we need to treat early with agents aimed at stemming the pathological process of the disease. Ultimately, there is little clinical utility in the development of effective treatments without the capacity for early diagnosis, or in the development of techniques for early diagnosis of the disease without the availability of effective treatments. For Alzheimer's disease, there must be a dialectic relationship between research on diagnosis and research on treatment. We are in a critical transition period that has as yet yielded neither adequate early diagnostic strategies nor robust therapeutic interventions. Ideally, the pace of progress in therapeutics will match that of diagnostics. If the development of predictive (genetic) or diagnostic tests outpaces that of therapeutics, we will face difficult social and ethical issues (see Chapter 12). We need to ensure that diagnostic information is used in humane, socially responsible ways. To allow such information to potentially harm our patients would be contrary to the clinical goals of early, accurate diagnosis. The chapters that follow will summarize the current status of diagnostic approaches to AD, and will provide a comprehensive perspective from which to evaluate future efforts.

Acknowledgments

We thank Dr. Barry Fogel for his very helpful comments.

References

1. Evans DA, Funkenstein HH, Albert MS, Scherr PA, Cook NR, Chown MJ. Prevalence of Alzheimer's disease in a community population of older persons: higher than previously reported. *JAMA* 1989;262:2551–2556.

2. Ritchie K, Kildea D. Is senile dementia "age related" or "aging related"?: evidence from a meta-analysis of dementia prevalence in the oldest old. *Lancet* 1995; 346:931–934.

3. Small GW, Rabins PV, Barry PP, Buckholtz NS, DeKosky ST, Ferris SH, Finkel SI, Gwyther LP, Khachaturian ZS, Lebowitz BD, McRae TD, Morris JC, Oakley F, Schneider LS, Streim JE, Sunderland T, Teri LA, Tune LE. Diagnosis and treatment of Alzheimer disease and related disorders. *JAMA* 1997;278:1363–1371.

4. Jorm AF. *The Epidemiology of Alzheimer's Disease and Related Disorders.* London: Chapman & Hall, 1990.

5. Bachman DL, Wolf PA, Linn RT, Knoefel JE, Cobb JL, Belanger AJ, White LR, D'Agostino RB. Incidence of dementia and probable Alzheimer's disease in a general population: the Framingham Study. *Neurology* 1993;42:515–519.

6. Paykel ES, Brayne C, Huppert FA, Gill C, Barkley C, Gelhaar E, Beardsall L, Girling DM, Pollitt P, O'Connor D. Incidence of dementia in a population older than 75 years in the United Kingdom. *Arch. Gen. Psychiatry* 1994;51:325–332.

7. Schumock GT. Economic considerations in the treatment and management of Alzheimer's disease. *Am. J. Health Syst. Pharm.* 1998;55(Suppl. 2):S17–S21.

8. Breitner JCS. Clinical genetics and genetic counseling in Alzheimer's disease. *Ann. Intern. Med.* 1991;115:601–606.

9. De Souza EB, Whitehouse PJ, Kuhar MJ, Price DL, Vale WW. Reciprocal changes in corticotropin-releasing factor (CRF)-like immunoreactivity and CRF receptors in cerebral cortex of Alzheimer's disease. *Nature* 1986;319:593–594.

10. Cohen BM, Zubenko GS, Babb SM. Abnormal platelet membrane composition in Alzheimer's-type dementia. *Life Sci.* 1987;40:2445–2451.

11. Tanzi RE, Gusella JF, Watkins PC, Bruns GAP, St. George-Hyslop P, Van Keuren ML, Patterson D, Pagan S, Kurnit DM, Neve RL. Amyloid β protein gene: cDNA, mRNA distribution, and genetic linkage near the Alzheimer locus. *Science* 1987; 235:880–884.

12. Zubenko GS, Teply I. Longitudinal study of platelet membrane fluidity in Alzheimer's disease. *Biol. Psychiatry* 1988;24:918–924.

13. Johnson KA, Holman L, Rosen J, Nagel S, English RJ, Growdon JH. Iofetamine I 123 single proton emission computed tomography is accurate in the diagnosis of Alzheimer's disease. *Arch. Intern. Med.* 1990;150:752–756.

14. Matsubara E, Hirai S, Amari M, et al. Alpha 1-antichymotrypsin as a possible biochemical marker for Alzheimer-type dementia. *Ann. Neurol.* 1990;28:561–567.

15. de la Monte SM, Volicer L, Hauser SL, Wands JR. Increased levels of neuronal thread protein in cerebrospinal fluid of patients with Alzheimer's disease. *Ann. Neurol.* 1992;32:733–742.

16. Holman BL, Johnson KA, Gerada B, Carvalho PA, Satlin A. The scintigraphic appearance of Alzheimer's disease: a prospective study using technetium-99m-HMPAO SPECT. *J. Nucl. Med.* 1992;33:181–185.

17. Jack CR Jr, Petersen RC, O'Brien PC, Tangalos EG. MR-based hippocampal volumetry in the diagnosis of Alzheimer's disease. *Neurology* 1992;42:183–188.
18. Jobst KA, Smith AD, Barker CS, Wear A, King EM, Smith A, Anslow PA, Molyneux AJ, Shepstone BJ, Soper N, et al. Association of atrophy of the medial temporal lobe with reduced blood flow in the posterior parietotemporal cortex in patients with a clinical and pathological diagnosis of Alzheimer's disease. *J. Neurol.Neurosurg. Psychiatry* 1992;55:190–194.
19. Jobst KA, Smith AD, Szatmari M, Molyneux A, Esiri ME, King E, Smith A, Jaskowski A, McDonald B, Wald N. Detection in life of confirmed Alzheimer's disease using a simple measurement of medial temporal lobe atrophy by computed tomography. *Lancet* 1992;340:1179–1183.
20. Etcheberrigaray R, Ito E, Oka K, Tofel-Grehl B, Gibson GE, Alkon DL. Potassium channel dysfunction in fibroblasts identifies patients with Alzheimer's disease. *Proc. Natl. Acad. Sci. U.S.A.* 1993;90:8209–8213.
21. Johnson K, Kijewski MF, Becker A, Garda B, Satlin A, Holman BL. Quantitative brain SPECT in Alzheimer's disease and normal aging. *J. Nucl. Med.* 1993; 34:2044–2048.
22. Killiany RJ, Moss MB, Albert MS, Sandor T, Tieman J, Jolesz F. Temporal lobe regions on magnetic resonance imagiing identify patients with early Alzheimer's disease. *Arch. Neurol.* 1993;50:949–954.
23. Masur DM, Sliwinski M, Lipton RB, Blau AD, Crystal HA. Neuropsychological prediction of dementia and the absence of dementia in healthy elderly persons. *Neurology* 1994;44:1427–1432.
24. Nakamura T, Shoji M, Harigaya Y, Watanabe M, Hosoda K, Cheung TT, Shaffer LM, Golde TE, Younkin LH, Younkin SG, et al. Amyloid beta protein levels in cerebrospinal fluid are elevated in early-onset Alzheimer's disease. *Ann. Neurol.* 1994;36:903–911.
25. Parker WD Jr, Mahr NJ, Filley CM, Parks JK, Hughes D, Young DA, Cullum CM. Reduced platelet cytochrome *c* oxidase activity in Alzheimer's disease. *Neurology* 1994;44:1086–1090.
26. Parker WD Jr, Parks J, Filley CM, Kleinschmidt-DeMasters BK. Electron transport chain defects in Alzheimer's disease brain. *Neurology* 1994;44:1090–1096.
27. Petersen RC, Smith GE, Ivnik RJ, Kokmen E, Tangalos EG. Memory function in very early Alzheimer's disease. *Neurology* 1994;44:867–872.
28. Scinto LF, Daffner KR, Dressler D, Ransil BJ, Rentz D, Weintraub S, Mesulam M, Potter H. A potential noninvasive neurobiological test for Alzheimer's disease. *Science* 1994;226:1051–1054.
29. Simonian NA, Hyman BT. Functional alterations in Alzheimer's disease: selective loss of mitochondrial-encoded cytochrome oxidase mRNA in the hippocampal formation. *J. Neuropathol. Exp. Neurol.* 1994;53:508–512.
30. Arai H, Terajima M, Miura M, Higuchi S, Muramatsu T, Machida N, Seiki H, Takase S, Clark CM, Lee VM-Y, Trojanowski JQ, Sasaki H. Tau in cerebrospinal fluid: a potential diagnostic marker in Alzheimer's disease. *Ann. Neurol.* 1995; 38:649–652.
31. DeCarli C, Murphy DGM, McIntosh AR, Teichberg D, Schapiro MB, Horwitz B. Discriminant analysis of MRI measures as a method to determine the presence of dementia of the Alzheimer type. *Psychiatry Res.* 1995;57:119–130.

32. Jacobs DM, Sano M, Dooneief G, Marder K, Bell KL, Stern Y. Neuropsychological detection and characterization of preclinical Alzheimer's disease. *Neurology* 1995;45:957–962.

33. Laakso MP, Soininen H, Partanen K, Helkala EL, Hartikainen P, Vainio P, Hallikainen M, Hanninen T, Riekkinen PJ. Volumes of hippocampus, amygdala and frontal lobes in the MRI-based diagnosis of early Alzheimer's disease: correlation with memory functions. *J. Neural Transm. Dis. Dement. Sect.* 1995;9:73–86.

34. Levy-Lahad E, Wijsman EM, Nemens E, Anderson L, Goddard KAB, Weber JL, Bird TD, Schellenberg G.D. A familial Alzheimer's disease locus on chromosome 1. *Science* 1995;269:970–973.

35. Licastro F, Morini MC, Polazzi E, Davis LJ. Increased serum alpha 1-antichymotrypsin in patients with probable AD: an acute phase reactant without the peripheral acute phase response. *J. Neuroimmunol.* 1995;57:71–75.

36. Linn RT, Wolf PA, Bachman DL, Knoefel JE, Cobb JL, Belanger AJ, Kaplan EF, D'Agostino RB. The "preclinical phase" of probably Alzheimer's disease. *Arch. Neurol.* 1995;52:485–490.

37. Motter R, Vigo-Pelfrey C, Kholodenko D, Barbour R, Johnson-Wood K, Galasko D, Chang L, Miller B, Clark C, Green R, Olsen D, Soutwick P, Wolfert R, Munroe R, Lieberburg I, Seubert P, Schenck, D. Reduction of β-amyloid peptide in the cerebrospinal fluid of patients with Alzheimer's disease. *Ann. Neurol.* 1995; 38:643–648.

38. Petersen RC, Smith GE, Ivnik RJ, Tangalos EG, Schaid DJ, Thibodeau SN, Kokmen E, Waring SC, Kurland LT. Apolipoprotein E status as a predictor of the development of Alzheimer's disease in memory-impaired individuals. *JAMA* 1995;273:1274–1278.

39. Roses AD. Apolipoprotein E genotyping in the differential diagnosis, not prediction, of Alzheimer's disease. *Ann. Neurol.* 1995;38:6–14.

40. Sherrington R, Rogaev EI, Liang Y, Rogaeva EA, Levesque G, Ikeda M, Chi H, Lin C, Li G, Holman K, Tsuda T, Mar L, Foncin J-F, Bruni AC, Montesi MP, Sorbi S, Rainero I, Pinessi L, Nee L, Chumakov I, Pollen D, Brookes A, Sanseau P, Polinsky RJ, Wasco W, Da Silva HAR, Haines JL, Pericak-Vance MA, Tanzi RE, Roses AD, Fraser PE, Rommens JM, St. George-Hyslop PH. Cloning of a gene bearing missense mutations in early-onset familial Alzheimer's disease. *Nature* 1995;375:754–760.

41. Small GS, Mazziotta JC, Collins MT, Baxter LR, Phelps ME, Mandelkern MA, Kaplan A, LaRue A, Adamson CF, Chang L, Guze BH, Corder EH, et al. Apolipoprotein E type 4 allele and cerebral glucose metabolism in relatives at risk for familial Alzheimer's disease. *JAMA* 1995;273:942–947.

42. Van de Voorde A, Vanmechelen E, Vandemeeren M, et al. Detection of tau in cerebrospinal fluid. In Iqbal K, Mortimer JA, Winblad B, Wisniewski HM, editors. *Research Advances in Alzheimer's Disease and Related Disorders.* Chichester: John Wiley & Sons Ltd., 1995:189–195.

43. Vigo-Pelfrey C, Seubert P, Blomquist C, et al. Tau in cerebrospinal fluid: an antemortem marker for Alzheimer's disease? In Iqbal K, Mortimer JA, Winblad B, Wisniewski HM, editors. *Research Advances in Alzheimer's Disease and Related Disorders.* Chichester: John Wiley & Sons Ltd., 1995:197–205.

44. Eckert A, Forstl H, Zerfass R, Hartmann H, Muller WE. Lymphocytes and neu-

rophils as peripheral models to study the effects of beta-amyloid on cellular signalling in Alzheimer's disease. *Life Sci.* 1996;59:5–6.

45. Fox NC, Warrington EK, Freeborough PA, Hartikainen P, Kennedy AM, Stevens JM, Rossor MN. Presymptomatic hippocampal atrophy in Alzheimer's disease: a longitudinal MRI study. *Brain* 1996;119:2001–2007.

46. Gibson GE, Zhang H, Toral-Barza L, Szolosi S, Tofel-Grehl B. Calcium stores in cultured fibroblasts and their changes with Alzheimer's disease. *Biochem. Biophys. Acta* 1996;1316:71–77.

47. Kennard ML, Feldman H, Yamada T, Jeffries WA. Serum levels of the iron binding protein p97 are elevated in Alzheimer's disease. *Nat. Med.* 1996;2: 1230–1235.

48. Reiman EM, Caselli RJ, Yun LS, Chen K, Bandy D, Minoshima S, Thibodeau SN, Osborne D. Preclinical evidence of Alzheimer's disease in persons homozygous for the ε4 allele for apolipoprotein E. *N. Engl. J. Med.* 1996;334:752–758.

49. Saunders AM, Hulette C, Welsh-Bohmer KA, Schmechel DE, Crain B, Burke JR, Alberts MJ, Strittmatter WJ, Breitner JCS, Rosenberg C, Scott SV, Gaskell PC Jr, Pericak-Vance MA, Roses AD. Specificity, sensitivity, and predictive value of apolipoprotein-E genotyping for sporadic Alzheimer's disease. *Lancet* 1996; 348:90–93.

50. Tierney MC, Szalai JP, Snow WG, Fisher RH, Nores A, Nadon G, Dunn E, St. George-Hyslop PH. Prediction of probable Alzheimer's disease in memory-impaired patients: a prospective longitudinal study. *Neurology* 1996;46:661–665.

51. de la Monte SM, Ghanbari K, Frey WH, Beheshti I, Averback P, Hauser SL, Ghanbari HA, Wands JR. Characterization of the AD7C-NTP cDNA expression in Alzheimer's disease and measurement of a 41-kD protein in cerebrospinal fluid. *J. Clin. Invest.* 1997;100:3093–3104.

52. Growdon JH, Graefe K, Tennis M, Hayden D, Schoenfeld D, Wray SH. Pupil dilation to tropicamide is not specific for Alzheimer's disease. *Arch. Neurol.* 1997; 54:841–844.

53. Higuchi S, Matsushita S, Hasegawa Y, Muramatsu T, Arai H, Hayashida M. Apolipoprotein E ε4 allele and pupillary response to tropicamide. *Am. J. Psychiatry* 1997;154:694–696.

54. Jack CR Jr, Petersen RC, Xu YC, Waring SC, O'Brien PC, Tangalos EG, Smith GE, Ivnik RJ, Kokmen E. Medial temporal atrophy on MRI in normal aging and very mild Alzheimer's disease. *Neurology* 1997;49:786–794.

55. Kalman J, Kanka A, Magloczky E, Szoke A, Jardanhazy T, Janka Z. Increased mydriatic response to tropicamide is a sign of cholinergic hypersensitivity but not specific to late-onset sporadic type of Alzheimer's disease. *Biol. Psychiatry* 1997; 41:909–911.

56. Kaye JA, Swihart T, Howieson D, Dame A, Moore MM, Karnos T, Camicioli R, Ball M, Oken B, Sexton G. Volume loss of the hippocampus and temporal lobe in healthy elderly persons destined to develop dementia. *Neurology* 1997;48: 1297–1304.

57. Riemenschneider M, Buch K, Schmolke M, Kurz A, Guder WG. Diagnosis of Alzheimer's disease with cerebrospinal fluid tau protein and aspartate aminotransferase. *Lancet* 1997;350:784.

58. Roses AD. Genetic testing for Alzheimer's disease: practical and ethical issues. *Arch. Neurol.* 1997;54:1226–1229.

59. Kaneyuki H, Mitsuno S, Nishida T, Yamada M. Enhanced miotic response to topical dilute pilocarpine in patients with Alzheimer's disease. *Neurology* 1998;50: 802–804.

59a. Kanai M, Matsubara E, Isoe K, Urakami K, Nakashima K, Arai H, Sasaki H, Abe K, Iwatsubo T, Kosaka T, Watanabe M, Tomidokoro Y, Shizuka M, Mizushima K, Nakamura T, Igeta Y, Ikeda Y, Amari M, Kawarabayashi T, Ishiguro K, Harigaya Y, Wakabayashi K, Okamoto K, Hirai S, Shoji M. Longitudinal study of cerebrospinal fluid levels of tau, A β 1-40, and A β 1-42(43) in Alzheimer's disease: a study in Japan. *Ann. Neurol.* 1998;44:17–26.

59b. Growdon JH. To tap or not to tap: cerebrospinal fluid biomarkers in Alzheimer's disease (editorial; comment). *Ann. Neurol.* 1998;44:6–7.

59c. Hulstaert F, Blennow K, Ivanoiu A, Schoonderwaldt HC, Riemenschneider M, De Deyn PP, Bancher C, Cras P, Wiltfang J, Mehta PD, Iqbal K, Pottel H, Vanmechelen E, Vanderstichele H. Improved discrimination of AD patients using beta-amyloid (1-42) and tau levels in CSF. *Neurology* 1999;52:1555–1562.

60. Larson EB, Reitler BV, Sumi SM, Canfield CG, Chann NM. Diagnostic tests in the evaluation of dementia: a prospective study of 200 elderly outpatients. *Arch. Intern. Med.* 1986;146:1917–1922.

61. Clarfield AM. The reversible dementias: do they reverse? *Ann. Intern. Med.* 1988; 109:476–486.

62. McKhann G, Drachman D, Folstein M, Katzman R, Price D, Stadlan EM. Clinical diagnosis of Alzheimer's disease: report of the NINCDS-ADRDA work group under the auspices of the department of health and human services task force on Alzheimer's disease. *Neurology* 1984;34:939–944.

63. Morris JC, Heyman A, Mohs RC, Hughes JP, van Belle G, Fillenbaum G, Mellits ED, Clark C. The consortium to establish a registry for Alzheimer's disease (CERAD). Part I. Clinical and neuropsychological assessment of Alzheimer's disease. *Neurology* 1989;3:1159–1165.

64. American Psychiatric Association. *Diagnostic and Statistical Manual of Mental Disorders*, 4th ed. Washington, DC: *American Psychiatric Association,* 1994.

65. Khachaturian Z. Diagnosis of Alzheimer's disease. *Arch. Neurol.* 1985;42: 1097–1105.

66. Mirra SS, Heyman A, McKeel D, Sumi SM, Crain BJ, Brownlee LM, Vogel FS, Hughes JP, van Belle G, Berg L. The consortium to establish a registry for Alzheimer's disease (CERAD). Part II. Standardization of the neuropathologic assessment of Alzheimer's disease. *Neurology* 1991;41:479–486.

67. Mirra SS, Hart MN, Terry RD. Making the diagnosis of Alzheimer's disease: a primer for practicing pathologist. *Arch. Pathol. Lab. Med.* 1993;117: 132–144.

68. Sulkava R, Haltia M, Paetau A, Wikstron J, Palo J. Accuracy of clinical diagnosis in primary degenerative dementia: correlation with neuropathologic findings. *J. Neurol. Neurosurg. Psychiatry* 1983;46:9–13.

69. Joachim CL, Morris JH, Selkoe DJ. Clinically diagnosed Alzheimer's disease: autopsy results in 150 cases. *Ann. Neurol.* 1988;24:50–56.

70. Tierney MC, Fisher RH, Lewis AJ, Zorzitto ML, Snow WG, Reid DW,

Nieuwstraten P. The NINCDS-ADRDA Work Group criteria for the clinical diagnosis of probable Alzheimer's disease: a clinicopathologic study of 57 cases. *Neurology* 1988;38:359–364.

71. Kukull WA, Larson EB, Reifler BV, Lampe TH, Yerby MS, Hughes JP. The validity of 3 clinical diagnostic criteria for Alzheimer's disease. *Neurology* 1990; 40:1364–1369.

72. Risse SC, Raskind MA, Nochlin D, Sumi SM, Lampe TH, Bird TD, Cubberley L, Peskind ER. Neuropathological findings in patients with clinical diagnosis of probable Alzheimer's disease. *Am. J. Psychiatry* 1990;147:168–172.

73. Mendez M, Mastri AR, Sung JH, Frey WH. Clinically diagnosed Alzheimer's disease: neuropathologic findings in 650 cases. *Alzheimer Dis. Assoc. Disord.* 1992;6:35–43.

74. Blacker D, Albert MS, Bassett SS, Go RCP, Harrell LE, Folstein MF. Reliability and validity of NINCDS-ADRDA criteria for Alzheimer's disease. *Arch. Neurol.* 1994;51:1198–1204.

75. Galasko D, Hansen LA, Katzman R, Wiederholt W, Masliah E, Terry R, Hill LR, Lessin P, Thal LJ. Clinical-neuropathological correlations in Alzheimer's disease and related dementias. *Arch. Neurol.* 1994;51:888–895.

76. Gearing M, Mirra SS, Hedreen JC, Sumi SM, Hansen LA, Heyman A. The consortium to establish a registry for Alzheimer's disease (CERAD). Part X. Neuropathology confirmation of the clinical diagnosis of Alzheimer's disease. *Neurology* 1995;45:461–466.

77. Cogan DG. Visual disturbances with focal progressive dementing disease. *Am. J. Ophthalmol.* 1985;100:68–72.

78. Brun A. Frontal lobe degeneration of non-Alzheimer type. I. Neuropathology. *Arch. Gerontol. Geriatr.* 1987;6:193–208.

79. Hof PR, Bouras C, Constantinidis J, Morrison JH. Balint's syndrome in Alzheimer's disease: specific disruption of the occipito-parietal visual pathway. *Brain Res.* 1989;493:368–375.

80. Mesulam MM, Weintraub S. Spectrum of primary progressive aphasia. In Rosser MN, editor. *Unusual Dementia, Baillière's Clinical Neurology,* Vol 1. 1992:583–609.

81. Weintraub, S, Mesulam MM. Four neuropsychological profiles in dementia. In Boller F, Grafman J, editors. *Handbook of Neuropsychology, Volume 8.* Amsterdam: Elsevier Science Publishers BV, 1993:253–282.

82. Victoroff J, Ross GW, Benson DF, Verity MA, Vinters HV. Posterior cortical atrophy: neuropathological correlations. *Arch. Neurol.* 1994;51:269–274.

83. Ulrich J. Alzheimer changes in nondemented patients younger than sixty-five: possible early stages of Alzheimer's disease and senile dementia of Alzheimer's type. *Ann. Neurol.* 1985;17:273–277.

84. Crystal H, Dickson D, Fuld P, Masur D, Scott R, Mehler M, Masdeu J, Kawas C, Aronson M, Wolfson L. Clinico-pathologic studies in dementia: nondemented subjects with pathologically confirmed Alzheimer's disease. *Neurology* 38:1682–1687.

85. Katzman R, Terry R, DeTeresa R, Brown T, Davies P, Fuld P, Renbing X, Peck A. Clinical, pathological and neurochemical changes in dementia: a subgroup with preserved mental status and numerous neocortical plaques. *Ann. Neurol.* 1988; 23:138–144.

86. Hubbard BM, Fenton GW, Anderson JM. A quantitative histological study of early clinical and preclinical Alzheimer's disease. *Neuropathol. Appl. Neurobiol.* 1990; 16:111–121.

87. Morris JC, McKeel DW, Storandt M, Rubin EH, Price JL, Grant EA, Ball MJ, Berg L. Very mild Alzheimer's disease: informant-based clinical, psychometric and pathological distinction from normal aging. *Neurology* 1991;41:469–478.

88. Morris JC, Storandt M, McKeel DW, Rubin EH, Price JI, Grant EA, Berg L. Cerebral amyloid deposition and diffuse plaques in "normal" aging: evidence for presymptomatic and very mild Alzheimer's disease. *Neurology* 1996;46:707–719.

89. Johansson K, Bogdanovic N, Kalimo H, Winblad B, Viitanen M. Alzheimer's disease and apolipoprotein E ε4 allele in older drivers who died in automobile accidents. *Lancet* 1997;349:1143–1144.

90. Blessed G, Tomlinson BE, Roth M. The association between quantitative measures of dementia and of senile change in the gray matter of elderly subjects. *Br. J. Psychiatry* 1968;114:797–811.

91. Delaere P, Duyckaerts C, Brion JP, Poulian V, Hauw J-J. Tau, paired helical filaments and amyloid in the neocortex: a morphometric study of 15 cases with graded intellectual status in aging and senile dementia of Alzheimer type. *Acta Neuropathol.* 1989;77:645–653.

92. DeKosky ST, Scheff SW. Synapse loss in the frontal cortex biopsies in Alzheimer's disease: correlation with cognitive severity. *Ann. Neurol.* 1990;27:457–464.

93. Terry RD, Masliah E, Salmon DP, Butters N, DeTeresa R, Hill R, Hansen LA, Katzman R. Physical basis of cognitiive alterations in Alzheimer's disease: synapse loss is the major correlate of cognitive impairment. *Ann. Neurol.* 1991;30:572–580.

94. Arriagada PV, Growdon JH, Hedley-Whyte ET, Hyman BT. Neurofibrillary tangles but not senile plaques parallel duration and severity of Alzheimer's disease. *Neurology* 1992;42:631–639.

95. Nagy Z, Esiri MM, Jobst KA, Morris JH, King EMF, McDonald B, Litchfield S, Smith A, Barnetson L, Smith AD. Relative roles of plaques and tangles in the dementia of Alzheimer's disease: correlations using three sets of neuropathological criteria. *Dementia* 1995;6:21–31.

96. Gibb WRG, Lees AJ. Pathological clues to the cause of Parkinson's disease. In Marsden CD, Fahn S, editors. *Movement Disorders 3.* Oxford: Butterworth-Heinemann Ltd., 1994;147–166.

97. Hughes CP, Berg L, Danziger W, Coben LA, Martin RL. A new clinical scale for the staging of dementia. *Br. J. Psychiatry* 1982;140:566–572.

98. Gomez-Isla T, Price JL, McKeel DW Jr, Morris JC, Growdon JH, Hyman BT. Profound loss of layer II entorhinal cortex neurons occurs in very mild Alzheimer's disease. *J. Neurosci.* 1996;16:4491–4500.

99. Stern Y, Alexander GE, Prohovnik I, Mayeux R. Inverse relationship between education and parietotemporal perfusion deficit in Alzheimer's disease. *Ann. Neurol.* 1992;32:371–375.

100. Evans DA, Beckett LA, Albert MS, Hebert LE, Scherr PA, Funkenstein HH, Taylor JO. Level of education and change in cognitive function in a community population of older persons. *Ann. Epidemiol.* 1993;3:71–77.

101. Katzman R. Education and the prevalence of dementia and Alzheimer's disease. *Neurology* 1993;43:13–20.
102. Mortimer JA, Graves AB. Education and other socioeconomic determinants of dementia and Alzheimer's disease. *Neurology* 1993;43(Suppl 4):S-39–S44.
103. Alexander GE, Furey ML, Grady CL, Pietrini P, Brady DR, Mentis MJ, Schapiro MB. Association of premorbid intellectual function with cerebral metabolism in Alzheimer's disease: implications for the cognitive reserve hypothesis. *Am. J. Psychiatry* 1997;154:165–172.
104. Snowdon DA, Greiner LH, Mortimer JA, Riley KP, Greiner PA, Markesbery WR. Brain infarction and the clinical expression of Alzheimer disease: the nun study. *JAMA* 1997;277:813–817.
105. Haxby JV, Grady CL, Duara R, Schlageter N, Berg G, Rapoport SI. Neocortical metabolic abnormalities precede nonmemory cognitive defects in early Alzheimer's-type dementia. *Arch. Neurol.* 1986;43:882–885.
106. Katzman R, Aronson M, Fuld P, Kawas C, Brown T, Morgenstern H, Frishman W, Gidez L, Eder H, Ooi WL. Development of dementing illness in an 80-year old volunteer cohort. *Ann. Neurol.* 1989;25:317–324.
107. Coyle JT, Oster-Granite ML, Gearhart JD. The neurobiologic consequences of Down syndrome. *Brain Res. Bull.* 1986;16:773–787.
108. Lai F, Williams RS. A prospective study of Alzheimer disease in Down syndrome. *Arch. Neurol.* 1989;46:849–853.
109. Mann DMA, Yuonis N, Jones D, Stoddart RW. The time course of pathological events in Down's syndrome with particular reference to the involvement of microglial cells and deposits of B/A4. *Neurodegeneration* 1992;1:201–205.
110. Grundman M, Petersen RC, Morris JC, Ferris S, Sano M, Farlow MR, Doody RS, Galasko D, Ernesto C, Thomas RG, Thal LJ, the ADCS Cooperative Study. Rate of dementia of the Alzheimer type (DAT) in subjects with mild cognitive impairment. *Neurology* 1996;46:A403.
111. Tomlinson BE, Blessed G, Roth M. Observations of the brains of demented old people. *J. Neurol. Sci.* 1970;11:205–242.
112. Brun A, Gustafson I. Distribution of cerebral degeneration in Alzheimer's disease: a clinico-pathological study. *Arch. Psychiatry* 1976;223:15–33.
113. Hooper MW, Vogel FS. The limbic system in Alzheimer's disease: a neuropathologic investigation. *Am. J. Pathol.* 1976;85:1–19.
114. Wilcock GK, Esiri MM. Plaques, tangles, and dementia: a quantitative study. *J. Neurol. Sci.* 1982;56:343–356.
115. Foster NL, Chase TN, Mansi L, Brooks R, Fedio P, Patronas NJ, DiChiro G. Cortical abnormalities in Alzheimer's disease. *Ann. Neurol.* 1984;16:649–654.
116. Hyman BT, Van Hoesen GW, Damasio AR, Barnes CL. Alzheimer's disease: cell-specific pathology isolates the hippocampal formation. *Science* 1984;225:1168–1170.
117. Ball MJ, Fisman M, Hachinski V, Blume W, Fox A, Kral VA, Kirshen AJ, Fox H, Merskey H. A new definition of Alzheimer's disease: a hippocampal dementia. *Lancet* 1985;1:14–16.
118. Cutler NR, Haxby JV, Duara R, Grady CL, Kay AD, Kressler RM, Sundaram M, Rapaport SI. Clinical history, brain metabolism, and neuropsychological function in Alzheimer's disease. *Ann. Neurol.* 1985;18:298–309.

119. Arnold SE, Hyman BT, Flory J, Damasio AR, Van Hoesen GW. The topographical and neuroanatomical distribution of neurofibrillary tangles and neuritic plaques in the cerebral cortex of patients with Alzheimer's disease. *Cereb. Cortex* 1991;1:103–116.

120. Braak H, Braak E. Neuropathological staging of Alzheimer-related changes. *Acta Neuropathol.* 1991;82:239–259.

121. Price JL, Davis PB, Morris JC, White DL. The distribution of tangles, plaques and related immunohistochemical markers in healthy aging and Alzheimer's disease. *Neurobiol. Aging* 1991;12:295–312.

122. Neary D, Snowden JS, Northen B, Goulding P. Dementia of frontal lobe type. *J. Neurol. Neurosurg. Psychiatry* 1988;51:353–361.

123. Miller BL, Cummings JL, Villanueva-Meyer J, Boone K, Mehringer CM, Lesser IM, Mena I. Frontal lobe degeneration: clinical, neuropsychological and SPECT characteristics. *Neurology* 1991;41:1374–1382.

124. Lund and Manchester Groups. Consensus statement: clinical and neuropathological criteria for frontotemporal dementia. *J. Neurol. Neurosurg. Psychiatry* 1994; 57:416–418.

125. Sherrington R, Froelich S, Sorbi S, Campion D, Chi H, Rogaeva EA, Levesque G, Rogaev EI, Lin C, Liang Y, Ikeda M, Mar L, Brice A, Agid Y, Percy ME, Clerget-Darpoux F, Piacentini S, Marcon G, Nacmias B, Amaducci L, Frebourg T, Lannfelt L, Rommens JM, St. George-Hyslop PH. Alzheimer's disease associated with mutations in presenilin 2 is rare and variably penetrant. *Hum. Mol. Genet.* 1996;5:985–988.

126. Cruts M, Van Broeckhoven C. Presenilin mutations in Alzheimer's disease. *Hum. Mutat.* 1998;11:183–190.

127. Brodaty H. Consensus statement on predictive testing for Alzheimer's disease and associated disorders. *Alzheimer Dis. Assoc. Disord.* 1995;9:182–187.

128. Statement on the use of apolipoprotein E testing for Alzheimer disease. American College of Medical Genetics/American Society of Human Genetics Working Group on ApoE and Alzheimer disease. *JAMA* 1995;274:1627–1629.

129. Relkin NR, Kwon YJ, Tsai J, Grandy S. The National Institute on Aging/Alzheimer's Association recommendations on the application of apolipoprotein ε genotyping to Alzheimer's disease. *Ann NY Acad Sci* 1998;802:149–176.

130. Post SG, Whitehouse PJ, Binstock RH, Bird TD, Eckert SK, Farrer LA, Fleck LM, Gaines AD, Juengst ET, Karlinsky H, Miles S, Murray TH, Quaid KA, Relkin NR, Roses AD, St. George-Hyslop PH, Sachs GA, Steinbock B, Truschke EF, Zinn AB. The clinical introduction of genetic testing for Alzheimer's disease: an ethical perspective. *JAMA* 1997;277:832–836.

131. Mayeux R, Saunders AM, Shea S, Mirra S, Evans D, Roses AD, Hyman BT, Crain B, Tang M-X, Phelps CH. Utility of the apolipoprotein E genotype in the diagnosis of Alzheimer's disease. *N. Engl. J. Med.* 1998;338:506–511.

132. Wade JPH, Mirsen TR, Hachinski VC, Fisman M, Lau C, Merskey H. The clinical diagnosis of Alzheimer's disease. *Arch. Neurol.* 1987;44:24–29.

133. Brust JCM. Vascular dementia is overdiagnosed. *Arch. Neurol.* 1988;45:799–801.

134. Victoroff J, Mack WJ, Lyness SA, Chui HC. Multicenter clinicopathological correlation in dementia. *Am. J. Psychiatry* 1995;152:1476–1484.

135. Hulette C, Nochlin D, McKeel D, Morris JC, Mirra SS, Sumi SM, Heyman A. Clinical-neuropathologic findings in multii-infarct dementia: a report of six autopsied cases. *Neurology* 1997;48:668–672.
136. Hakim AM, Mathieson G. Dementia in Parkinson disease: a neuropathologic study. *Neurology* 1979;29:1209–1214.
137. Boller F, Passafiume D, Keefe NC, Rogers K, Morrow L, Kim Y. Visuospatial impairment in Parkinson's disease: role of perceptual and motor factors. *Arch. Neurol.* 1984;41:485–490.
138. Katzman R. Should a major imaging procedure (CT or MRI) be required in the workup of dementia?: an affirmative view. *J. Fam. Pract.* 1990;31:401–410.
139. Bird T. Apolipoprotein E genotyping in the diagnosis of Alzheimer's disease: a cautionary view. *Ann. Neurol.* 1995;38:2–3.

References Cited in Footnote on Page 4

a. West MJ, Coleman PD, Flood DG, Troncoso JC. Differences in the pattern of hippocampal neuronal loss in normal ageing and Alzheimer's disease. *Lancet* 1994; 344:769–772.
b. Scheltens Ph, Barkhof F, Leys D, Wolters E Ch, Ravid R, Kamphorst W. Histopathologic correlates of white matter changes on MRI in Alzheimer's disease and normal aging. *Neurology* 1995;45:883–888.
c. Morris JC, Storandt M, McKeel DW, et al. Cerebral amyloid deposition and diffuse plaques in "normal" aging: evidence for presymptomatic and very mild Alzheimer's disease. *Neurology* 1996;46:707–719.
d. Mukaetova-Ladinska EB, Harrington CR, Roth M, Wischik CM. Alterations in tau protein metabolism during normal aging. *Dementia* 1996;7:95–103.
e. Simic G, Kostovic I, Winblad B, Bogdanovic N. Volume and number of neurons of the human hippocampal formation in normal aging and Alzheimer's disease. *J. Comp. Neurol.* 1997;379:482–494.
f. Wang D, Munoz DG. Qualitative and quantitative differences in senile plaque dystrophic neurites of Alzheimer's disease and normal aged brain. *J. Neuropathol. Exp. Neurol.* 1995;54:548–556.
g. Troncoso JC, Cataldo AM, Nixon RA, Barnett JL, Lee MK, Checler F, Fowler DR, Smialek JE, Crain B, Martin LJ, Kawas CH. Neuropathology of preclinical and clinical late-onset Alzheimer's disease. *Ann. Neurol.* 1998;43:673–676.

2

Current Approaches to the Clinical Diagnosis of Alzheimer's Disease

Kirk R. Daffner

Introduction

Assessing the value of new diagnostic approaches to Alzheimer's disease (AD) requires an appreciation of the "standard" clinical diagnostic evaluation. In reality, there is no single, universally accepted clinical approach to the evaluation of demented patients. The workup is likely to vary from setting to setting. Different approaches may be found, for example, among primary care physicians, clinical neurologists in the community, and dementia researchers in academic centers. With the growth of managed care programs, more explicit standards may be established, perhaps with an increased emphasis on containing costs.

Two antithetical attitudes about diagnosis of dementia are common even within the medical community, each with damaging consequences. One is that changes in cognition and behavior seen in elderly individuals are simply a reflection of the normal aging process and thus can be readily dismissed. The second is that all disruptive cognitive decline in the elderly is due to Alzheimer's disease. The terms dementia and Alzheimer's disease often are used interchangeably. Either of these attitudes can lead to the unfortunate view that there is no need to make an effort to accurately diagnose dementia. Clearly, accuracy of diagnosis will become increasingly important as more treatments become available. Even now, accuracy of diagnosis remains an important goal. Perhaps most significantly, such efforts can help identify potentially reversible or treatable conditions that have contributed to cognitive decline and dementia. Accuracy of diagnosis can provide important prognostic information to families that allow for generating appropriate expectations

From: *Early Diagnosis of Alzheimer's Disease*
Edited by L. F. M. Scinto & K. R. Daffner © Humana Press, Inc., Totowa, NJ

and plans for the patient's future needs. In addition, it can allow family members to consider the implications that a particular diagnosis might have for them in terms of their own future. Finally, before the establishment of clear in vivo markers for Alzheimer's disease, trials to assess the efficacy of new medications for AD depend on the accurate clinical diagnosis to identify patients who most likely are suffering from Alzheimer's disease. Including misdiagnosed patients without Alzheimer's disease in such trials is likely to dilute the results of potentially efficacious treatments *(1)*.

In the absence of definitive diagnostic markers for Alzheimer's and other dementing illnesses, clinicians and researchers have turned to provisional strategies for trying to accurately assess a patient's clinical status and diagnosis. The need for developing rational guidelines to assist in the diagnosis of AD has become more apparent with the growing magnitude of the problem of dementia. Alzheimer's disease is the major cause of dementia in the United States, accounting for 55% to 70% of cases *(2–4)*. This disease alone constitutes a significant and increasing health care problem. Prevalence of AD has risen steadily as the average age of the population has increased. It is estimated that up to 10% of Americans 65 and older suffer from the disease *(5,6)*. For the population of 85 and older, estimates of prevalence have been as high as 47% *(7)*. As many as four million Americans may suffer from AD, with the cost in excess of 100 billion dollars per year *(8)*.

This chapter emphasizes practices that have been codified over the last 10–15 years by several prominent research and clinical groups. Many of these standards were originally developed to establish diagnostic criteria for research purposes such as the Diagnostic and Statistical Manual of the American Psychiatric Association (DSM) *(9)*, the task force report of the National Institutes of Neurologic and Communicative Diseases and Stroke-Alzheimer Disease and Related Disorders Association (NINCDS–ADRDA) *(10)*, and the Consortium to Establish a Registry for Alzheimer's Disease (CERAD) *(11–13)* but are now used as guidelines in clinical practice. Others *(14–17)* have been developed to help direct the practicing clinician (e.g., Quality Standards Subcommittee of the American Academy of Neurology). The extent to which practitioners actually follow these guidelines, however, has not been clearly established. Thus, this chapter provides information about "recommended" clinical workups, not about how often they are actualized in the community.

Initiation of a Dementia Evaluation

Evaluations for dementia are initiated under different circumstances. Most often, family members bring in a loved one because they are concerned about a decline in his/her cognitive or behavioral status. Patients who often lack insight due to their central nervous system (CNS) disease (or psychological defenses), are unlikely to recognize the need for such an evaluation. Other patients may accept some of the observations of decline made by their loved ones, but downplay their implications. Increasingly, patients themselves seem to be sharing concerns with their physicians about problems with forgetfulness, word-finding difficulties, or slowness in retrieving names. Some of these patients will be in the early stages of a dementing illness. Others may be particularly sensitive to the cognitive changes that are associated with "normal" aging or be suffering from depression *(18,19)*. Requests for evaluation may become increasingly common as information about dementia and Alzheimer's disease inundates the popular press. A third pathway for initiating an evaluation is established when interactions between a patient and medical staff raise concerns about the patient's mental state or ability to manage his or her affairs independently.

Workup of a potentially demented patient is a multidimensional process with two major branching points (American Academy of Neurology practice parameters algorithm) (Fig. 1). The first major step involves establishing whether or not an individual fits criteria for being clinically demented. The second major step occurs after establishing a diagnosis of dementia and involves a workup to evaluate possible underlying conditions that fall within the differential diagnosis. Establishing a diagnosis of dementia relies principally on a detailed history and mental state assessment. Identifying the most likely underlying causes of dementia relies on recognizing the salient patterns of cognitive decline as revealed by the history and mental state examination and obtaining appropriate diagnostic studies that look for potential contributions to the deterioration in the patient's cognitive or behavioral status.

Diagnostic Criteria

The defining criteria for dementia vary *(9,10,16,17)*. Our working definition is as follows: Dementia is a progressive, but not necessarily irreversible, decline in cognitive or behavioral functioning that interferes with daily living activities that are appropriate for one's age and background and is not simply due to a delirium, confusional state, or related alteration in sensorium. Both DSM-IV and NINCDS-ADRDA diagnostic criteria for dementia require a decline in memory and other cognitive processes such as language, visual-spatial abilities, or executive functions. DSM-IV criteria explicitly states that such cognitive deficits must "cause significant impairment in social or occupational functioning (e.g., going to school, working, shopping, dressing, bathing, handling finances, and other activities of daily living) and must represent a decline from a previous level of functioning" *(9)*. This criterion is not explicitly included in the NINCDS-ADRDA formula (Table 1). In both

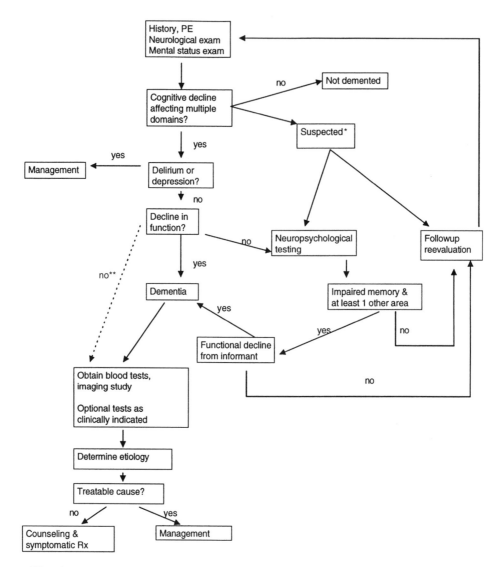

Fig. 1. Proposed algorithm for dementia diagnosis and workup. *Suspected and worrisome history without obvious abnormalities on office mental state testing. **Some physicians will work up patients who show no functional decline without doing neuropsychological testing. (Reprinted with permission from *Neurology* 1995; 45:212.)

schemes, dementia cannot be appropriately diagnosed in the context of an altered sensorium such as delirium or confusional state. It is also important to point out that the diagnosis of dementia is a clinical one. It reflects impairments in neuropsychological and functional status. As such, the diagnosis of dementia cannot be made by a pathologist, neuroradiologist, or blood test.

Table 1
Criteria for Dementia

DSM-IV Diagnostic Criteria

A. The development of multiple cognitive deficits manifested by both
   (1) memory impairment (impaired ability to learn new information or to recall previously learned information
   (2) one (or more) of the following cognitive disturbances:
      (a) aphasia (language disturbance)
      (b) apraxia (impaired ability to carry out motor activities despite intact motor function)
      (c) agnosia (failure to recognize or identify objects despite intact sensory function)
      (d) disturbance in executive functioning (i.e., planning, organizing, sequencing, abstracting)
B. The cognitive deficits in Criteria A1 and A2 each cause significant impairment in social or occupational functioning and represent a significant decline from a previous level of functioning.
C. The deficits do not occur exclusively during the course of a delirium.

Reprinted with permission from the *Diagnostic and Statistic Manual of Mental Disorders*, 4th edn. Washington, D.C.: American Psychiatric Association, 1994.

NINCDS–ADRDA Diagnostic Criteria

A. Decline in memory and other cognitive functions in comparison with the patient's previous level of functions as determined by
   (1) a history of decline in performance
   (2) abnormalities noted on clinical examination
   (3) abnormalities noted on neuropsychological tests
B. Diagnosis of dementia cannot be made when consciousness is impaired by delirium, drowsiness, stupor, or coma or when other clinical abnormalities prevent adequate evaluation of mental status.

Reprinted with permission from *Neurology,* 1984; 34:940.

Components of a Dementia Evaluation

History: Changes in Cognitive and Functional Status

Perhaps the most crucial aspect of establishing the diagnosis of dementia in a patient is obtaining a detailed history. Most often this requires a reliable informant, such as a family member or friend. The patient's dementing condition often prevents the individual from providing an accurate picture of his or her personal history. The clinician needs to inquire about the patient's premorbid, baseline cognitive and behavioral status, education, and highest level of personal achievements. For example, the manifestations of a decline in cognitive and functional status will be very different for a person who was highly educated and held positions of great responsibility compared to a person who at baseline had borderline intellectual capacities, a grade-school education, and worked menial jobs. One inquires about changes in mental abilities that can present as forgetfulness, episodes of getting lost, word-finding difficulties, paraphasic errors, and a tendency for the patient to repeat herself. One asks about changes in personality, mood, and behavior, including evidence of sadness, withdrawal, apathy, inappropriateness, impulsivity, irritability, suspiciousness, and altered appetitive behaviors. Is there evidence to suggest hallucinations, illusions, misperceptions, or delusions (e.g., that others are stealing things from the patient or that one's spouse is unfaithful)?

Inquiries should be made of observed changes in functional status and daily living activities including job performance if the patient is still working, household responsibilities and chores, family finances, self-care, personal hygiene, and episodes of incontinence. Informants should also be asked if they have noted changes in motor functioning such as focal weakness, tremor, stiffness, or gait disturbance. Establishing the onset and temporal pace of changes in mental state is helpful in elucidating potential underlying disease processes. When were the cognitive problems first noted? What were their initial features? Have the changes been insidiously progressive (suggestive of a degenerative disease) or stepwise (more suggestive of vascular insults)? Has the decline been rapid (suggestive of possible infectious process or toxic metabolic state) or more chronic in nature?

Past Medical History

Past medical history and ongoing medical conditions also may provide clues about processes contributing to a decline in cognitive functioning. Specifically, the clinician wants to inquire about a history of cerebrovascular disease, systemic illness, and risk factors for infections. Also pertinent are current and past medication use, a history of alcohol or substance abuse, major head trauma, depression or other psychiatric illness, poor nutritional status, and potential exposure to toxins. Finally, one wants to identify if there is a family history of dementing illness or other diseases that can affect the central nervous system. If so, what was the age of onset of the dementia in the family member, the clinical characteristics, and was there an autopsy that confirmed the suspected underlying pathology?

Mental State Evaluation

A mental state examination is an essential feature of a dementia assessment. This may be the most variable aspect of the evaluation among clinicians. There is no consensus among neurologists, psychiatrists, or primary care physicians of the "best" mental state screening examination or testing strategy to use. Most would agree on the need to assess the following domains: orientation, attention, recent memory, long-term memory, language, praxis, visual-spatial functions and executive functions (insight, judgment, planfulness). It is important for clinicians to have a means of estimating whether a patient's performance falls within age-appropriate norms. There are several standard mental state screening tools that clinicians use, including the Mini Mental State Exam (MMSE) *(20)* and the Blessed Dementia Scale [Information–Memory–Concentration subset (BDS-IMC)] *(21)* (Table 2A,B). Such instruments have certain clear advantages including being brief, standardized, and reasonably well-normed. In addition, there are published reports of cutoff values that are adjusted for various ages and educational backgrounds *(22,23)*. Such tests can serve as a screening device for dementia or cognitive impairment and provide a measure of intellectual decline over time *(24–27)*. However, they are often insensitive to early, subtle cognitive impairments, especially in well-educated, highly intelligent individuals *(28)*. In addition, they are insensitive to late changes in dementia severity *(29)*. Finally, they serve as global screening devices and provide very limited information about damage to specific neurocognitive systems and their associated neuroanatomical networks. Such patterns of cognitive impairment often provide important information for identifying the most likely underlying disease processes *(30–32)* (see Chapter 8). A very poor performance on a mental state screening test certainly can help identify patients suffering from a dementing illness. If there is a discrepancy between an informant's observations of cognitive and behavioral functioning and the patient's performance on mental state tests, it suggests the need for close follow-up and further investigation with more extensive neuropsychological testing.

Sensorimotor Examination

The sensorimotor neurological examination does not contribute to making a diagnosis of dementia per se. However, the pattern of neurological abnormalities often point to likely underlying diseases that may be contributing to the dementing process. For example, a clinician should look for evidence of upper motor neuron signs (e.g., hemiparesis, asymmetric deep tendon reflexes, extensor plantar responses) that would suggest the possibility of stroke or structural lesion. Extrapyramidal signs would raise the question of Parkinson's disease, progressive supranuclear palsy, or Lewy body dementia. Abnormalities of gait may be associated with cerebrovascular disease,

Table 2
Two Standard Mental State Screening Tests

A. Blessed Dementia Scale: Information–Memory–Concentration Subtest

Maximum Score*	Score	
		INFORMATION
2	( )	What is your (name) (age)?
7	( )	What is the (time) (time of day) (day) (date) (month) (season) (year)?
3	( )	Where are we: (name of place) (street) (town)?
1	( )	What type of place are we in (e.g. hospital)?
2	( )	Recognize 2 persons (e.g., relative, doctor, nurse)
		PERSONAL MEMORY
4	( )	What is your (date of birth) (place of birth) (school attended) (occupation)?
3	( )	What is the name of (sibling or spouse) (any town where patient worked) (employer)?
		NON-PERSONAL MEMORY
2	( )	What is the date of (WWI '14-'18) (WWII '39-'45)?
2	( )	Who is the (President) (Vice-President)?
		5-MINUTE RECALL
2	( )	(Mr.) John Brown
2	( )	42 West (Street)
1	( )	Cambridge, (MA)
		CONCENTRATION
2	( )	Months backwards
2	( )	Counting 1-20
2	( )	Counting 20-1
37		

(Reprinted with permission from *British Journal of Psychiatry* 1968;114).
* One point is given for every error made.

B. Mini-Mental State Examination

Maximum Score*	Score	
		ORIENTATION
5	( )	What is the (year) (season) (date) (day) (month)?
5	( )	Where are we: (state) (country) (town) (hospital (floor)?
		REGISTRATION
3	( )	Name three objects, one second to say each, then ask the patient to repeat all three after you have said them. Give one

(continued)

Table 2 *(continued)*

Maximum Score*	Score	
		point for each correct answer. Continue repeating all three objects until the patient learns all three. Count trials and record.
		ATTENTION AND CALCULATION
5	( )	Serial 7's. One point for each correct response. Stop after five answers. Alternatively, spell "world" backward.
		RECALL
3	( )	Ask for the three objects named in *Registration*. Give one point for each correct answer.
		LANGUAGE
2	( )	Name a pencil and watch.
1	( )	Repeat the following "No ifs, ands, or buts."
3	( )	Follow a 3-stage command: "Take paper in your right hand, fold it in half, and put it on the floor."
1	( )	Read and obey the following: CLOSE YOUR EYES.
1	( )	Write a sentence.
1	( )	Copy a design.
30		

(Reprinted with permission from *Journal of Psychiatric Research* 1975;12).
*One point is given for every correct response.

Parkinson's disease, and normal pressure hydrocephalus. Dysarthria would alert the clinician to possible extrapyramidal disorders, bilateral strokes, demyelinating disease, and motor neuron disease. Sensory abnormalities (e.g., peripheral neuropathy) may be associated with B_{12}, other vitamin deficiency states, thyroid disease, or a paraneoplastic syndrome. Cerebellar signs might raise concerns about cerebrovascular disease, spinocerebellar degeneration, a paraneoplastic syndrome, and Creutzfeldt-Jakob disease. In Alzheimer's disease, especially early in its course, the sensorimotor examination tends to be relatively benign. Some researches have pointed out that the presence of extrapyramidal signs in patients with a profile otherwise consistent with Alzheimer's disease suggests a worse prognosis *(33)*. Extrapyramidal signs may indicate the presence of Lewy body variant of AD *(34)*. In general, if a patient with dementia presents with focal or multifocal neurological signs, the clinician should investigate diseases other than AD that may be contributing to the patient's decline in status.

Laboratory Studies

Laboratory studies help to rule out potentially reversible causes of dementia. Initially, the literature suggested that reversible dementias occurred in 10–15% of cases; however, recent reports have pointed to a lower frequency *(35–38)*. The practice parameters of the American Academy of Neurology *(14)* recommend that a workup include the following: complete blood count, electrolytes, calcium, glucose, BUN, creatinine, liver function tests, thyroid function tests, B_{12}, and syphilis serology. Many would also include a sedimentation rate, urinalysis, and chest radiograph. A patient's history should help guide other tests that may need to be ordered. For example, a patient with a long history of smoking should have a chest radiograph if none has been done recently. Someone with a history of high-risk sexual behaviors or exposure to intravenous drugs should have HIV testing. Patients who may have been exposed to industrial toxins at work should be considered for 24-hour urine collection for heavy metals. Currently, acquisition of ApoE genotyping is not recommended for routine evaluations *(39–43)* and is discussed more thoroughly in Chapter 5.

Neuroimaging

Traditionally, neuroimaging [computed tomography (CT) scan or magnetic resonance imaging (MRI)] has been used to rule out potential structural abnormalities that may be causing or contributing to a decline in cognitive functioning. Specifically, the clinician is looking for evidence of tumor, subdural hematoma, hydrocephalus, large and small vessel strokes, and white matter disease. The MRI is much more sensitive than CT in detecting abnormalities in white matter *(44)*, although the clinical significance of such white matter changes is often unclear *(45)*. Atrophy is common in degenerative dementias such as Alzheimer's disease. However, such a finding is not diagnostic and cannot clearly distinguish demented patients from those undergoing normal aging *(46)*. Structural lesions, such as tumor, hydrocephalus, or subdural hematomas, are reported to be relatively uncommon in several recent series of patients being evaluated at out-patient dementia clinics *(36,37,47)*. By contrast, Bradshaw and colleagues *(48)* identified structural lesions in almost 10% of patients being evaluated for dementia, including 5% who had no associated focal signs or symptoms. Furthermore, Katzman *(49)* has noted that the incidence of structural lesions tends to be higher in large autopsy series of demented patients than in studies of patients being evaluated by outpatient dementia clinics. He raises the possibility of a selection bias in the outpatient series. Patients with structural lesions may have been identified by CT scan in the community and referred to a neurosurgeon rather than to a dementia clinic. Many would advocate that obtaining neuroimaging is worth the expense because structural lesions represent potentially treatable entities *(49)*. Others have argued against the routine acquisition of neuroimaging in patients with an insidiously progressive dementia beginning after the age of 60, who lack focal signs or symptoms, seizures or gait disturbance *(37,47)*. In fact, the American Academy of Neurology practice parameters do not designate neuroimaging as "standard procedure" but leaves it up to the judgment of the individual clinician *(14)*.

Recent approaches to identifying patients with Alzheimer's disease using morphometric analysis of temporal lobe structures are discussed in Chapter 6. PET, SPECT, and functional MRI are currently not part of a routine dementia workup. Their potential usefulness is discussed in Chapter 7. In current clinical practice, functional imaging may be particularly helpful in the workup of dementias with atypical presentations. Such studies can support the diagnosis of degenerative diseases that are less common than Alzheimer's disease such as a frontotemporal dementia, which is associated with hypoperfusion in the anterior regions of the brain *(50–52)*.

Neuropsychological Testing

Formal neuropsychological tests also are not part of the routine workup of patients with possible dementia. Such testing can provide a quantitative assessment of a range of cognitive domains. Establishing a patient's performance during an initial assessment allows for quantitative measurement of decline in cognitive status over time. Progressive impairments of cognitive abilities, especially if they exceed age-matched norms, are very suggestive of an underlying dementing process. Neuropsychological assessment is particularly helpful for a patient whose results on an initial evaluation and mental state screen are ambiguous, and the suspicion of an early dementing process remains. Such assessment can help establish areas of cognitive impairment before decline in functional status that accompanies clinical dementia. As noted, certain patterns of cognitive impairment have implications for which neuroanatomical networks are likely disturbed by the underlying disease process, which in turn have implications about the most likely underlying etiology *(30–32)* (see Chapter 8). For example, patients with probable AD whose pathology often begins in the temporolimbic cortex that subserves memory tend to demonstrate significant impairments in the realm of memory before crossing the "threshold" into a clinical dementia *(53–58)*.

Neuropsychological assessment also can be extremely helpful in patients whose baseline cognitive and educational status was in either the very superior or borderline range. There are strategies for estimating premorbid cognitive abilities against which to compare current intellectual functioning *(59,60)*. Education-adjusted norms are available for some cognitive tests *(61,62)*. Unexpected or excessive scatter in performance on different cognitive tests raises questions about a patient's current intellectual status that would require monitoring. Finally, neuropsychological tests are also particularly helpful in documenting atypical patterns of dementia, in which, for example, memory problems are not the most salient feature.

CSF Evaluation

Lumbar puncture with cerebrospinal fluid (CSF) analysis is no longer part of the routine evaluation of dementia. This procedure is appropriate if there are concerns about any of the following: CNS infection (e.g., fever, headache), carcinomatous meningitis, reactive syphilis serology, subacute onset, or other atypical presentations of dementia, or if dementia occurs under the age of 50 *(14,63,64)*. In addition, lumbar puncture is indicated when there is evidence that a patient may be suffering from an inflammatory or vasculitic process or when the patient is immunosuppressed. A recent report suggested that the diagnosis of Creutzfeldt-Jakob disease could be confirmed with reasonably high sensitivity and specificity in demented patients without a history of recent infarction or encephalitis who were found to have the protein 14-3-3 in their CSF *(65, 65a, 65b, 65c)*. The potential usefulness of CSF levels of tau protein, β-amyloid, or $α_1$-antichymotrypsin for the diagnosis of Alzheimer's disease are discussed in Chapter 9.

EEG

An electroencephalogram (EEG) is also not currently part of a standard dementia evaluation. Although the EEG of a demented patient often reveals a slowed background, this pattern lacks specificity. It can also be seen in "normal" aging and be found in a variety of dementing illnesses. Quantitative EEG analysis has pointed to patterns of abnormal electrical activity that are seen more commonly in Alzheimer's disease than normal aging *(66,67)*. However, to date such analyses have not yielded sufficient sensitivity and specificity to justify the routine use of such tests in the diagnostic evaluation of dementia *(68)*. It may turn out that the overlap in findings between AD patients and normal aging controls in quantitative EEG and other tests is largely due to the fact that some of the "normal" subjects had underlying AD pathology that disrupted normal functioning without yet causing a clinical dementia. As with many other techniques, ordering an EEG should be guided by the history and neurological examination. Specifically, an EEG is helpful in evaluating for possible toxic-metabolic encephalopathy, seizures, encephalitis, or Creutzfeldt-Jakob disease *(69,70)*.

Cerebral Biopsy

Currently, brain biopsy in patients with dementia is pursued very infrequently. In experienced centers, mortality is probably under 1% and postoperative morbidity is relatively low *(70–72)*. However, most clinicians would not recommend such an invasive procedure unless the results would lead to a change in the therapy or management of the individual patient. Thus, biopsy is considered in cases in which there is a concern about possible atypical infectious, inflammatory, vasculitic, or demyelinating processes. Unfortunately, 20–25% of cerebral biopsies for dementia do not yield a specific diagnosis *(70)*.

First Major Decision Point: Abnormal Versus Normal Status

The evaluation of dementia can proceed in a relatively orderly fashion. The first major task is to determine if a patient is exhibiting abnormal cognitive abilities and a decline in function. As noted, an appreciation of the patient's baseline mental state and achievements is crucial in making such an assessment. In addition, a clinician needs to be aware of changes associated with normal aging to determine whether a patient exceeds these bounds. On average, many cognitive functions decline in later life, including speed of mental processing and responding, digit span, visual-perceptual abilities, mental flexibility and abstractions *(73–76)*. Acquisition of the new information also is diminished. However, once encoded, there does not tend to be a significant loss of information over time regardless of a patient's level of education *(77)*.

Most importantly, these age-related cognitive changes do not lead to significant interference with the maintenance of an independent and productive life. The mental state screening tests discussed earlier are a means of rapidly assessing a patient's current level of performance and can be compared to established norms. If the patient's performance on mental state examination is borderline or questionable, or if by history the patient appears to be exhibiting a decline in functioning, even with an apparently normal screening mental status examination, the provider should strongly consider formal neuropsychological tests and arrange follow-up in 6 to 12 months to assess whether the decline is progressive.

If there is clear evidence of cognitive impairments, the next task is to determine if the mental state changes reflect a delirium, altered sensorium, or acute confusional state. The salient abnormality in such conditions is inattention, in which the patient exhibits an inability to maintain a coherent stream of thought or behavior. The most common etiology of an acute confusional state in the elderly is a toxic-metabolic encephalopathy due to side effects from medications, systemic illness, or end organ failure. As noted, a diagnosis of dementia is inappropriate if mental state changes occur in the setting of an acute confusional state. Clinicians need to treat the underlying conditions and reevaluate the patient's mental capacities once the confusional state has resolved. Of particular note, demented individuals are themselves very vulnerable to developing acute confusional states *(78,79)*. They are exquisitely sensitive to a perturbation of their internal or external environments. This condition has been called a "beclouded dementia," indicating that there is a delirium superimposed upon an underlying dementia *(80)*. Such individuals never return to a "normal" cognitive state. Obtaining a careful history regarding the patient's recent "baseline" status (before becoming more acutely confused) can be very informative. Specifically, one wants to know if the change in mental state emerged against a background of a previously well-functioning or cognitively compromised individual.

Second Major Decision Point: Differential Diagnosis

Once the diagnosis of dementia has been made, the clinician needs to establish the most likely underlying etiology of the condition. Traditionally, this involves trying to "rule out" potentially treatable or reversible etiologies of dementia that may be identified by the workup discussed earlier. Specifically, one aims to exclude encephalopathies due to metabolic problems (e.g., thyroid deficiency) or side effects from medications, CNS infections, vitamin deficiencies, or structural lesions (e.g., hydrocephalus, tumor, subdural hematoma). These conditions tend to account for small percentage of patients presenting with dementia *(36–38)*. When these conditions have been excluded, the two largest remaining disease categories are the degenerative dementias (of which Alzheimer's disease is by far the most common) and vascular dementia.

Major Patterns of Dementia

Diagnostic accuracy may be improved if the clinician is also attentive to the *pattern* of mental state dysfunction exhibited by a patient, which within the context of the patient's specific history, point to a circumscribed set of disease processes that are most likely to be contributing *(30,31)*. By employing this strategy, the clinician not only attempts to "rule out" certain entities but also to identify clinical patterns with a high likelihood of being associated with specific kinds of underlying pathologies.

Progressive Amnestic Dementia
(Probable Alzheimer's Disease)

The most common pattern is a progressive amnestic dementia, in which deterioration in memory functions is the salient feature. The course is insidiously progressive, with memory impairments usually being the initial source of disruption of daily activities. Informants often provide a history of progressive problems with recalling recent events, misplacing objects, repeating questions, becoming disoriented or lost, producing the wrong words, or exhibiting fluent but "empty" speech. Early on, there may be subtle changes in personality in the form of increased disengagement or withdrawal from activities, but grossly inappropriate behaviors are unusual *(81,82)*.

On mental state testing, the dominant problems involve the storage, retention or retrieval components of memory. Language and visuospatial functions also are usually abnormal and over time insight, attention and executive functions deteriorate. Atrophic changes on CT or MRI are most common. When functional imaging is done, the most likely pattern reflects abnormalities in temporoparietal regions bilaterally.

This dementia profile is the most frequent one seen in the elderly and is most often associated with the plaque and tangle pathology of Alzheimer's disease. The National Institute of Neurological and Communicative Disorders and Stroke-Alzheimer's Disease and Related Disorders Association (NINCDS–ADRA) *(10)* has codified the clinical criteria associated with the high likelihood of Alzheimer's pathology (Table 3). The major elements defining "probable Alzheimer's disease" (PrAD) include:

1. Presence of dementia
2. Progressive worsening of memory and other cognitive functions
3. Deficits in two or more areas of cognition
4. No disturbance of consciousness
5. Age of onset between 40 and 90
6. Absence of systemic or CNS disorders that could account for the dementia

The diagnosis of "possible Alzheimer's disease" is appropriate when a patient exhibits an atypical presentation or clinical course, progressive decline of a single cognitive deficit, or in the presence of a second systemic or brain disorder sufficient to produce the dementia that is not considered to be the cause of the dementia. "Definite Alzheimer's disease" can only be diagnosed when in life the patient had met criteria for probable Alzheimer's disease and at autopsy (or by biopsy) there is appropriate histopathological evidence of Alzheimer's pathology. DSM-IV criteria for "dementia of the Alzheimer's type" (DAT) are simi-

Table 3
NINCDS-ADRDA Criteria for Clinical Diagnosis of Alzheimer's Disease

I. The criteria for the clinical diagnosis of *probable* Alzheimer's disease include:
  1. Dementia established by clinical examination and documented by the Mini-Mental State Test, Blessed Dementia Scale, or some similar examination, and confirmed by neuropsychological tests
  2. Deficits in two or more areas of cognition
  3. Progressive worsening of memory and other cognitive functions
  4. No disturbance of consciousness
  5. Onset between ages 40 and 90, most often after age 65
  6. Absence of systemic disorders or other brain diseases that in and of themselves could account for the progressive deficits in memory and cognition

II. The diagnosis of *probable* Alzheimer's disease is supported by:
  1. Progressive deterioration of specific cognitive functions such as language (aphasia), motor skills (apraxia), and perception (agnosia)
  2. Impaired activities of daily living and altered patterns of behavior
  3. Family history of similar disorders, particularly if confirmed neuropathologically
  4. Laboratory results of:
     a. Normal lumbar puncture as evaluated by standard techniques
     b. Normal pattern or nonspecific changes in EEG, such as increased slow-wave activity
     c. Evidence of cerebral atrophy on CT with progression documented by serial observation

III. Other clinical features consistent with the diagnosis of *probable* Alzheimer's disease, after exclusion of causes of dementia other than Alzheimer's disease include:
  1. Plateaus in the course of progression of the illness
  2. Associated symptoms of depression, insomnia, incontinence, delusions, illusions, hallucinations; catastrophic verbal, emotional, or physical outbursts; sexual disorders; and weight loss
  3. Other neurologic abnormalities in some patients, especially those with more advanced disease and including motor signs such as increased muscle tone, myoclonus, or gait disorder
  4. Seizures in advanced disease
  5. CT normal for age

IV. Features that make the diagnosis of *probable* Alzheimer's disease uncertain or unlikely include:
  1. Sudden, apoplectic onset
  2. Focal neurological findings such as hemiparesis, sensory loss, visual field deficits, and incoordination early in the course of the illness
  3. Seizures or gait disturbances at the onset or very early in the course of the illness

V. Clinical diagnosis of *possible* Alzheimer's disease:
  1. May be made on the basis of the dementia syndrome; in the absence of other

(continued)

Table 3 *(continued)*

      neurological, psychiatric, or systemic disorders sufficient to cause dementia; and in the presence of variations in the onset, presentation, or clinical course

    2. May be made in the presence of a second systemic or brain disorder sufficient to produce dementia, which is not considered to be the cause of the dementia

    3. Should be used in research studies when a single, gradually progressive, severe cognitive deficit is identified in the absence of other identifiable cause

VI. Criteria for diagnosis of *definite* Alzheimer's disease are:

    1. The clinical criteria for probable Alzheimer's disease

    2. Histopathologic evidence obtained from a biopsy or autopsy

VII. Classifications of Alzheimer's disease for research purposes should specify features that may differentiate subtypes of the disorder, such as:

    1. Familial occurrence

    2. Onset before age 65

    3. Presence of trisomy-21

    4. Coexistence of other relevant conditions such as Parkinson's disease

Reprinted with permission from *Neurology* 1984;34:940.

lar to the NINCDS–ADRDA criteria. First, one needs to ensure that a patient fits the criteria for dementia as noted on Table 1. Furthermore, according to DSM-IV, the course of DAT is characterized by gradual onset, continuing cognitive decline, and is not due to other CNS or systemic conditions that cause progressive deficits in memory and cognition (Table 4).

Other degenerative diseases that have been associated with a progressive amnestic dementia include diffuse Lewy body disease, Pick's disease, and focal neuronal atrophy *(34,83–85)*. However, these pathological processes are much less common than Alzheimer's disease. In addition, there are a number of nondegenerative processes that have been associated with the "amnestic syndrome." Most often, however, these are not progressive processes. They include anoxia, carbon monoxide poisoning, posterior cerebral artery strokes, anterior cerebral artery aneurysm with bleed or surgery, Korsakoff's syndrome, head trauma, and herpes encephalitis.

Dementias With a Prominent Dysexecutive Syndrome

A second major dementia pattern involves patients who exhibit salient changes in personality and behavior, accompanied by compromised attention, motivation, judgment, insight, and other "executive" functions. This clinical entity has been given several names including frontotemporal dementia (FTD), dementia of the frontal lobe type, and comportmental dementia *(30,50,86–88)*.

Table 4
DSM-IV Diagnostic Criteria for Dementia of the Alzheimer's Type

---

A. The development of multiple cognitive deficits manifested by both
    (1) memory impairment (impaired ability to learn new information or to recall previously learned information)
    (2) one (or more) of the following cognitive disturbances:
        (a) aphasia (language disturbance)
        (b) apraxia (impaired ability to carry out motor activities despite intact motor function)
        (c) agnosia (failure to recognize or identify objects despite intact sensory function)
        (d) disturbance in executive functioning (i.e., planning, organizing, sequencing, abstracting)
B. The cognitive deficits in Criteria A1 and A2 each cause significant impairment in social or occupational functioning and represent a significant decline from a previous level of functioning.
C. The course is characterized by gradual onset and continuing cognitive decline.
D. The cognitive deficits in Criteria A1 and A2 are not due to any of the following:
    (1) other central nervous system conditions that cause progressive deficits in memory and cognition (e.g., cerebrovascular disease, Parkinson's disease, Huntington's disease, subdural hematoma, normal-pressure hydrocephalus, brain tumor)
    (2) systemic conditions that are known to cause dementia (e.g., hypothyroidism vitamin B12 or folic acid deficiency, niacin deficiency, hypercalcemia, neurosyphilis, HIV infection)
    (3) substance-induced conditions
E. The deficits do not occur exclusively during the course of a delirium.
F. The disturbance is not better accounted for by another Axis I disorder (e.g., Major Depressive Disorder, Schizophrenia).

Reprinted with permission from the *Diagnostic and Statistical Manual of Mental Disorders,* 4th edn. American Psychiatric Association, 1994.

In addition, there are overlapping features with the so-called "subcortical dementias" *(89,90).* This overlap is likely due to the intense connections between the frontal lobes and subcortical regions *(91,92),* as noted in Figure 2.

A history from a reliable informant often reveals major changes in the patient's personality and social conduct, with inappropriate, embarrassing, or impulsive behaviors. Such disruptions often punctuate behaviors that are otherwise characterized by apathy and withdrawal. Changes in appetitive behavior such as eating or sexual activity are common. Patients tend to present in the presenile years (less than 65 years of age). Mental state examination often reveals compromise of the so-called executive functions, including attention, judgment, and insight. Compared to patients with probable AD, patients with

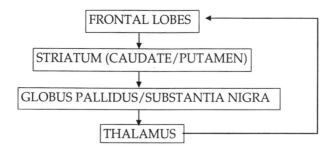

Fig. 2. Schematic view of the frontal networks.

frontotemporal dementia reportedly do better on tests of constructions and calculations *(93)*. Performance in other realms may also be impaired because of a lack of motivation or mental activation. Memory is compromised mainly at the encoding or retrieval stages. With cueing, recognition memory is often relatively well preserved. There is diminished spontaneous verbal output that over time may progress to mutism. CT or MRI tend to show involutional changes in the frontal regions and functional imaging may show diminished perfusion in frontal lobes and anterior temporal regions *(50,51)*. The Lund and Manchester research groups have proposed specific criteria for the diagnosis of frontotemporal dementia, based on behavioral, affective, and cognitive impairments and the results of investigations *(50)*. Table 5 summarizes the diagnosis criteria. The frontotemporal dementias reportedly account for 10–20% of cases of degenerative dementias *(87)*. A recent epidemiological study of the Dutch population suggested that 38% of patients with FTD had a strong family history of dementia (vs. 15% of controls) *(93a)*. Approximately 43% of FTD patients with a family history of dementia were found to have a mutation in the tau gene located on chromosome 17 *(93b)*. Intense interest has developed in investigating the relationship between non-Alzheimer's degenerative dementias and abnormalities linked to chromosome 17 *(93c)*.

On a pathological plane, this dementia syndrome is most often associated with marked atrophy of the frontal lobes and anterior temporal regions and histologically with neuronal loss and gliosis *(30,88)*. Also, 20% of cases also have Pick bodies and ballooned cells, which are pathognomonic for Pick's disease *(88)*. The preponderance of pathology in the frontal lobes and anterior temporal regions accounts for the profile of cognitive and personality changes. This pattern of dementia is rarely associated with the plaque and tangle pathology that defines Alzheimer's disease *(88)*. Lewy body dementia (in which there is widespread distribution of Lewy bodies in brainstem, basal forebrain, and cortex) can present with prominent behavioral changes and has recently been re-

Table 5
Lund/Manchester Criteria: Clinical Diagnostic Features
of Frontotemporal Dementia

CORE DIAGNOSTIC FEATURES
Behavioral disorder
   Insidious onset and slow progression
   Early loss of personal awareness (neglect of personal hygiene and grooming)
   Early loss of social awareness (lack of social tact, misdemeanors such as shoplift-
      ing)
   Early signs of disinhibition (such as unrestrained sexuality, violent behavior, inap-
      propriate jocularity, restless pacing)
   Mental rigidity and inflexibility
   Hyperorality (oral/dietary changes, overeating, food fads, excessive smoking and
      alcohol consumption, oral exploration of objects)
   Stereotyped and perseverative behavior (wandering, mannerisms such as clapping,
      singing, dancing, ritualistic preoccupation such as hoarding, toileting, and dress-
      ing)
   Utilization behavior (unrestrained exploration of objects in the environment)
   Distractibility, impulsivity, and impersistence
   Early loss of insight into the fact that the altered condition is due to a pathological
      change of own mental state

Affective symptoms
   Depression, anxiety, excessive sentimentality, suicidal and fixed ideation, delusion
      (early and evanescent)
   Hypchondriasis, bizarre somatic preoccupation (early and evanescent)
   Emotional unconcern (emotional indifference and remoteness, lack of empathy
      and sympathy, apathy)
   Amimia (inertia, aspontaneity)

Speech disorder
   Progressive reduction of speech (aspontaneity and economy of utterance)
   Stereotypy of speech (repetition of limited repertoire of words, phrases, or themes)
   Echolalia and perseveration
   Late mutism

Spatial orientation and praxis preserved
   (intact abilities to negotiate the environment)

Physical signs
   Early primitive reflexes
   Early incontinence
   Late akinesia, rigidity, tremor
   Low and labile blood pressure

Investigations
   Normal EEG despite clinically evident dementia
   Brain imaging (structural or functional, or both): predominant frontal or anterior
      temporal abnormality, or both

(continued)

Table 5 *(continued)*

Neuropsychology (profound failure on "frontal lobe" tests in the absence of severe amnesia, aphasia, or perceptual spatial disorder)

SUPPORTIVE DIAGNOSTIC FEATURES
Onset before 65
Positive family history of similar disorder in a first degree relative
Bulbar palsy, muscular weakness and wasting, fasciculations (motor neuron disease).

DIAGNOSTIC EXCLUSION FEATURES
Abrupt onset with ictal events
Head trauma related to onset
Early severe amnesia
Early spatial disorientation, lost in surroundings, defective localization of objects
Early severe apraxia
Logoclonic speech with rapid loss of train of thought
Myoclonus
Cortical bulbar and spinal deficits
Cerebellar ataxia
Choreoathetosis
Early, severe pathological EEG
Brain imaging (predominant postcentral structural or functional deficit. Multifocal cerebral lesions on CT or MRI)
Laboratory tests indicating brain involvement or inflammatory disorder (such as multiple sclerosis, syphilis, AIDS, and herpes simplex encephalitis)

RELATIVE DIAGNOSTIC EXCLUSION FEATURES
Typical history of chronic alcoholism
Sustained hypertension
History of vascular disease (such as angina, claudication)

Reprinted with permission from the *Journal of Neurology, Neurosurgery and Psychiatry* 1994;57:416–418.

ported as a fairly common form of degenerative dementia with autopsy series suggesting that it may be seen in 15–25% of cases *(94–96)*. Lewy body dementia has been associated with fluctuating cognitive impairment, transient episodes of marked confusion, a high incidence of visual and/or auditory hallucinations and delusions. It is most often accompanied by extrapyramidal signs or heightened sensitivity to a neuroleptic medication.

Dementias that exhibit prominent impairments in attention and executive functioning probably have the widest differential diagnosis and constitute many of the potentially reversible conditions. Table 6 provides a list of nondegenerative diseases with prominent changes in attention and behavior that includes the dementia of depression (also known as "pseudodementia"). It has

Table 6
Nondegenerative Disease With Prominent Changes in Attention and Behavior

Toxic-metabolic disease (e.g., hypothyroidism, or side effects from medications)
Alcohol-related dementia
Space-occupying lesions (especially to the frontal lobe, such as subdural hematoma or tumor)
The dementia of depression (also known as "pseudodementia")

been estimated that the dementia of depression accounts for about 5% of dementias in general and about 25% of the potentially reversible causes of dementia *(36)*. On mental state examination, there are often impairments in attention, concentration, processing speed, and spontaneous behavioral output. Motivation tends to be limited and the patient may complain of not knowing the answers, rather than offering incorrect responses. Difficulties with memory tend to be at the level of encoding and for some retrieval, with relatively preserved recognition memory after delay. There is no aphasia, although word retrieval may be slow. Somatic complaints are not uncommon. There may or may not be vegetative symptoms or past psychiatric history of depression. Clinicians should have a low threshold for treating depression, preferably with medications like the serotonin reuptake inhibitors (SSRIs) that have relatively low anticholinergic side-effects. Unfortunately, some patients who initially present with depression go on to exhibit a progressive dementia despite appropriate treatment for their mood disorder *(97–99)*. In such cases, the depression was probably an early manifestation of their degenerative process. It has been shown that patients suffering from degenerative dementias are at increased risk for developing symptoms of depression that often manifest themselves early in the course of their illness *(100–102)*.

Dementia Associated with Sensorimotor Signs

A third major pattern in dementia is one in which cognitive decline is accompanied by sensory and motor signs. Most often, the salient mental state changes of these dementias also involve complex attention, behavior, and personality. Changes in executive functions are not universal, but depend on where the brunt of the neuropathology is located. Table 7 lists a number of disease processes that tend to have this dementia profile. The disease entity in this category with the highest prevalence is vascular dementia. Unfortunately, it is not uncommon for clinicians to "automatically" render the diagnosis of vascular dementia after a demented patient's MRI or CT scan returns with some evidence of strokes or small vessel disease. Many autopsy series suggest that the accuracy of clinical diagnoses of vascular dementia can be quite low (21–82%) *(103,104)*. A large per-

Table 7
Dementias Associated With Sensorimotor Signs

Vascular dementia
Infection (e.g., HIV, syphilis, Creutzfeldt-Jacob disease)
Metabolic abnormalities (e.g., B_{12} deficiency)
Inherited disorders of metabolism (e.g., metachromatic leukodystrophy, Kuf's disease)
Normal pressure hydrocephalus
Multiple sclerosis
Inflammatory/autoimmune disease (e.g., SLE)
Degenerative diseases with extrapyramidal features (e.g., Parkinson's disease,
   Huntington's disease, progressive supranuclear palsy, and Wilson's disease)
Motor neuron disease with frontotemporal dementia

---

centage of patients diagnosed with vascular dementia are determined at autopsy to have Alzheimer's pathology, with or without significant cerebrovascular insults *(105,106)*. Although earlier reports of the prevalence of vascular dementia varied widely, recent reviews suggest a prevalence in the United States of around 10% *(15,70,107)*. Symptoms of dementia are reportedly more likely to develop after a critical volume of tissue is infarcted (over 50 mL) or if small strokes are strategically placed that disrupt cognitive abilities *(108)*. Table 8 summarizes the DSM-IV diagnostic criteria for vascular dementia. Diagnosis of vascular dementia is supported by the sudden development of impairments in one or more cognitive domains, a stepwise deteriorating course, focal neurological signs, risk factors for stroke, and a history or imaging evidence of strokes.

If a patient has a history of an insidiously progressive amnestic dementia and is found to have a stroke with sensorimotor signs, a clinician should still consider the diagnosis Alzheimer's disease as likely, but recognize that the cerebrovascular disease may be making an additional contribution to the patient's cognitive impairments. Strokes may reduce "cognitive reserve" in patients and lead to earlier, more dramatic presentations of clinical problems in patients with underlying AD pathology *(109)*. A diagnosis of vascular dementia is probably most tenuous in a demented patient with prominent memory problems, no history suggestive of clinical strokes, and an MRI scan that reveals mild white matter changes and a few T2 signal abnormalities.

As noted on Table 7, there are numerous dementias that are associated with sensorimotor signs of which we will briefly mention HIV associated dementia, neurosyphilis, normal pressure hydrocephalus, multiple sclerosis, and extrapyramidal syndromes. These dementias tend to present with apathy, social withdrawal, blunted affect, diminished behavioral output, and compromised attention. For example, changes in mental state changes can be the presenting

Table 8
DSM IV Diagnostic Criteria for Vascular Dementia

A. The development of multiple cognitive deficits manifested by both
   1) memory impairment (impaired ability to learn new information or to recall previously learned information)
   2) one (or more) of the following cognitive disturbances:
      (a) aphasia (language disturbance)
      (b) apraxia (impaired ability to carry out motor activities despite intact sensory function)
      (c) agnosia (failure to recognize or identify objects despite intact sensory function)
      (d) disturbance in executive functioning (i.e., planning, organizing, sequencing, abstracting)
B. The cognitive deficits in Criteria A1 and A2 each cause significant impairment in social or occupational functioning and represent a significant decline from a previous level of functioning.
C. Focal neurological signs and symptoms (e.g., exaggeration of deep tendon reflexes, extensor plantar response, pseudobulbar palsy, gait abnormalities, weakness of an extremity) or laboratory evidence indicative of cerebrovascular disease (e.g., multiple infarctions involving cortex and underlying white matter) that are judged to be etiologically related to the disturbance.
D. The deficits do not occur exclusively during the course of a delirium.

Reprinted with permission from the *Diagnostic and Statistical Manual of Mental Disorders*, 4th edn, American Psychiatric Association, 1994.

symptoms of HIV infection, although much more commonly there are systemic signs to point to this diagnosis *(110,111)*. Peripheral neuropathy and myelopathy are also commonly seen in HIV infection. The pathology associated with tertiary syphilis tends to be most severe in the frontal and temporal lobes, with associated personality changes, impaired judgment, and altered mood *(112,113)*. Sensorimotor abnormalities commonly accompany the dementia, including dysarthria and changes in gait and reflexes.

Normal pressure hydrocephalus (NPH) is believed to account for about 10% of the reversible dementing illnesses *(36)*. The well-known triad associated with NPH includes gait disturbance, incontinence, and progressive decline in cognitive functioning *(114)*. The pattern of mental state changes seen in NPH usually involves slowed processing speed, impaired complex attention, and diminished executive functioning *(115–117)*. Aphasia and apraxia are unusual and would suggest other contributing etiologies. There is ongoing debate about the best strategies for identifying patients who will benefit most from the placement of a shunt. Normal-sized sulci, periventricular edema, CSF flow void on MRI in the cerebral aqueduct, third and fourth ventricles, and clinical response to the removal of approximately 30 mL of CSF have been reported to be predictive of better outcomes *(118–120)*. Cisternography does not appear to add much to the information obtained by clinical history and imaging studies *(121)*.

Patients with multiple sclerosis often suffer from cognitive, emotional, and behavioral problems that tend to add to their disability and problems functioning at home and work *(122–124)*. Dementia has been reported in up to a third of patients with Parkinson's disease *(125–128)*. Some patients have coexisting Alzheimer's pathology, which probably accounts for their decline in mental state functioning. Others present with a disruption of frontal networks ("subcortical dementia syndrome") with bradyphrenia, impaired activation, and forgetfulness. These difficulties may reflect diminished dopamine availability to caudate nucleus and prefrontal regions. Medications and coexisting depression also may play an important role. Huntington's disease, progressive supranuclear palsy, and Wilson's disease all have associated mental state changes, which in part reflect the disruption of frontal networks *(89,129–136)*. The associated extrapyramidal features tend to point to the diagnosis in these cases. From 2% to 3% of patients with motor neuron disease present with dementia that has nearly identical features to the frontotemporal dementia that was described earlier *(137,138)*.

Progressive Focal Neuropsychological Deficits

The last major dementia pattern involves progressive neuropsychological deterioration that remains relatively well circumscribed and without prominent memory problems at least in the first 2 years of the illness *(30,139)*. These rare entities serve to remind us that degenerative processes are often relatively selective in their distribution of pathology early in their course. The clinical symptomatology associated with these dementia profiles can be interpreted as reflecting the relatively focal distribution of pathological damage to the nervous system. Primary progressive aphasia has received the most attention *(139–145)*. Other degenerative diseases within this dementia category have been termed slowly progressive apraxia, progressive prosopagnosia, progressive semantic dementia, and posterior cortical atrophy *(146–153)*.

Summary

This chapter has reviewed the clinical approach to the evaluation of a demented patient. The major branching points along the decision tree of working up the patient were reviewed. We emphasized the importance of clinical judgment in this process, which depends so heavily on a detailed history, mental status examination, and neurological assessment. We discussed the value of a variety of laboratory tests used by clinicians to assess potentially reversible contributions to a patient's decline in mental state and functional status and noted some of the controversies that have arisen over their cost:benefit ratio.

The chapter reviewed diagnostic criteria, guidelines, and practice parameters offered by major clinical and research bodies. In studies that have employed such guidelines, the accuracy rates for the diagnosis of probable Alzheimer's disease has ranged from 64% to 100%, as determined at autopsy using a variety of standard neuropathological criteria *(1,12,30,154–159)*. Most of the studies achieved a positive predictive value in the mid to high 80s. Such results are very encouraging and are as good as or better than those yielded by many of the experimental diagnostic strategies being investigated. In fact, most of the experimental diagnostic assays have used clinical research criteria as a provisional "gold standard" to diagnose their patients with AD, presumably until a large enough series of their patients has been brought to autopsy.

Limits of Current Approaches to the Clinical Evaluation of Alzheimer's Disease

If using standard clinical tools can yield such high accuracy rates for diagnosis of AD, why is there a need for other approaches? This important question can be addressed in several ways. First, we are unaware of any systematic study regarding the extent to which most practitioners actually follow the guidelines reviewed in this chapter. There is likely to be a gap between the practice patterns of clinician-researchers in Alzheimer's disease centers and physicians in the community. Practitioners in research centers see a very large volume of demented patients. The impressive accuracy rates reported by such centers may not be due to the fact that the clinicians followed standard guidelines. Rather these particular clinicians may have a wealth of experience upon which they developed the kind of clinical expertise that yields excellent diagnostic results. The extension of such expertise into the community is an important goal, but one that may be very difficult to achieve. We suspect that clinicians in these centers devote more time than average to patients and their families and obtain a detailed history, mental state, and neurological examination. Patients in such centers tend to be followed closely over time. The pattern that emerges with longitudinal evaluations can confirm the initial diagnostic impressions or raise questions about the patient's profile that would lead to even closer scrutiny. Autopsies are often sought, which allows feedback to clinicians on the accuracy of their diagnoses. This kind of intensive, time-consuming review process is unlikely to be carried out in the average community practice.

The accuracy rates in the community have not been as high as in research centers dedicated to the study of Alzheimer's disease and related clinical entities *(160)*. Moreover, autopsy studies on the accuracy of clinical diagnoses in settings that have not utilized careful diagnostic criteria have revealed success rates as low as 55% *(5)*. Given the prevalence of Alzheimer's disease, such a low "hit-rate" suggests a diagnostic accuracy of close to chance. Many of these studies were done during an era in which there was less awareness about the criteria for dementia in general and AD specifically *(16,70)*. Presumably, current accuracy rates would be better, although the economic pressures of modern medicine that encourage clinicians to spend less time with patients than in the past may counter trends toward improvement in diagnosis.

With the exception of the report by Morris and colleagues *(156)*, most autopsy series that have demonstrated very high diagnostic accuracy rates have studied patients who were in the moderate to severe stages of the illness. Also, these studies have identified highly selected patients and excluded those with any unusual or complicating features that often arise in clinical practice. Enthusiasm about the accuracy of clinical assessment needs to be tempered by the fact that success rates may be much lower for groups of patients that suffer from a mixture of dementing illnesses, especially those who are in the earliest stages. More importantly, existing diagnostic criteria are not applicable to patients in the preclinical stages of the disease. As treatments become available, identifying AD patients in these stages will become increasinglyimportant.

In summary, studies have demonstrated that clinical assessment, using well established guidelines, can yield very high diagnostic accuracy rates, especially for patients who have reached the moderately severe stages of dementia. The extent to which the average clinician actually follows these guidelines and the degree to which the superb results reported are dependent upon the expertise of a select group of highly trained clinicians have not been determined. The concerns raised in this chapter point to the need to develop additional strategies for identifying AD patients in the preclinical and early stages of the illness. Ideally these strategies would be accessible to clinicians in both research centers and the community.

References

1. Gearing M, Mirra SS, Hedreen JC, Sumi SM, Hansen LA, Heyman A. The consortium to establish a registry for Alzheimer's disease (CERAD). *Neurology* 1995:45:461–466.
2. Katzman R. Alzheimer's disease. *N. Engl. J. Med.* 1986;314:964–973.
3. Kokmen E, Beard CM, Offord KP, Kurland LT. Prevalence of medically diagnosed dementia in a defined United States population: Rochester, Minnesota. *Neurology* 1989;39:773–776.

4. Smith JS, Kilch LG. The investigation of dementia: results in 200 consecutive admissions. *Lancet* 1981;2:824–827.

5. Rocca WA, Amaducci LA, Schoenberg BS. Epidemiology of clinically diagnosed Alzheimer's disease. *Ann. Neurol.* 1986;19:415–424.

6. Pfeffer RI, Afifi AA, Chance JM. Prevalence of Alzheimer's disease in a retirement community. *Am. J. Epidemiol.* 1987;125:420–436.

7. Evans DA, Funkenstein HH, Albert MS, Scherr PA, Cook NR, Chown MJ. Prevalence of Alzheimer's disease in a community population of older persons: higher than previously reported. *JAMA* 1989;262:2551–2556.

8. Schumock GT. Economic considerations in the treatment and management of Alzheimer's disease. *Am. J. Health Syst. Pharm.* 1998;55(Suppl. 2):S17–S21.

9. American Psychiatric Association. *Diagnostic and Statistical Manual of Mental Disorders,* 4th ed. Washington, DC: American Psychiatric Association, 1994.

10. McKhann G, Drachman D, Folstein M, Katzman R, Price D, Stadlan EM, et al Clinical diagnosis of Alzheimer's disease: report of the NINCDS-ADRDA work group under the auspices of department of health and human services task force on Alzheimer's disease. *Neurology* 1984;34:939–944.

11. Morris JC, Heyman A, Mohs RC, Hughes JP, van Belle G, Fillenbaum G, et al The consortium to establish a registry for Alzheimer's disease (CERAD). Part I. Clinical and neuropsychological assessment of Alzheimer's disease. *Neurology* 1989;3:1159–1165.

12. Mirra SS, Heyman A, McKeel D, Sumi SM, Crain BJ, Brownlee LM, et al. The consortium to establish a registry for Alzheimer's disease (CERAD). Part II. Standardization of the neuropathologic assessment of Alzheimer's disease. *Neurology* 1991;41:479–486.

13. Morris JC, Edland S, Clark C, Galasko D, Koss E, Mohs R, et al. The consortium to establish a registry for Alzheimer's disease (CERAD). Part IV. Rates of cognitive change in the longitudinal assessment of probable Alzheimer's disease. *Neurology* 1993;43:2457–2465.

14. American Academy of Neurology. Practice parameter for the diagnosis and evaluation of dementia (summary statement). *Neurology* 1994;44:2203–2206.

15. Corey-Bloom J, Thal LJ, Galasko D, Folstein M, Drachman D, Raskind M, Lanska DJ. Diagnosis and evaluation of dementia. *Neurology* 1995;45:211–218.

16. Council on Scientific Affairs, American Medical Association. Dementia. *JAMA* 1986;256:2234–2238.

17. Consensus Conference. Differential diagnosis of dementing diseases. *JAMA* 1987;258:3411–3416.

18. McGlone J, Gupta S, Humphrey D, Oppenheimer S, Mirsen T, Evans DR. Screening for early dementia using memory complaints from patients and relatives. *Arch. Neurol.* 1990;47:1189–1193.

19. Flicker C, Ferris SH, Reisberg B. A longitudinal study of cognitive function in elderly persons with subjective memory complaints. *J. Am. Geriatr. Soc.* 1993;41:1029–1032.

20. Folstein MF, Folstein SE, McHaugh PR. Mini-mental state: a practical method for grading the cognitive state of patients for the clinician. *J. Psychiatr. Res.* 1975;12:189–198.

21. Blessed G, Tomlinson BE, Roth M. The association between quantitative measures of dementia and of senile change in the gray matter of elderly subjects. *Br. J. Psychiatry* 1968;114:797–811.
22. Magaziner J, Bassett SS, Hebel JR. Predicting performance on the Mini-Mental State Examination: use of age- and education-specific equations. *J. Am. Geriatr. Soc.* 1987;35:996–1000.
23. Crum RM, Anthony JC, Bassett SS, Folstein MF. Population-based norms for the Mini-Mental State Examination by age and education level. *JAMA* 1993;269:2386–91.
24. Huff FJ, Growdon JH, Corkin S, Rosen TJ. Age at onset and rate of progression of Alzheimer's disease. *J. Am. Geriatr. Soc.* 1987;35:27–30.
25. Huff FJ, Growdon JH, Corkin S, Rosen TJ. Deterioration of Blessed information-memory-concentration test in Alzheimer's disease. *Psychiatry Res.* 1992;4:167–168.
26. Katzman R, Brown T, Thal LJ, Fuld PA, Aronson M, Butters N, et al. Comparison of rate of annual change of mental status score in four independent studies of patients with Alzheimer's disease. *Ann. Neurol.* 1988;24:384–389.
27. Salmon DP, Thal LJ, Butters N, Heindel WC. Longitudinal evaluation of dementia of the Alzheimer type: a comparison of 3 standardized mental status examinations. *Neurology* 1990;40:1225–1230.
28. Nelson A, Fogel BS, Faust D. Bedside cognitive screening instruments: a critical assessment. *J. Nerv. Ment. Dis.* 1986;174:73–83.
29. Panisset M, Roudier M, Saxton J, Boller F. Severe impairment battery: a neuropsychological test for severely demented patients. *Arch. Neurol.* 1994;51:41–45.
30. Weintraub S, Mesulam MM. Four neuropsychological profiles in dementia. In Boller F, Grafman J, editors. *Handbook of Neuropsychology, Volume 8.* Amsterdam: Elsevier Science Publishers BV, 1993:253–282.
31. Daffner KR. Alzheimer's disease and related disorders. In Samuels MA, Feske S, editors. *Office Practice of Neurology.* New York: Churchill Livingstone, 1996: 710–715.
32. Chui HC. Dementia: a review emphasizing clinicopathologic correlation and brain-behavior relationships. *Arch. Neurol.* 1989;46:806–814.
33. Mayeux R, Stern Y, Spanto S. Heterogeneity in dementia of the Alzheimer type: evidence of subgroups. *Neurology* 1985;35:453–461.
34. Hansen L, Salmon D, Galasko D, Masliah E, Katzman R, DeTeresa R, et al. The Lewy body variant of Alzheimer's disease: a clinical and pathologic entity. *Neurology* 1990;40:1–8.
35. Marsden CD, Harrison MJG. Outcome of investigation of patients with presenile dementia. *BMJ* 1972;2:249–252.
36. Clarfield AM. The reversible dementias: do they reverse? *Ann. Intern. Med.* 1988;109:476–486.
37. Larson EB, Reitler BV, Sumi SM, Canfield CG, Chann NM. Diagnostic tests in the evaluation of dementia: a prospective study of 200 elderly outpatients. *Arch. Intern. Med.* 1986;146:1917–1922.
38. Weytingh MD, Bossuyt PMM, van Crevel H. Reversible dementia: more than 10% or less than 1%: a quantitative review. *J. Neurol.* 1995;242:466–471.
39. Brodaty H. Consensus statement on predictive testing for Alzheimer disease and associated disorders. *Alzheimer Dis. Assoc. Disord.* 1995;9:182–187.

40. Bird T. Apolipoprotein E genotyping in the diagnosis of Alzheimer's disease: a cautionary view. *Ann. Neurol.* 1995;38:2–3.

41. Relkin NR, Kwon YJ, Tsai J, Grandy S. The National Institute on Aging/ Alzhemer's Association recommendations on the application of apolipoprotein ε genotyping to Alzheimer's disease. *Ann NY Acad Sci* 1996;802:149–173.

42. Post SG, Whitehouse PJ, Binstock RH, et al The clinical introduction of genetic testing for Alzheimer's disease: an ethical perspective. *JAMA* 1997;277:832–836.

43. Farrer L, Brin M, Elsas L, Goate A, Kennedy J, Mayeux R, et al. Statement on the use of apolipoprotein E testing for Alzheimer disease (AD). *JAMA* 1995;274: 1627–1629.

44. Johnson KA, Davis KR, Buonanno FS, Brady TJ, Rosen J, Growdon JH. Comparison of magnetic resonance and roentgen ray computed tomography in dementia. *Arch. Neurol.* 1987;44:1075–1080.

45. Hunt AL, Orrison WW, Yeo RA, Haaland KY, Rhyne RL, Garry PJ, et al. Clinical significance of MRI white matter lesions in the elderly. *Neurology* 1989;39: 1470–1474.

46. Benson DF. Neuroimaging and dementia. *Neurol. Clin.* 1986;4:341–353.

47. Clarfield AM, Larson EB. Should a major imaging procedure (CT or MRI) be required in the workup of dementia?: an opposing view *J. Fam. Pract.* 1990;31: 405–410.

48. Bradshaw JR, Thomson JLG, Campbell MJ. Computed tomography in the investigation of dementia. *BMJ* 1983;286:277–280.

49. Katzman R. Should a major imaging procedure (CT or MRI) be required in the workup of dementia?: an affirmative view. *J. Fam. Pract.* 1990;31:401–410.

50. The Lund and Manchester Groups. Consensus Statement: clinical and neuropathological criteria for frontotemporal dementia. *J. Neurol., Neurosurg. Psychiatry* 1994;57:416–418.

51. Starkstein SE, Migliorelli R, Teson A, Sabe L, Vazquez S, Turjanski M, et al. Specificity of changes in cerebral blood flow in patients with frontal lobe dementia. *J. Neurol. Neurosurg. Psychiatry* 1994;57:790–796.

52. Miller BL, Cummings JL, Villanueva-Meyer J, Boone K, Mehringer CM, Lesser IM, et al. Frontal lobe degeneration: clinical, neuropsychological and SPECT characteristics. *Neurology* 1991;41:1374–1382.

53. Tierney MC, Szalai JP, Snow WG, Fisher RH, Nores A, Nadon G, et al. Prediction of probable Alzheimer's disease in memory-impaired patients: a prospective longitudinal study. *Neurology* 1996;46:661–665.

54. Masur DM, Sliwinski M, Lipton RB, Blau AD, Crystal HA. Neuropsychological prediction of dementia and the absence of dementia in healthy elderly persons. *Neurology* 1994;44:1427–1432.

55. Jacobs DM, Sano M, Dooneief G, Marder K, Bell KL, Stern Y. Neuropsychological detection and characterization of preclinical Alzheimer's disease. *Neurology* 1995;45:957–962.

56. Linn RT, Wolf PA, Bachman DL, Knoefel JE, Cobb JL, Belanger AJ, et al. The "preclinical phase" of probable Alzheimer's disease. *Arch. Neurol.* 1995;52: 485–490.

57. Arriagada PV, Growdon JH, Hedley-Whyte ET, Hyman BT. Neurofibrillary tan-

gles but not senile plaques parallel duration and severity of Alzheimer's disease. *Neurology* 1992;42:631–639.

58. Locascio JJ, Growdon JH, Corkin S. Cognitive test performance in detecting, staging, and tracking Alzheimer's disease. *Arch. Neurol.* 1995;52:1087–1099.

59. Paque L, Warrington EK. A longitudinal study of reading ability in patients suffering from dementia. *J. Int. Neuropsychol. Soc.* 1995;1:517–524.

60. Grober E, Sliwinski M, Korey SR. Development and validation of a model for estimating premorbid verbal intelligence in the elderly. *J. Clin. Exp. Neuropsychol.* 1991;13:933–949.

61. Ivnik RJ, Malec JF, Smith GE. Mayo's older Americans normative studies, WAIS-R, WMS-R, and AVLT norms for ages 56 through 97. *Clin. Neuropsychol.* 1992;6:1–104.

62. Ivnik RJ, Malec JF, Smith GE, Tangalos EG, Petersen RC. Neuropsychological tests' norms above age 55: COWAT, BNT, MAE Token, WRAT-R Reading, AMNART, STROOP, TMT, and JLO. *Clin. Neuropsychol.* 1996;10:262–278.

63. Becker PM, Feussner JR, Mulrow CD, Williams BC, Vokaty KA. The role of lumbar puncture in the evaluation of dementia: the Durham Veterans Administration/Duke University study. *J. Am. Geriatr. Soc.* 1985;33:392–396.

64. Hammerstrom DC, Zimmer B. The role of lumbar puncture in the evaluation of dementia: the University of Pittsburgh study. *J. Am. Geriatr. Soc.* 1985;33: 397–400.

65. Hsich G, Kenney K, Gibbs CJ, Lee KH, Harrington MG. The 14-3-3 brain protein in cerebrospinal fluid as a marker for transmissible spongiform encephalopathies. *N. Engl. J. Med.* 1996;335:924–930.

65a. Rosemann H, Meiner Z, Kahana E, Halimi M, Lenetsky E, Abramsky O, Gabizon R. Detection of 14-3-3 protein in the CSF of genetic Creutzfeldt-Jakob disease. *Neurology.* 1997;49:593–595.

66b. Zerr I, Bodemer M, Gefeller O, Otto M, Poser S, Wiltfang J, Windl O, Kretzschmar HA, Weber T. Detection of 14-3-3 protein in the cerebrospinal fluid supports the diagnosis of Creutzfeldt-Jakob disease. *Ann. Neurol.* 1998;43:32–40.

67c. Weber T, Otto M, Bodemer M, Zerr I. Diagnosis of Creutzfeldt-Jakob disease and related human spongiform encephalopathies. *Biomed. Pharmacother.* 1997;51: 381–387.

66. Duffy FH, Albert MS, McAnulty G. Brain electric activity in patients with senile and presenile dementia of the Alzheimer type. *Ann. Neurol.* 1984;16:439–448.

67. Leuchter AF, Spar JE, Walter DO, Weiner H. Electroencephalographic spectra and coherence in the diagnosis of Alzheimer's-type and multi-infarct dementia. *Arch. Gen. Psychiatry* 1987;44:993–998.

68. American Academy of Neurology. Therapeutics and technology assessment subcommittee: assessment: EEG brain mapping. *Neurology* 1989;39:1100–1101.

69. Brown P, Cathala F, Sadowsky D, Gajdusek DC. Creutzfeldt-Jakob disease in France II: clinical characteristics of 124 consecutive cases during the decade, 1968–1977. *Ann. Neurol.* 1979;6:430–437.

70. Katzman R, Lasker B, Bernstein N. Advances in the diagnosis of dementia: accuracy of diagnosis and consequences of misdiagnosis of disorders causing dementia. In Terry RD, editor. *Aging and the Brain.* New York: Raven Press, 1988:17–62.

71. Neary D, Snowden JS, Bowen DM, Sims NR, Mann DMA, Yates PO, et al. Cerebral biopsy in the investigation of presenile dementia due to cerebral atrophy. *J. Neurol. Neurosurg. Psychiatry* 1986;49:157–162.

72. Hulette CM, Earl NL, Crain BJ. Evaluation of cerebral biopsies for the diagnosis of dementia. *Arch. Neurol.* 1992;49:28–31.

73. Flicker C, Ferris SH, Crook T, Bartus RT, Reisberg B. Cognitive function in normal aging and early dementia. In Traber J, Gispen WH, editors. *Senile Dementia of the Alzheimer Type.* NY: Springer-Verlag, 1985:2–17.

74. Craik FIM. Age differences in human memory. In Birren JE, Schaie KW, editors. *Handbook of the Psychology of Aging.* New York: Van Nostrand Reinhold, 1977:384–420.

75. Craik FIM. Memory functions in normal aging. In Yanagihara T, Petersen RC, editors. *Memory Disorders: Research and Clinical Practice.* New York: Marcel Dekker, 1992:347–367.

76. Ardilia A, Rosselli M. Neuropsychological characteristics of normal aging. *Dev. Neuropsychol.* 1989;5:307–320.

77. Petersen RC, Smith G, Kokmen E, Ivnik RJ, Tangalos EG. Memory function in normal aging. *Neurology* 1992;42:396–401.

78. Francis J, Martin D, Kapor WN. A prospective study of delirium in hospitalized elderly. *JAMA* 1990;263:1097–1101.

79. Schor JD, Levkoff SE, Lipsitz LA, Reilly CH, Cleary PD, Rowe JW, et al. Risk factors for delirium in hospitalized elderly. *JAMA* 1992;267:827–831.

80. Adams RD. Delirium and other acute confusional states. In Adams RD, Victor M, Ropper AH, editors., *Principles of Neurology,* 6th ed. New York: McGraw-Hill, 1997:405–416.

81. Bozzola FG, Gorelick PB, Freels S. Personality changes in Alzheimer's disease. *Arch. Neurol.* 1992;49:297–300.

82. Patterson MB, Schnell AH, Martin RJ, Mendez MF, Smyth KA, Whitehouse PJ. Assessment of behavioral and affective symptoms in Alzheimer's disease. *J. Geriatr. Psychiatry Neurol.* 1990;3:21–30.

83. Clark A, White III CL, Manz HJ, Parhad IM, Curry B, Whitehouse PJ, et al. Primary degenerative dementia without Alzheimer pathology. *Can. J. Neurol. Sci.* 1986;13:462–470.

84. Eggerston DE, Sima AAF. Dementia with cerebral Lewy bodies: a mesocortical dopaminergic deficit? *Arch. Neurol.* 1986;43:524–527.

85. Knopman DS, Mastric AR, Frey II WH, Sung JH, Rustan T. Dementia lacking distinctive histologic features: a common non-Alzheimer degenerative dementia. *Neurology* 1990;40:251–256.

86. Gustafson L. Frontal lobe degeneration of non-Alzheimer type. II. Clinical picture and differential diagnosis. *Arch. Gerontol. Geriatr.* 1987;6:209–223.

87. Neary D, Snowden JS, Northen B, Goulding P. Dementia of frontal lobe type. *J. Neurol. Neurosurg. Psychiatry* 1988;51:353–361.

88. Brun A. Frontal lobe degeneration of non-Alzheimer type. I. Neuropathology. *Arch. Gerontol. Geriatr.* 1987;6:193–208.

89. Albert ML, Feldman RG, Willis AL. The "subcortical dementia" of progressive supranuclear palsy. *J. Neurol. Neurosurg. Psychiatry* 1974;37:121–130.

90. Cummings JL, Benson DF. Subcortical dementia: review of an emerging concept. *Arch. Neurol.* 1984;41:874–879.

91. Alexander GE, DeLong MR, Strick PL. Parallel organization of functionally segregated circuits linking basal ganglia and cortex. *Annu. Rev. Neurosci.* 1986;9:357–381.

92. Cummings JL. Frontal-subcortical circuits and human behavior. *Arch. Neurol.* 1993;50:873–880.

93. Mendez MF, Cherrier M, Perryman KM, Pachana N, Miller BL, Cummings JL. Frontotemporal dementia versus Alzheimer's disease: differential cognitive features. *Neurology* 1996;47:1189–1194.

93a. Stevens M, van Duijn CM, Kamphorst W, de Knijff P, Heutink P, van Gool WA, Scheltens P, Ravid R, Oostra BA, Niermeijer MF, van Swieten JC. Familial aggregation in frontotemporal dementia. *Neurology* 1998;50:1541–1545.

93b. Rizzu P, Van Swieten JC, Joosse M, Hasegawa M, Stevens M, Tibben A, Niermeijer MF, Hillebrand M, Ravid R, Oostra BA, Goedert M, van Duijn CM, Heutink P. High prevalence of mutations in the microtubule-associated protein tau in a population study of frontotemporal dementia in the Netherlands. *Am. J. Hum. Genet.* 1999;64:414–421.

93c. Foster NL, Wilhelmsen, K, Sima AAF, Jones MZ, D'Amato CJ, Gilman S. Frontotemporal dementia and parkinsonism linked to chromosome 17: a consensus conference. Conference Participants. *Ann. Neurol.* 1997;41:706–715.

94. McKeith IG, Fairbairn AF, Bothwell RA, Moore PB, Ferrier IN, Thompson P, et al. An evaluation of the predictive validity and inter-rater reliability of clinical diagnostic criteria for senile dementia of Lewy body type. *Neurology* 1994; 44:872–877.

95. Perry RH, Irving D, Blessed G, Fairbairn A, Perry EK. Senile dementia of Lewy body type: a clinically and neuropathologically distinct type of Lewy body dementia in the elderly. *J. Neurol. Sci.* 1990;95:119–139.

96. McKeith IG, Galasko D, Kosaka K, Perry EK, et al. Consensus guidelines for the clinical and pathologic diagnosis of dementia with Lewy bodies (DLB): report of the consortium on DLB international workshop. *Neurology* 1996;47:1113–1124.

97. Reding M, Haycox J, Wigforss K, Brush D, Blass JP. Follow-up of patients referred to a dementia service. *J. Am. Geriatr. Soc.* 1984;32:265–268.

98. McCallister TW, Price TRP. (1982) Severe depressive pseudodementia with and without dementia. *Am. J. Psychiatry* 1982;139:5.

99. Kral VA. The relationship between senile dementia (Alzheimer type) and depression. *Can. J. Psychiatry* 1983;28:304–306.

100. Patterson C. The diagnosis and differential diagnosis of dementia and pseudodementia in the elderly. *Can. Fam. Physician* 1986;32:2607–2610.

101. Lopez OL, Boller F, Becker JT, Miller M, Reynolds III CF. Alzheimer's disease and depression: neuropsychological impairment and progression of disease. *Am. J. Psychiatry* 1990;147:855–860.

102. Rovner BW, Broadhead J, Spencer M, Carson K, Folstein M. Depression and Alzheimer's disease. *Am. J. Psychiatry* 1989;146:350–353.

103. Erkinjuntti T, Haltia M, Palo J, Sulkava R, Paetau A. Accuracy of the clinical diagnosis of vascular dementia: a prospective clinical and postmortem neuropathological study. *J. Neurol. Neurosurg. Psychiatry* 1988;51:1037–1044.

104. Molsa PK, Paljarvi L, Rinne JO, Rinne UK, Sako E. Validity of clinical diagnosis in dementia: a prospective clinico-pathological study. *J. Neurol. Neurosurg. Psychiatry* 1985;48:1085–1090.

105. Brust JCM. Vascular dementia is overdiagnosed. *Arch. Neurol.* 1988;45:799–801.

106. Wade JPH, Mirsen TR, Hachinski VC, Fisman M, Lau C, Merskey H. The clinical diagnosis of Alzheimer's disease. *Arch. Neurol.* 1987;44:24–29.

107. O'Brien MD. Vascular dementia is underdiagnosed. *Arch. Neurol.* 1988;45: 797–798.

108. Tomlinson BE, Blessed S, Roth M. Observations on the brains of demented old people. *J. Neurol. Sci.* 1970;11:205–242.

109. Snowdon DA, Greiner LH, Mortimer JA, Riley KP, Greiner PA, Markesbery WR. Brain infarction and the clinical expression of Alzheimer's disease. *JAMA* 1997;277:813–817

110. Navia BA, Jordan BD, Price RW. The AIDS dementia complex: I. Clinical features. *Ann. Neurol.* 1986;19:517–524.

111. Perry SW. Organic mental disorders caused by HIV: update on early diagnosis and treatment. *Am. J. Psychiatry* 1990;147:696–710.

112. Merritt HH, Adams RD, Solomon H. *Neurosyphilis.* Oxford: New York.

113. Adams RD, Victor M, Ropper AH. Infections of the nervous system (bacterial, fungal, spirochetal, parasitic) and sarcoid. In *Principles of Neurology,* 6th ed. New York: McGraw-Hill, 1997:695–741.

114. Adams RD, Fisher CM, Hakim S, Ojemann RG, Sweet WH. Symptomatic occult hydrocephalus with "normal" cerebrospinal-fluid pressure: a treatable syndrome. *N. Engl. J. Med.* 1965;273:117–126.

115. Fisher CM. The clinical picture in occult hydrocephalus. *Clin. Neurosurg.* 1977; 24:240–284.

116. Caltagirone C, Gainotti G, Masullo C, Villa G. Neuropsychological study of normal pressure hydrocephalus. *Acta Psychiatr. Scand.* 1982;65:93–100.

117. Stambrook M, Gill DD, Cardoso E, Moore AD. Communicating (normal-pressure) hydrocephalus. In Parks RW, Zec RF, Wilson RS, editors. *Neuropsychology of Alzheimer's Disease and Other Dementias.* New York: Oxford University Press, 1993:283–307.

118. Thomsen AM, Brogesen SE, Bruhn P, Gjerris F. Prognosis of dementia in normal-pressure hydrocephalus after a shunt operation. *Ann. Neurol.* 1986; 20:304–310.

119. Bradley WG, Whittmore AR, Kortman KE, Watanabe AS, Homyak M, Teresi LM, et al. Marked cerebrospinal fluid void: indicator of successful shunt in patients with suspected normal-pressure hydrocephalus. *Radiology* 1991;178:459–466.

120. Wikkelso C, Andersson H, Blomstrand C, Lindqvist G, Svendsen P. Normal pressure hydrocephalus: predictive value of the cerebrospinal fluid tap-test. *Acta Neurol. Scand.* 1986;73:566–573.

121. Vanneste J, Augustijn P, Davies GAG, Dirven C, Tan WF. Normal pressure hydrocephalus: is cisternography still useful in selecting patients for a shunt? *Arch. Neurol.* 1992;49:366–370.

122. Mindin SL, Schiffer RB. Affective disorders in multiple sclerosis. *Arch. Neurol.* 1990;47:98–104.

123. van den Burg W, van Zomeren AH, Minderhound JM, Prange AJA, Meijer NSA. Cognitive impairment in patients with multiple sclerosis and mild physical disability. *Arch. Neurol.* 1987;44:494–501.

124. Rabins PV, Brooks BR, O'Donnell P, Pearlson GD, Moberg P, Jubelt B, et al. Structural brain correlates of emotional disorder in multiple sclerosis. *Brain* 1986;109:585–597.

125. Huber SJ, Cumming JL, *Parkinson's Disease, Neurobehavioral Aspects.* New York: Oxford University Press, 1992.

126. Mayeux R, Stern Y, Rosenstein R, Marder K, Hauser A, Cote L, et al. An estimate of the prevalence of dementia in idiopathic Parkinson's disease. *Arch. Neurol.* 1988;45:260–262.

127. Stern Y, Richards M, Sano M, Mayeux R. Comparison of cognitive changes in patients with Alzheimer's and Parkinson's disease. *Arch. Neurol.* 1993;50: 1040–1045.

128. Lieberman A, Dziatolowski M, Kupersmith M, Serby M, Goodgold A, Korein J, et al. Dementia in Parkinson's disease. *Ann. Neurol.* 1979;6:355–359.

129. Shoulson I. Huntington's disease: cognitive and psychiatric features. *Neuropsychiatry Neuropsychol. Behav. Neurol.* 1990;3:15–22.

130. Folstein SE, Folstein MF. Psychiatric features of Huntington's disease: recent approaches and findings. *Psychiatr. Dev.* 1983;2:193–205.

131. Butters N, Wolfe J, Granholm E, Martone M. An assessment of verbal recall, recognition and fluency abilities in patients with Huntington's disease. *Cortex* 1986;22:11–32.

132. Brouwers P, Cox C, Martin A, Chase T. Differential perceptual–spatial impairment in Huntington's and Alzheimer's dementias. *Arch. Neurol.* 1984;41:1073–1076.

133. Grafman J, Litvan I, Gomez C, Chase TN. Frontal lobe function in progressive supranuclear palsy. *Arch. Neurol.* 1990;47:553–558.

134. Goffinet AM, De Volder AG, Gillain C, Rectem D, Bol A, Michel C, et al. Positron tomography demonstrates frontal lobe hypometabolism in progressive supranuclear palsy. *Ann. Neurol.* 1989;25:131–139.

135. Dening TR, Berrios GE. Wilson's disease: psychiatric symptoms in 195 cases. *Arch. Gen. Psychiatry* 1989;46:1126–1134.

136. Rosselli M, Lorenzana P, Rosselli A, Vergara I. Wilson's disease, a reversible dementia: case report. *J. Clin. Exp. Neuropsychol.* 1987;9:399–406.

137. Talbot PR, Goulding PJ, Lloyd JJ, Snowden JS, Neary D, Testa HJ. Inter-relation between "classic" motor neuron disease and frontotemporal dementia: neuropsychological and single photon emission computed tomography study. *J. Neurol. Neurosurg. Psychiatry* 1995;58:541–547.

138. Neary D, Snowden JS, Mann DMA, Northen B, Goulding PJ, Macdermott N. Frontal lobe dementia and motor neuron disease. *J. Neurol. Neurosurg. Psychiatry* 1990;53:23–32.

139. Mesulam MM, Weintraub S. Spectrum of primary progressive aphasia. In Rossor MN, editor. *Unusual Dementia, Bailliere's Clinical Neurology,* Vol 1. 1992: 583–609.

140. Mesulam MM. Slowly progressive aphasia without generalized dementia. *Ann. Neurol.* 1982;11:592–598.

141. Mesulam MM. Primary progressive aphasia: differentiation from Alzheimer's disease. *Ann. Neurol.* 1987;2:533–534.

142. Heath PD, Kennedy P, Kapur N. Slowly progressive aphasia without generalized dementia. *Ann. Neurol.* 1983;13:687–688.

143. Grossman M, Mickanin J, Onishi K, et al. Progressive non-fluent aphasia: language, cognitive, and PET measures contrasted with probable Alzheimer's disease. *J. Cognitive Neurosci.* 1996;8:135–154.

144. Green J, Morris JC, Sandson J, McKeel DW, Miller JW. Progressive aphasia: a precursor of global dementia? *Neurology* 1990;40:423–429.

145. Karbe H, Kertesz A, Polk M. Profile of language impairment in primary progressive aphasia. *Arch. Neurol.* 1993;50:193–201.

146. Cogan DG. Visual disturbances with focal progressive dementing disease. *Am. J. Ophthal.* 1985;100:68–72.

147. Benson DF, Davis RJ, Snyder BD. Posterior cortical atrophy. *Arch Neurol.* 1988;45:789–793.

148. Tyrell PJ, Warrington EK, Frackowiak RSJ, Rossor MN. Progressive degeneration of the right temporal lobe studied with positron emission tomography. *J. Neurol. Neurosurg. Psychiatry* 1990;53:1046–1050.

149. Victoroff J, Ross GW, Benson DF, Verity MA, Vinters HV. Posterior cortical atrophy: neuropathological correlations. *Arch. Neurol.* 1994;51:269–274.

150. De Renzi E. Slowly progressive visual agnosia or apraxia without dementia. *Cortex* 1986;22:171–180.

151. Dick JPR, Snowden J, Northen B. et al. Slowly progressive apraxia. *Behav. Neurol.* 1989;2:101–114.

152. Evans JJ, Heggs AJ, Antoun N, Hodges JR. Progressive prosopagnosia associated with selective right temporal lobe atrophy: a new syndrome? *Brain* 1995;118:1–13.

153. Snowden JS, Goulding PJ, Neary D. Semantic dementia: a form of circumscribed cerebral atrophy. *Behav. Neurol* 1989;2:167–182.

154. Kukull WA, Larson EB, Reifler BV, Lampe TH, Yerby M, Hughes J. The validity of 3 clinical diagnostic criteria for Alzheimer's disease. *Neurology* 1990;40:1364–1369.

155. Tierney MC, Fisher RH, Lewis AJ, Zorzitto ML, Snow WG, Reid DW, et al. The NINCDS-ADRDA Workgroup criteria for the clinical diagnosis of probable of Alzheimer's disease: a clinicopathologic study of 57 cases. *Neurology* 1988;38:359–364.

156. Morris JC, McKeel DW, Fulling K, Torack RM, Bere L. Validation of clinical diagnostic criteria for Alzheimer's disease. *Ann. Neurol.* 1988;24:17–22.

157. Price BH, Gurvit H, Weintraub S. Neuropsychological patterns and language deficits in twenty consecutive cases of autopsy-confirmed Alzheimer's disease. *Arch. Neurol.* 1993;50:931–937.

158. Risse SC, Raskind MA, Nochlin D, Sumi SM, Lampe TH, Bird TD, et al. Neuropathological findings in patients with clinical diagnoses of probable Alzheimer's disease. *Am. J. Psychiatry* 1990;147:168–172.

159. Mendez M, Mastri AR, Sung JH, Frey WH. Clinically diagnosed Alzheimer's disease: neuropathologic findings in 650 cases. *Alzheimer Dis. Assoc. Disord.* 1992; 6:35–43.

3

Pathological Diagnosis of Alzheimer's Disease

Changiz Geula

Introduction

The diagnosis of dementia of the Alzheimer type in living patients is a clinical judgment based upon careful neurological and neuropsychological examination combined with results from other clinical tests. Because of the existence of other dementing disorders with similar clinical presentation to that of Alzheimer's disease (AD) (some of which are of unknown pathological origin) *(1,2)*, the clinical diagnosis of AD must be confirmed by neuropathological examination. Thus, at present, the most reliable (if not the only) definitive diagnosis of AD is neuropathological. For this reason, a great deal of effort has been directed, particularly in recent years, toward standardization of criteria for the pathological diagnosis of AD.

This chapter first presents the pathological entities upon which a diagnosis of AD is rendered. Next, the most commonly used neuropathological criteria for this diagnosis are reviewed. Finally, some of the complexities in the application of these criteria are discussed.

Pathological Hallmarks of Alzheimer's Disease

In the first report on the disease which now bears his name, Alois Alzheimer *(3)* described two types of lesions in the brain of his patient: "tangled bundle of fibrils" and "miliary foci resulting from the deposit of a unique substance." The terms commonly used today to designate these lesions are the neurofibrillary tangle (NFT) and the senile plaque (SP), respectively. The presence, characteristic distribution, and density of these lesions are used by pathologists for the diagnosis of AD.

From: *Early Diagnosis of Alzheimer's Disease*
Edited by L. F. M. Scinto & K. R. Daffner © Humana Press, Inc., Totowa, NJ

Senile Plaque

The plaque is a complex structure found in the neuropil and consists of amyloid, abnormal neurites and glial cells *(4)*. The β-amyloid (Aβ), which is present in all plaques, is a protein of 1–43 amino acids *(5,6)*. It is clipped out of a larger amyloid precursor protein through a set of complex processes that are under intensive investigation at the present time *(7)*. Aβ can exist in various physical conformations, which include soluble, aggregated (but nonfibrillar), and aggregated fibrillar forms *(8,9)*. In addition to Aβ, abnormal (dystrophic) neurites are associated with a subset of SP (Fig. 1E–G) and represent degenerated processes of neurons (mainly dendrites) and consist of bundles of fibrillar elements *(4,10)*. The plaques with neurites often have microglia and astrocytes associated with them *(4)*.

Plaques occur in various types. The first classification of plaques was proposed by Terry and Wisniewski *(4)* who described three types of SP based on electron-microscopic observations. The primitive SP has some amyloid as well as dystrophic neurites, the latter being invisible in the light microscope. The classical SP has a compact core of amyloid surrounded by a zone of abnormal neurites. Finally, the burned out or compact SP is a large mass of amyloid and no neurites are associated with it. These three types of SP can be visualized in sections processed with Bielschowsky silver stain (or a modification thereof) or thioflavine S stain. The amyloid associated with these SP is also congophilic (can be visualized using the Congo red stain under polarized light).

More recently, SPs have been divided into types based on the presence or absence of various features at the light microscopic level. The first of these classifications became possible with the advent of specific antibodies to Aβ. Immunohistochemistry using these antibodies results in staining of a very large number of plaques, more than any other procedure used *(11–13)*. These immunostained SPs are of two types *(11,14)*. The *diffuse* SPs are round or amorphous deposits of aggregated (nonfibrillar) Aβ with a granular reaction product and without clear borders (Fig.1A). The *compact* SPs, on the other hand, are clearly defined, round deposits of fibrillar Aβ (Fig. 1B,C), which also stain positively for thioflavine S and Congo red. The presence of a heavy central deposit of amyloid in compact SP, often visualized using thioflavine S or silver stain, defines a *cored* (Fig. 1C–E) as distinguished from uncored SP. Finally, the presence of dystrophic (abnormal) neurites distinguishes *neuritic* SP (Fig. 1E–G) from SP without neurites *(10,13,15)*. It is currently believed that the various plaque types represent maturational stages of a single pathological process *(16)*. According to this hypothesis, amyloid is first deposited in the form of diffuse

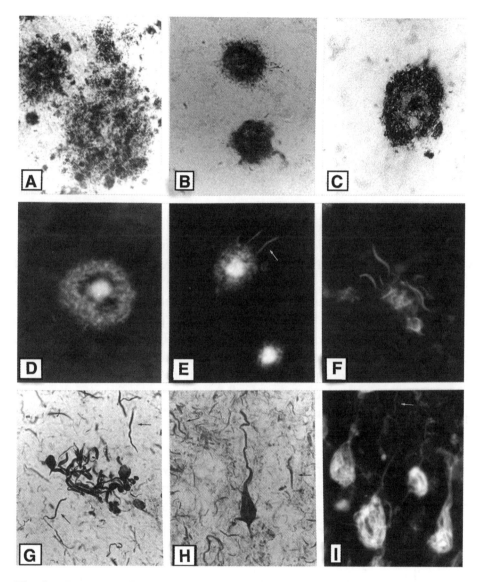

Fig. 1. Examples of the pathological lesions observed in the brains of patients suffering from Alzheimer's disease. (**A**) Diffuse Aβ-positive plaques visualized using immunohistochemical techniques. (**B**) Aβ-positive compact plaques. (**C**) Aβ-positive compact plaque with a dense amyloid core (cored plaque). (**D**) A cored plaque visualized using the thioflavine S stain. (**E**) Thioflavine S stained cored plaques with a few associated dystrophic neurites (*arrow*). (**F**) Thioflavine S stained neuritic plaque. (**G**) Dystrophic neurites associated with a plaque visualized immunohistochemically using an antibody against a hyperphosphorylated epitope of tau (PHF-1). Neuropil threads (*arrows*) are also PHF-1 positive. (**H**) A PHF-1-positive neurofibrillary tangle and neuropit threads (*arrows*). (**I**) Thioflavine S stained tangles and neuropil threads (*arrow*).

SP. Gradually, this amyloid is transformed to fibrils, which are thought to be toxic to neurons and disruptive to neuronal processes present in the neuropil *(8)*. Still later, dystrophic neurites become associated with the SP, presumably representing degeneration of neuronal components damaged by amyloid.

Although SPs are observed throughout the brain in AD, the heaviest deposits are found within the cerebral cortex. The densest accumulation of SPs are observed in association cortical regions, followed by paralimbic and core limbic regions, respectively *(13,17,18)*. A dense accumulation of SP, particularly the neuritic variety *(10)*, is thought to be a specific marker of Alzheimer's disease since it does not occur in other neurodegenerative disorders *(19,20)*.

Neurofibrillary Tangle

Tangles are intracellular accumulations of neurofibrillar elements within the cytoplasm. Ultrastructurally, NFT are made of paired helical filaments (PHF), which measure about 220 Å at their widest, and are constricted at about 800 Å intervals to a width of about 100 Å. Some straight filaments are also associated with NFT *(4)*. NFT are argentophilic, thioflavine S-positive (Fig. 1I), and stain immunohistochemically with antibodies against PHF as well as other antigens (e.g., A68) *(21–23)*. A major component of NFT is abnormally phosphorylated tau (a microtubule associated protein) and antibodies against this element can also be used to stain tangles (Fig. 1H). It is important to note that the neurites within SP and the NFT are composed of nearly identical components *(4,10)* (Fig. 1G). The NFT is thought to damage neurons by disrupting transport of various cellular components and by displacing cytoplasmic elements and thus leading to the degeneration of the neurons within which it is formed.

NFT are found in many neuronal types throughout the AD brain and especially within the cortex. Large neurons are particularly vulnerable to NFT formation. Within the cortex, NFT appear first, and are found in highest density in limbic and paralimbic regions such as the hippocampus and the entorhinal cortex, followed by the association cortical regions *(13,17,18)*. NFT does not appear to be a specific feature of AD since it also occurs in some other neurodegenerative disorders *(19)*.

Other Pathology

Most cortical areas in AD brains with a high density of tangles also display significant loss of neurons *(24,25)*. Significant neuronal loss is also present in many subcortical nuclei with diffuse projections to the cerebral cortex, resulting in marked cortical denervation in AD *(26)*. Among these subcortical nuclei, the cholinergic system of the basal forebrain displays the earliest and most widespread pathology *(26)*. Tangle-bearing regions of cortex also display substantial loss of synapses *(27,28)* and decreases in neuronal dendritic extent *(24,29)*. An inevitable consequence of this pathology is the disruption of neural circuits and isolation of affected areas from the rest of the cortex.

A number of other pathological elements are present in AD brains. Of these, the most prominent are the *neuropil threads* (NT) (Fig. 1G–I), which are considered an extension of the cytoskeletal pathology in AD. NT are relatively short threadlike, argentophilic, and thioflavine S-positive fibers in the neuropil *(4,30)*. They possess staining and antigenic characteristics nearly identical to the NFT and SP neurites, and are commonly thought of as degenerating processes (axons and dendrites) of neurons with tangles *(30)*. *Granulovacuolar degeneration* is found in pyramidal neurons of the Ammon's horn of hippocampus, and is composed of a vacuole, bounded by a unit membrane containing clear material and a core of finely granular, highly insoluble, dense matter *(4,30,31)*. *Hirano body* is an eosinophilic, paracrystalline, rodlike body filled with filaments *(4,30)* found within or sometimes adjacent to pyramidal cells. It is by far the most common in the hippocampal pyramidal cell layer. Finally, *amyloid (congophilic) angiopathy*, which consists of deposits of fibrillar Aβ in small to medium-sized leptomeningial and cortical vessels *(30)*, is present, to varying degrees, in the cerebral cortex of a significant number of AD patients. Recent reports suggest that non-AD-related vascular pathology (e.g., atherosclerosis) may play a role in amyloid deposition in cerebral vessels in AD *(32)*. The AD brain also presents with a large array of other abnormalities the enumeration of which is beyond the scope of this chapter.

Although of great potential significance, the "other" alterations summarized here are not commonly used for the pathological diagnosis of AD.

Contribution of Plaques and Tangles to Dementia

Initial studies reported significant correlations between the presence and density of cortical SP and NFT and the severity of dementia in AD *(21,33)*. A large number of more recent investigations, however, have indicated divergent relationships. More specifically, the distribution and total density of SP have been found to display little relationship with the presence, and particularly the severity, of dementia *(18,34–36)*. Some studies, however, have reported a correlation between the density of neuritic plaques and severity of dementia *(23,35)*. In contrast to SP, the density of NFT has been found to display a strong relationship with the presence and severity of dementia *(18,37,38)*.

A simple interpretation of the above findings would be that SP does not figure prominently in the etiology of dementia in AD. However, such a simple interpretation may be premature for several reasons. *First,* the presence of SP, particularly its neuritic variety, appears to be a more specific feature of AD than that of NFT. *Second,* a number of in vivo and in vitro studies have indicated that the Aβ found in SP can be directly toxic to neurons *(8,39,40).* More importantly, in some of these studies, Aβ has been shown to be able to cause phosphorylation of tau similar to that observed in NFT *(8,40).* Thus, it may be argued that the sequence of the pathological cascade in AD begins with the deposition of Aβ, followed by abnormal phosphorylation of tau, formation of tangles within neurons, neuronal death, and the resultant dementia. *Third,* no measure of Aβ deposition has been found to correlate with age or duration of disease in AD. This has been interpreted to indicate that Aβ is continually deposited and resolved (removed) from AD cortex *(34).* If true, this interpretation would suggest that the number of Aβ-positive SPs observed in an AD brain is not an indication of the total Aβ burden throughout the disease process, rendering correlations with cognitive status meaningless. It should be noted that a recent study with careful control of many variables (such as postmortem interval and age) and inclusion of subjects with a wide spectrum of cognitive performance, did find a strong correlation between SP and severity of dementia *(41).*

Some of the other alterations observed in AD brains, such as loss of neurons, synapses, and dendrites, have also been shown to display significant correlations with the severity and duration of dementia *(25,27,42,43).* The loss of neurons and synapses most likely represent the proximal cause of the dementia observed in AD.

Pathology of Normal Aging and Mild Dementia

A large number of investigations have indicated that SP and NFT can also occur in the brains of cognitively normal elderly *(12,22,44,45).* SP and, in particular, Aβ immunoreactive SP are commonly found in the cerebral cortex of many normal aged brains. In some of these brains, the density of Aβ deposits has been found to be similar to that present in AD. NFT are also present in the normal aged brain. However, they are found less frequently, in much lower density and with very restricted distribution as compared with SP. SP neurites, which appear to involve the same pathological process as the NFT, are rare in the normal aged brain. In fact, a number of studies have indicated that the frequency and distribution of neuritic SP may be the main pathological element that distinguishes AD from normal aging *(10,12,23,35).*

Careful neuropsychological studies have indicated that many nondemented community dwelling elderly individuals suffer from mild cognitive abnormalities *(46–48)*. The presence of pathology in nondemented elderly may serve as a substrate for these mild cognitive abnormalities. In fact, a number of recent studies have indicated that aged individuals with high frequency of SP, particularly of the diffuse type, are very mildly demented (i.e., possibly in the earliest stages of AD) *(22,36,49–51)*. By contrast, the distribution of NFT has been shown to be relatively restricted in the brains of mildly demented individuals, found predominantly within the entorhinal cortex. NFT seem to appear first in the entorhinal region and later in the hippocampus and neocortical areas *(22,36,52)*. In fact, this focal appearance of NFT and its gradual and later presence in other areas have been used to identify the possible stages in the progression of AD-like pathology in normal, mildly demented, and AD brains *(37)*. In addition to NFT accumulation, the entorhinal cortex displays significant neuronal loss in mildly demented individuals *(43)*.

In summary, SP formation appears to represent an early pathological event, which may contribute to the formation of NFT. Accumulation of NFT, on the other hand, is probably a later event in the cascade of AD pathology, which coincides with the clinical manifestation and severity of dementia.

Pathological Diagnostic Criteria

Ruling Out Other Pathology

Perhaps the most important task in the process of pathological diagnosis of AD is ruling out other pathology *(53–55)*. Grossly, the AD brain should be weighed and checked for obvious lesions such as subdural hematomas, cortical infarcts, tumors, or hemorrhages. Ventricular size is variable in AD, but invariably there is general atrophy and enlargement of sulci. White matter and deep gray matter should be checked for presence of cystic or lacunar infarcts or other vascular lesions. Other causes of dementia should be ruled out. These include lobar atrophy, Pick's disease, vascular (or multiinfarct) dementia, Creutzfeldt-Jakob disease, diffuse Lewy body disease, and progressive supranuclear palsy. Only after the presence of other pathology has been carefully determined should an assessment of the pathological hallmarks of AD be undertaken.

Pathological diagnosis of AD is often complicated by the presence of other pathology. In a subpopulation of pathologically confirmed cases of AD, abundant pathology characteristic of other neurodegenerative disorders, such as Parkinson's disease, are also present, allowing simultaneous diagnosis of both diseases in the same individual *(1,2,56,57)*. Additional complications are presented by the presence of dementing disorders, which are relatively more difficult to diagnose, such as multiinfarct dementia *(58,59)*. Some of these additional pathologies have been shown to contribute to the dementia seen in AD patients and to influence the density of plaques and tangles *(56)*.

A number of pathological criteria have been proposed for the diagnosis of AD *(53,60,61)*. Of these, two have been extensively used. The first is the criteria recommended by the neuropathology panel of a workshop on the diagnosis of AD sponsored by several components of the National Institutes of Health, spearheaded by the National Institute on Aging (NIA) and summarized by Khachaturian *(53)*. The second and more recent are the criteria recommended by the Consortium to Establish a Registry for Alzheimer's Disease (CERAD) *(61)*. A third set of criteria was recommended by the Working Group on Diagnostic Criteria of the NIA and the Reagan Institute (RI) very recently *(62)*, and therefore is not yet widely used.

NIA Consensus Criteria

According to these criteria, the minimum number of areas to be examined include three regions of neocortex (frontal, temporal, and parietal lobes), the amygdala, the hippocampus (presumably including the entorhinal cortex), and a number of subcortical areas. Examination of tissue per ×200 microscopic field is made of 5–15 μm sections stained for Bielschowsky silver, thioflavine S, or Congo red. The diagnosis is based on the age of the subject, the number of SPs, and the presence of NFT in the neocortex. In patients less than 50 years of age, more than 2–5 SPs or neuritic SPs and tangles should be observed per field anywhere in the neocortex. In individuals aged 50–65 years, tangles may be present, but 8 or more SPs per field are necessary for the diagnosis of AD. In patients aged 66–75 years, tangles may be present and more than 10 SPs must be observed per field. In patients older than 75 years, tangles may sometimes not be found but the number of SPs must be more than 15 per field. It is stated that in the presence of a clinical history of AD, these criteria should be revised downward, although it is not clear to what extent *(53)*.

CERAD Criteria

The CERAD neuropathology criteria use the presence and density of neuritic SP to establish the diagnosis of AD *(55,61)*. Regions that must be examined include middle frontal gyrus, superior and middle temporal gyri, inferior parietal lobule, hippocampus, entorhinal cortex, and midbrain, including the substantia nigra. However, the final diagnosis is based only on observations from the neocortical areas sampled. The density of neuritic SP in a ×100 microscopic field is recorded as "sparse," "moderate," or "severe." This semiquantitative measure of neuritic SP in the most severely affected "neo-cortical" region is combined with the age of the subject to yield the age-related plaque score. This score is then integrated with clinical information for the diagnosis of "definite," "probable," or "possible" AD.

NIA–RI Criteria

The NIA-RI criteria represent a reassessment of the original NIA Consensus criteria. The pathological diagnosis of AD is based on the presence of both plaques and tangles. Areas to be sampled include four neocortical regions (superior temporal gyrus, inferior parietal lobule, midfrontal cortex, and occipital cortex), hippocampal formation at the level of the lateral geniculate nucleus, hippocampal formation, and the entorhinal cortex at the level of the uncus, the substantia nigra, and the locus ceruleus. The NIA–RI diagnostic scheme is based on the fact that dementia in the elderly may arise from more than one disorder, several of which may coexist in the same individual. Based on semiquantitative measures of the density and distribution of both neuritic SP and NFT, the NIA–RI criteria provides the "likelihood" (high, intermediate, or low) that the observed clinical dementia is due to AD lesions. The identification of coexisting pathology is emphasized. It is also recommended that the presence of diffuse SP be noted, even though it is acknowledged that the contribution of these lesions to dementia is at present uncertain *(62)*.

Evaluation of Pathological Diagnostic Criteria

All of the criteria described above are based on the combined experience of many expert neuropathologists as well as published reports in the literature *(53,61,62)* and therefore are considered accurate. However, a certain degree of arbitrariness is inevitable in any such criteria. This is particularly true of the NIA Consensus criteria, which rely on absolute minimum numbers of SP for diagnosis. It is likely that these minimum required quantities represent best estimates rather than absolute measures.

Given the strong correlation between the density of NFT and the presence and severity of dementia in AD, it is interesting that two of the pathological criteria described above are based so heavily on the density of SP *(54)*. The NIA consensus criteria do factor in the *presence* of NFT in the diagnostic criteria. However, the *number* of NFT are used only in the diagnosis of young cases (younger than 50 years). In the CERAD criteria, the NFT are not used in the process of diagnosis. In the NIA–RI criteria, on the other hand, the density of NFT is used more directly in the diagnosis.

In terms of the brain regions to be examined for quantitative or semiquantitative analysis, the NIA and NIA–RI criteria incorporate a balanced approach, including assessment of neocortical as well as limbic and paralimbic regions. The CERAD diagnostic criteria, however, are based on the semiquantitative analysis of the neocortex only. The exclusion of the limbic and paralimbic cortical structures, particularly the hippocampus and the entorhinal cortex, is contrary to the suggestion of some investigators that AD is primarily a limbic/paralimbic disorder *(26,63)*. For example, it has been suggested that NFT formation in the entorhinal cortex disconnects the hippocampus from the cerebral cortex, hence resulting in the deficits in memory observed in AD *(64,65)*.

One factor that complicates any diagnostic criteria is the presence of nonneuritic SP and some NFT in the brains of normal aged and mildly demented individuals. The NIA criteria do not include an explicit distinction between neuritic and nonneuritic SP in its quantification scheme except for younger cases (below 50 years). Thus, it is possible that a non-AD aged individual, possibly with mild cognitive abnormalities, is diagnosed as AD because of the presence of a high density of nonneuritic SP. The CERAD and NIA–RI criteria use only the neuritic type of SP for the diagnosis of AD. This avoids the complications posed by the pathology of normal aging and mild dementia, since, as we have seen, neuritic types of SP are found predominantly (if not exclusively) in AD brains. Obviously, the issue of the pathology of normal aging and mild cognitive abnormality is rendered unimportant when clinical dementia is present and other pathology nonexistent. It gains considerable importance, however, in research settings within which the use of pathologically normal aged brains as well as brains in the early stages of disease are a necessity for comparison with AD brains.

Another factor that must be considered in relation to the diagnostic criteria is the reliability with which these criteria are applied. Several studies have dealt directly with this issue. The results showed that neuropathology laboratories use a wide variety of stains to visualize SP and NFT, some of these techniques being quite different from those recommended by the pathological criteria listed above. When the same tissue was sent to different neuropathologists for staining and quantitation of SP and NFT, reasonable interrater agreement was obtained for semiquantitative analysis, but quantitative measures yielded significant differences between raters. These differences reflected variations in stain sensitivity, staining technique, and the interpretation of histological findings *(66)*. When the same tissue was first stained and then evaluated by two different neuropathologists, higher interrater reliability was achieved *(67)*. A surprising finding of a survey of a large number of neuropathologists conducted in 1989 was that a significant proportion did not use the recommended pathological criteria at the time, nor based their diagnosis on semiquantitative or quantitative measures *(68)*. The awareness for the necessity of more uniform criteria has most likely increased from that in 1989. However, the trend revealed by the above survey indicates that no matter how specific and reliable a set of criteria may be, its widespread use cannot be guaranteed.

Pathological Variants of Alzheimer's Disease

There is considerable heterogeneity in neuropathological findings of AD. Few AD brains are likely to show the exact same density or pattern of distribution of SP and NFT. Any criteria proposed for the pathological diagnosis of AD must accommodate this heterogeneity. A major challenge in devising pathological diagnostic criteria is to account for divergent pathology in some cases of clinically diagnosed AD. Several possible pathological variants of AD are discussed below.

Tangle-Only Variant

In some cohorts, approximately 5–10% of clinically diagnosed AD-type dementia cases show NFT only, and then only in limbic/paralimbic regions and some subcortical areas *(69–71)*. Some neocortical regions, such as the inferior temporal cortex, may contain a few NFT in some cases. However, NFT are generally absent from the neocortex. Very rare Aβ-positive diffuse SP are seen in some cases. No neuritic SP is present. Most of these cases are of late onset. It has been proposed that this type of clinicopathological presentation be recognized as an NFT-only or NFT-predominant variant of AD *(69)*. Others have used the term "atypical AD" to refer to such cases *(55)*. The CERAD and NIA Consensus diagnostic criteria would diagnose such cases as non-AD type of dementia since they rely primarily on the presence and density of SP to make a diagnosis. The NIA–RI criteria would postulate that there is a low (or perhaps moderate) likelihood that AD pathology contributes to dementia in such cases.

As mentioned earlier, SP appears to be a more specific marker of AD as compared with NFT. Thus, it could be argued that cases which do not present with a high density of SP, such as the NFT-only cases, should not be diagnosed as AD. The striking clinical similarity observed in some of these cases to that of typical AD, however, poses problems for this argument.

Neocortical Plaque-Only Variant

As many as 30% of the brains from cases with clinically diagnosed AD-type dementia display only SP in neocortical regions; no neocortical NFT are present *(72,73)*. The majority of these SPs are of the diffuse type and significantly fewer neuritic SPs are observed as compared with typical AD. NFT are present in these cases, but are confined to limbic/paralimbic regions. Demented patients presenting with this type of pathology are typically of the late-onset variety. These cases are indistinguishable from typical AD in all other parameters (clinical, morphological, and neurochemical) other than the pathology described above. For this reason, it has been suggested that these cases may represent a neocortical plaque-only variant of AD.

The NIA Consensus pathological criteria explicitly recognize the neocortical SP-only presentation as AD in that its criteria for diagnosis of AD in older cases state that NFT may sometimes not be present while SP must be present in high density. The CERAD criteria, however, would categorize at least some of these cases as non-AD dementia based upon the low numbers of neocortical neuritic SP. According to the NIA–RI criteria, the likelihood that AD lesions contribute to dementia in such cases is low.

Lewy Body Variant

Lewy bodies (LB) are intracytoplasmic inclusions *(74)*. They appear as a dense eosinophilic core surrounded by a less densely stained peripheral halo. The LB is a pathological hallmark of brains of patients suffering from Parkinson's disease (PD), within which LB are found most prominently in the substantia nigra (SN) and other subcortical nuclei. Sparsely distributed cortical LB are also found in most PD cases. The cortical LB are observed mostly in nonpyramidal neurons of layers V and VI *(74)*.

A more widespread distribution of LB, particularly within the cerebral cortex, is a hallmark of the dementing disorder termed *diffuse Lewy body disease* (DLBD) *(75)*. In a significant number of brains from demented cases in which LB are diffusely distributed, AD pathology is also present *(74,76,77)*. This has prompted some investigators to suggest the existence of a Lewy body variant (LBV) of AD *(74,78)*. However, the designation of LBV as a separate pathological entity has been criticized *(79)*. It has been proposed that this type of pathology represents the coexistence of AD and DLBD *(79)* or AD and PD *(57,77)*. Proponents of the LBV designation have pointed out, however, that DLBD has a much earlier onset than LBV and is characterized by severe PD signs and, while mild extrapyramidal signs are present in LBV, tremor rigidity and akinesia, which are the clinical hallmarks of PD, are not observed *(74,75)*.

Cases that show diffusely distributed LB and AD pathology present with important features *(74,78,80)*. In general, NFT are rare in the neocortex, and are found in limbic/paralimbic regions but with slightly lower density as compared with AD. SP are found in abundance in neocortical regions. However, most SP are of the nonneuritic and diffuse variety. This pattern of pathology is identical to that described for the plaque-only variant of AD. In fact, a significant percentage (as high as 75%) of cases with diffuse LB and AD lesions present with the plaque-only distribution of pathology. Thus, it may be suggested that the plaque-only variant and the suggested LBV are one and the same. However, at least 25% of brains from plaque-only cases do not contain LB *(80),* suggesting the existence of a pure plaque-only variety.

The prescreening for other pathological causes of dementia suggested by the diagnostic criteria discussed above would most likely result in the exclusion of the cases under discussion as typical AD cases. According to the NIA consensus criteria, the most comfortable classification of these cases would be as coexistent DLBD and AD, because of the presence of LBs and high cortical SP counts. The CERAD criteria, however, would not consider such cases as AD owing to the small number of neocortical neuritic plaques. The NIA–RI criteria would postulate that AD lesions have a low to intermediate likelihood to contribute to dementia in such cases, while perhaps LBs are more likely to do so.

It is important to note that the three possible variants of AD discussed above share one neuropathological feature in common with typical AD: *all are characterized by a relatively high density of NFT in limbic/paralimbic regions.* It remains to be determined if the presence of this one feature is sufficient for producing the dementia characteristic of AD.

Conclusions

At present, the only definitive diagnosis of AD is neuropathological. This fact has heightened the need for standardized diagnostic neuropathological criteria. Despite important strides, the need for more specific and comprehensive criteria persists. Future efforts, no doubt, will result in significant improvements in this area. Such efforts will need to accomplish the following:

1. Address more completely the pathological distinction between normal aging, mild dementia, and AD.
2. Take advantage of *all* of the pathological features of AD (various types of plaques, tangles, neuropil threads, etc.).
3. Address the issue of pathological heterogeneity.

Acknowledgments

The preparation of this chapter was made possible, in part, by grants from the National Institute on Aging (AG10262, AG14706).

References

1. Mendez MF, Mastri AR, Sung JH, and Frey WH. Clinically diagnosed Alzheimer disease: neuropathologic findings in 650 cases. *Alz. Dis. Assoc. Disord.* 1992;6:35–43.
2. Joachim CL, Morris JH, Selkoe DJ. Clinically diagnosed Alzheimer's disease: autopsy results in 150 cases. *Ann. Neurol.* 1988;24:50–56.
3. Alzheimer A. A unique illness involving the cerebral cortex. In Rothenberg DA, Hochberg FH, editors. *Neurological Classics in Modern Translation.* London: Hafner Press,1977:41–43.
4. Terry RD, Wisniewski HM. Ultrastructure of senile dementia and of experimental analogues. In Gaitz CM, editor. *Aging and the Brain.* New York: Plenum, 1972:89–116.
5. Mak K, Yang F, Vinters HV, Frautschy SA, Cole GM. Polyclonals to beta-amyloid (1-42) identify most plaque and vascular deposits in Alzheimer cortex, but not striatum. *Brain Res.* 1994;667:138–142.
6. Iizuka T, Shoji M, Harigaya Y, Kawarabayashi T, Watanabe M, Kanai M, Hirai S. Amyloid B-protein ending at Thr-43 is a minor component of some diffuse plaques in the Alzheimer's disease brain, but is not found in cerebrovascular amyloid. *Brain Res.* 1995;702:275–278.
7. Selkoe DJ. Normal and abnormal biology of the β-amyloid precursor protein. *Annu. Rev. Neurosci.* 1994;17:489–517.
8. Lorenzo A, Yankner BA. B-Amyloid neurotoxicity requires fibril formation and is inhibited by Congo red. *Proc. Natl. Acad. Sci. U.S.A.* 1994;91:12243–12247.
9. Pike CJ, Walencewicz AJ, Glabe CG, Cotman CW. In vitro aging of beta-amyloid protein causes peptide aggregation and neurotoxicity. *Brain Res.* 1991;563:311–314.
10. Trojanowski JQ, Shin RW, Schmidt ML, Lee VM. Relationship between plaques, tangles, and dystrophic processes in Alzheimer's disease. *Neurobiol. Aging* 1995;16:335–345.
11. Mann DMA, Brown AMT, Prinja D, Jones D, Davies CA. A morphological analysis of senile plaques in the brains of non-demented persons of different ages using silver, immunocytochemical and lectin histochemical staining techniques. *Neuropathol. Appl. Neurobiol.* 1990;16:17–25.
12. Arriagada PV, Marzloff K, Hyman BT. Distribution of Alzheimer-type pathologic changes in nondemented elderly individuals matches the pattern in Alzheimer's disease. *Neurology* 1992;42:1681–1688.
13. Geula C, Mesulam M-M, Saroff DM, Wu C-K. Relationship between plaques, tangles, and loss of cortical cholinergic fibers in Alzheimer's disease. *J. Neuropathol. Exp. Neurol.* 1998;57:63–75.
14. Wisniewski HM, Bancher C, Barcikowska M, Wen GY, Currie J. Spectrum of morphological appearance of amyloid deposits in Alzheimer's disease. *Acta Neuropathol.* 1989;78:337–347.
15. Yamaguchi H, Nakazato Y, Shoji M, Takatama M, Hirai S. Ultrastructure of diffuse plaques in senile dementia of the Alzheimer type: comparison with primitive plaques. *Acta Neuropathol.* 1991;82:13–20.
16. Dickson DW. The pathogenesis of senile plaques. *J. Neuropathol. Exp. Neurol.* 1997;56:321–339.
17. Arnold SE, Hyman BT, Flory J, Damasio AR, Van Hoesen GW. The topographical

and neuroanatomical distribution of neurofibrillary tangles and neuritic plaques in the cerebral cortex of patients with Alzheimer's disease. *Cereb. Cortex* 1991;1: 103–116.

18. Arriagada PV, Growdon JH, Hedley-Whyte ET, Hyman BT. Neurofibrillary tangles but not senile plaques parallel duration and severity of Alzheimer's disease. *Neurology* 1992;42:631–639.

19. Selkoe DJ. The molecular pathology of Alzheimer's disease. *Neuron* 1991;6:487–498.

20. Hardy J, Allsop D. Amyloid deposition as the central event in the aetiology of Alzheimer's disease. *TIPS* 1991;12:383–388.

21. Delaere P, Duyckaerts C, Brion JP, Poulian V, Hauw J-J. Tau, paired helical filaments and amyloid in the neocortex: a morphometric study of 15 cases with graded intellectual status in aging and senile dementia of Alzheimer type. *Acta Neuropathol.* 1989;77: 645–653.

22. Price JL, Davis PB, Morris JC, White DL. The distribution of tangles, plaques and related immunohistochemical markers in healthy aging and Alzheimer's disease. *Neurobiol. Aging* 1991;12:295–312.

23. Mena R, Wischik CM, Novak M, Milstein C, Cuello C. A progressive deposition of paired helical filaments (PHF) in the brain characterizes the evolution of dementia in Alzheimer's disease. *J. Neuropathol. Exp. Neurol.* 1991;50:474–490.

24. Coleman PD, Flood DG. Neuron numbers and dendritic extent in normal aging and Alzheimer's disease. *Neurobiol. Aging* 1987;8:521–545.

25. Gomez-Isla T, Hollister R, West H, Mui S, Growdon JH, Petersen RC, Parisi JE, Hyman BT. Neuronal loss correlates with but exceeds neurofibrillary tangles in Alzheimer's disease. *Ann. Neurol.* 1997;41:17–24.

26. Geula C, Mesulam M-M. Cholinergic systems and related neuropathological predilection patterns in Alzheimer disease. In Terry RD, Katzman R, Bick KL, editors. *Alzheimer Disease.* New York: Raven Press, 1994:263–291.

27. Terry RD, Masliah E, Salmon DP, Butters N, DeTeresa R, Hill R, Hansen LA, Katzman R. Physical basis of cognitive alterations in Alzheimer's disease: synapse loss is the major correlate of cognitive impairment. *Ann. Neurol.* 1991;30:572–580.

28. Scheff SW, DeKosky ST, Price DA. Quantitative assessment of cortical synaptic density in Alzheimer's disease. *Neurobiol. Aging.* 1990;11:29–37.

29. Catala I, Ferrer I, Galofre E, Fabregues I. Decreased numbers of dendritic spines on cortical pyramidal neurons in dementia: a quantitative Golgi study on biopsy samples. *Hum. Neurobiol.* 1988;6:255–259.

30. Terry RD, Masliah E, Hansen LA. Structural basis of cognitive alterations in Alzheimer's disease. In Terry RD, Katzman R, Bick KL, editors. *Alzheimer Disease.* New York: Raven Press, 1994:179–196.

31. Xu M, Shibayama H, Kobayashi H, Yamada K, Ishihara R, Zhao P, Takeuchi T, Yoshida K, Inagaki T, Nokura K. Granulovacuolar degeneration in the hippocampal cortex of aging and demented patients: a quantitative study. *Acta Neuropathol.* 1992;85:1–9.

32. Ellis RJ, Olichney JM, Thal LJ, Mirra SS, Morris JC, Beekly D, Heyman A. Cerebral amyloid angiopathy in the brains of patients with Alzheimer's disease: the CERAD experience, Part XV. *Neurology* 1996;46:1592–1596.

33. Blessed G, Tomlinson BE, Roth M. The association between quantitative measures

of dementia and of senile change in the cerebral gray matter of elderly subjects. *Br. J. Psychiat.* 1968;114:797–811.

34. Hyman BT, Marzloff K, Arriagada PV. The lack of accumulation of senile plaques or amyloid burden in Alzheimer's disease suggests a dynamic balance between amyloid deposition and resolution. *J. Neuropathol. Exp. Neurol.* 1993;52:594–600.

35. Nagy Z, Esiri MM, Jobst KA, Morris JH, King EM, McDonald B, Litchfield S, Smith A, Barnetson L, Smith AD. Relative roles of plaques and tangles in the dementia of Alzheimer's disease: correlations using three sets of neuropathological criteria. *Dementia* 1995;6:21–31.

36. Crystal H, Dickson D, Fuld P, Masur D, Scott R, Mehler M, Masdeu J, Kawas C, Aronson M, Wolfson L. Clinico-pathologic studies in dementia: nondemented subjects with pathologically confirmed Alzheimer's disease. *Neurology* 1988;38:1682–1687.

37. Braak H, Braak E. Neuropathological staging of Alzheimer's disease. *Acta Neuropathol.* 1991;82:239–259.

38. Bierer LM, Hof PR, Purohit DP, Carlin L, Schmeidler J, Davis KL, Perl DP. Neocortical neurofibrillary tangles correlate with dementia severity in Alzheimer's disease. *Arch. Neurol.* 1995;52:81–88.

39. Busciglio J, Lorenzo A, Yeh J, Yankner BA. beta-Amyloid fibrils induce tau phosphorylation and loss of microtubule binding. *Neuron* 1995;14:879–888.

40. Geula C, Wu C-K, Saroff D, Lorenzo A, Yuan M, Yankner BA. Aging renders the brain vulnerable to amyloid B neurotoxicity. *Nature Medi.* 1998;4:827–831.

41. Cummings BJ, Pike CJ, Shankle R, Cotman CW. B-amyloid deposition and other measures of neuropathology predict cognitive status in Alzheimer's disease. *Neurobiol. Aging* 1996;17:921–933.

42. Samuel W, Terry RD, DeTeresa R, Butters N, Masliah E. Clinical correlates of cortical and nucleus basalis pathology in Alzheimer dementia. *Arch. Neurol.* 1994;51:772–778.

43. Gomez-Isla T, Price JL, McKeel DWJ, Morris JC, Growdon JH, Hyman BT. Profound loss of layer II entorhinal cortex neurons occurs in very mild Alzheimer's disease. *J. Neurosci.* 1996;16:4491–4500.

44. Giannakopoulos P, Hof PR, Mottier S, Michel JP, Bouras C. Neuropathological changes in the cerebral cortex of 1258 cases from a geriatric hospital: retrospective clinicopathological evaluation of a 10-year autopsy population. *Acta Neuropathol.* 1994;87:456–468.

45. Giannakopoulos P, Hof PR, Giannakopoulos AS, Herrmann FR, Michel JP, Bouras C. Regional distribution of neurofibrillary tangles and senile plaques in the cerebral cortex of very old patients. *Arch. Neurol.* 1995;52:1150–1159.

46. Rentz D, Daffner K, Calvo V, Scinto L. The limits of screening tests for selecting normal community dwelling elders. *Soc. Neurosci. Abst.* 1997;21:533.

47. Graham JE, Rockwood K, Beattie BL, Eastwood R, Gauthier S, Tuokko H, McDowell I. Prevalence and severity of cognitive impairment with and without dementia in an elderly population. *Lancet* 1997;349:1793–1796.

48. Linn RT, Wolf PA, Bachman DL, Knoefel JE, Cobb JL, Belanger AJ, Kaplan EF, D'Agostino RB. The "preclinical phase" of probable Alzheimer's disease. A 13-year prospective study of the Framingham cohort. *Arch. Neurol.* 1995;52:485–490.

49. Morris ME, Baimbridge KG, Elbeheiry H, Obrocea GV, Rosen AS. Correlation of anoxic neuronal responses and calbindin-D- 28k localization in stratum pyramidal of rat hippocampus. *Hippocampus* 1995;5:25–39.
50. Morris JC, Storandt M, McKeel DW Jr, Rubin EH, Price JL, Grant EA, Berg L. Cerebral amyloid deposition and diffuse plaques in "normal" aging: evidence for presymptomatic and very mild Alzheimer's disease. *Neurology* 1996;46:707–719.
51. Morris JC, McKeel DW Jr, Storandt M, Rubin EH, Price JL, Grant EA, Ball MJ, Berg L. Very mild Alzheimer's disease: informant-based clinical, psychometric, and pathologic distinction from normal aging. *Neurology* 1991;41:469–478.
52. Braak E, Braak H, Mandelkow EM. A sequence of cytoskeleton changes related to the formation of neurofibrillary tangles and neuropil threads. *Acta Neuropathol.* 1994;87:554–567.
53. Khachaturian Z. Diagnosis of Alzheimer's disease. *Arch. Neurol.* 1985;42:1097–1105.
54. Markesbery WR. The diagnosis of Alzheimer's disease. *Arch. Pathol. Lab. Med.* 1993;117:129–131.
55. Mirra SS, Hart MN, Terry RD. Making the diagnosis of Alzheimer's disease: a primer for practicing pathologists. *Arch. Pathol. Lab. Med.* 1993;117:132–144.
56. Nagy Z, Esiri MM, Jobst KA, Morris JH, King EM, McDonald B, Joachim C, Litchfield S, Barnetson L, Smith AD. The effects of additional pathology on the cognitive deficit in Alzheimer disease. *J. Neuropathol. Exp. Neurol.* 1997;56:165–170.
57. Hulette C, Mirra S, Wilkinson W, Heyman A, Fillenbaum G, Clark C. The consortium to establish a registry for Alzheimer's disease (CERAD). Part IX. A prospective cliniconeuropathological study of Parkinson's features in Alzheimer's disease. *Neurology* 1995;45:1991–1995.
58. Kosunen O, Soininen H, Paljarvi L, Heinonen O, Talasniemi S, Riekkinen PJ Sr. Diagnostic accuracy of Alzheimer's disease: a neuropathological study. *Acta Neuropathol.* 1996;91:185–193.
59. Hulette C, Nochlin D, McKeel D, Morris JC, Mirra SS, Sumi SM, Heyman A. Clinical-neuropathologic findings in multi-infarct dementia: a report of six autopsied cases. *Neurology* 1997;48:668–672.
60. Mizutani T. Neuropathological diagnosis of senile dementia of the Alzheimer type (SDAT): proposal of diagnostic criteria and report of the Japanese research meeting on neuropathological diagnosis of SDAT. *Neuropathology* 1994;14:91–103.
61. Mirra SS, Heyman A, McKeel D, Sumi SM, Crain BJ, Brownlee LM, Vogel FS, Hughes JP, van Belle G, Berg L. The Consortium to Establish a Registry for Alzheimer's Disease (CERAD). Part II. Standardization of the neuropathologic assessment of Alzheimer's disease. *Neurology* 1991;41:479–486.
62. The National Institute on Aging, and Reagan Institute Working Group on Diagnostic Criteria for the Neuropathological Assessment of Alzheimer's Disease. Consensus recommendations for the postmortem diagnosis of Alzheimer's disease. *Neurobiol. Aging* 1997;18(4 Suppl):S1–S2.
63. Braak H, Braak E. Alzheimer's disease affects limbic nuclei of the thalamus. *Acta Neuropathol.* 1991;81:261–268.
64. Hyman BT, Van Hoesen GW, Damasio AR, Barnes CL. Alzheimer's disease: cell-specific pathology isolates the hippocampal formation. *Science* 1984;225:1168–1170.

65. Van Hoesen GW, Hyman BT, Damasio AR. Cell-specific pathology in neural systems of the temporal lobe in Alzheimer's disease. *Prog. Brain Res.* 1986;70:321–335.

66. Mirra SS, Gearing M, McKeel DW Jr, Crain BJ, Hughes JP, van Belle G, Heyman A. Interlaboratory comparison of neuropathology assessments in Alzheimer's disease: a study of the Consortium to Establish a Registry for Alzheimer's Disease (CERAD). *J. Neuropathol. Exp. Neurol.* 1994;53:303–315.

67. Chui HC, Tierney M, Zarow C, Lewis A, Sobel E, Perlmutter LS. Neuropathologic diagnosis of Alzheimer disease: interrater reliability in the assessment of senile plaques and neurofibrillary tangles. *Alz. Dis. Assoc. Disord.* 1994;7:48–54.

68. Wisniewski HM, Robe A, Zigman W, Silverman W. Neuropathological diagnosis of Alzheimer disease. *J. Neuropathol. Exp. Neurol.* 1989;48:606–609.

69. Bancher C, Jellinger KA. Neurofibrillary tangle predominant form of senile dementia of Alzheimer type: a rare subtype in very old subjects. *Acta Neuropathol.* 1994;88:565–570.

70. Itoh Y, Yamada M, Yoshida R, Suematsu N, Oka T, Matsushita M, Otomo, E. Dementia characterized by abundant neurofibrillary tangles and scarce senile plaques: a quantitative pathological study. *Eur. Neurol.* 1996;36:94–97.

71. Ulrich J, Spillantini MG, Goedert M, Dukas M, Stahelin HB. Abundant neurofibrillary tangles without senile plaques in a subset of patients with senile dementia. *Neurodegeneration* 1992;1:257–264.

72. Braak H, Braak E. Neurofibrillary changes confined to the entorhinal region and an abundance of cortical amyloid in cases of presenile and senile dementia. *Acta Neuropathol.* 1990;80:479–486.

73. Terry RD, Hansen LA, DeTeresa R, Davies P, Tobias H, Katzman R. Senile dementia of the Alzheimer type without neocortical neurofibrillary tangles. *J. Neuropathol. Exp. Neurol.* 1987;46:262–268.

74. Hansen LA. Pathology of other dementias. In Terry RD, Katzman R, Bick KL, editors. *Alzheimer Disease.* New York: Raven Press, 1994:167–177.

75. Perry RH, Irving D, Blessed G, Fairbairn A, Perry E.K. Senile dementia of Lewy body type: a clinically and neuropathologically distinct form of Lewy body dementia in the elderly. *J. Neurol. Sci.* 1990;95:119–139.

76. Dickson DW, Crystal H, Mattiace LA, Kress Y, Schwagerl A, Ksiezak-Reding H, Davies P, Yen SH. Diffuse Lewy body disease: light and electron microscopic immunocytochemistry of senile plaques. *Acta Neuropathol.* 1989;78:572–584.

77. Lippa CF, Smith TW, Swearer JM. Alzheimer's disease and Lewy body disease: a comparative clinicopathological study. *Ann. Neurol.* 1994;35:81–88.

78. Hansen L, Salmon D, Galasko D, Masliah E, Katzman R, DeTeresa R, Thal L, Pay MM, Hofstetter R, Klauber M, Rice V, Butters N, Alford M. The Lewy body variant of Alzheimer's disease: a clinical and pathologic entity. *Neurology* 1990;40:1–8.

79. Dickson DW. Lewy body variant. *Neurology* 1996;40:1147–1148.

80. Hansen LA, Masliah E, Galasko D, Terry RD. Plaque-only Alzheimer disease is usually the Lewy body variant, and vice versa. *J. Neuropathol. Exp. Neurol.* 1993; 52:648–654.

4

The Pathophysiology of Alzheimer's Disease

Dennis J. Selkoe

Introduction

Progress in accurately diagnosing and effectively treating Alzheimer's disease (AD) must rest on a fundamental understanding of its pathophysiology. The application of molecular genetic, biochemical, and morphological techniques to this disorder during the last two decades has produced a large and complex body of data that is steadily being integrated into a temporal sequence of pathogenetic events. Although our understanding of the mechanism of the disease is still evolving, there is growing agreement among many investigators about the major steps in the cascade that precede the symptoms of the disease. In this chapter, we review the salient features of our current understanding of AD pathophysiology and explore how this new knowledge improves early diagnosis and illuminates the pathway to therapeutics.

The neuropathology of Alzheimer's disease has provided the starting point for defining its causes and mechanism. Much of the progress in identifying factors underlying AD began with the biochemical dissection of its histological phenotype in the early 1980s. Both the neurofibrillary tangles and the senile (amyloid) plaques that represent the classical diagnostic features of the pathology have been subjected to intensive scrutiny by structural, biochemical, and molecular biological approaches. Studies in a number of laboratories have firmly established that the principal if not sole constituent of the abnormal paired helical filaments (PHF) that comprise neurofibrillary tangles are modified, highly phosphorylated forms of the microtubule associated protein, tau *(1–6.)* PHF composed of modified tau proteins are present not only in tangles but in many of the dystrophic neurites that cluster around extracellular amyloid deposits (i.e., neuritic plaques) and are also more widely distributed throughout much of the cortical neuropil (i.e., neuropil threads or curly fibers). Despite the widespread abundance of a modified form of this cy-

From: *Early Diagnosis of Alzheimer's Disease*
Edited by L. F. M. Scinto & K. R. Daffner © Humana Press, Inc., Totowa, NJ

toskeletal protein in almost all AD brains, cloning of the gene encoding tau has so far resulted in no evidence of defects in this gene in inherited forms of AD. This observation is in keeping with the knowledge that neurofibrillary tangles composed of highly similar if not identical forms of modified tau proteins can be detected in numerous etiologically distinct human brain diseases, including subacute sclerosing panencephalitis, variants of Hallervorden-Spatz disease, the Parkinson-dementia complex of Guam, and dementia pugilistica. In other words, PHF formation appears to be part of the response of human neurons and their processes to a variety of disparate insults.

Although the identification of hyperphosphorylated tau proteins in tangles and dystrophic neurites has not been linked to the etiology of AD, this discovery nevertheless has considerable diagnostic implications. More than a dozen published studies have shown that the levels of tau protein in the cerebrospinal fluid are elevated in a majority of subjects with AD compared to age-matched normal individuals. The sensitivity and specificity of tau elevation as an adjunct to the diagnosis of AD is discussed in Chapter 9.

Biochemical dissection of the extracellular amyloid deposits that are found in the centers of neuritic plaques and in some meningeal and cortical microvessels led to the identification of the amyloid β-protein (Aβ) as the principal constituent of both types of deposits *(7–10)*. Aβ comprises a heterogeneous group of ~4 kDa peptides, with the major species being 40 or 42 residues long. The amino acid sequence of Aβ is quite hydrophobic, helping to explain the strong tendency of this small protein to self-aggregate and form clusters of fibrils that precipitate from solution (see, e.g., *11–15)*. Aβ is the subunit of the amyloid fibrils characteristic of AD and is structurally entirely distinct from other amyloid-forming proteins in various systemic amyloidoses. It is also structurally unrelated to the prion protein implicated in the etiology of Creutzfeld-Jakob disease (CJD), a protein that can also form insoluble extracellular filaments. However, amyloid fibrils composed of prion protein fragments are generally far less abundant in CJD brains than are Aβ fibrils in AD brains. Indeed, all Alzheimer subjects have moderate or, more often, high numbers of amyloid plaques in areas of the brain important for memory and cognition.

Biology of the Amyloid β-Protein and Its Precursor Polypeptide

Aβ has provided a starting point for molecular biological and genetic studies that led to the eventual identification of the first specific molecular cause of AD—missense mutations in and around the Aβ region of the β-amyloid precursor protein (APP). APP, an intriguing and now much studied polypeptide

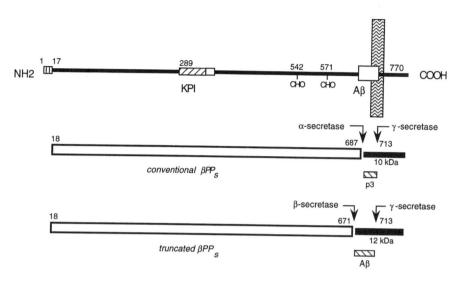

Fig. 1. Schematic diagrams of the β-amyloid precursor protein and its principal metabolic derivatives. **(Top)** The largest of the known APP alternate transcripts, comprising 770 amino acids. Regions of interest are indicated at their correct relative positions. A 17-residue signal peptide occurs at the amino terminus (box with vertical lines). Two alternatively spliced exons of 56 and 19 amino acids are inserted at residue 289; the first contains a serine protease inhibitor domain of the Kunitz type (KPI). Two sites of *N*-glycosylation (CHO) are found at residues 542 and 571. A single membrane-spanning domain at amino acids 700–723 is indicated by the vertical hatched bar. The amyloid β-protein (Aβ) fragment *(white box)* includes 28 residues just outside the membrane plus the first 12–14 residues of the transmembrane domain. **(Middle)** The *arrow* indicates the site (after residue 687) of a constitutive proteolytic cleavage made by an unknown protease(s) designated α-secretase that enables secretion of the large, soluble ectodomain of βAPP (APP$_s$) into the medium and retention of the 83-residue carboxy-terminal fragment ~10-kDa) in the membrane. The 10-kDa fragment can undergo cleavage by an unknown protease(s) called γ-secretase at residue 711 or residue 713 to release the p3 peptides. **(Bottom)** The alternative proteolytic cleavage after residue 671 by an unknown enzyme(s) called β-secretase that results in the secretion of a truncated APP$_s$ molecule and the retention of a 99-residue (~12-kDa) carboxy-terminal fragment. The 12-kDa fragment can also undergo cleavage by γ-secretase to release the Aβ peptides.

(Fig. 1), is a large glycoprotein anchored in various cellular membranes (including the plasma membrane) by a single transmembrane region. It thus projects from the cell surface (and also into the lumens of many intracellular vesicles) in a fashion resembling well-characterized receptors such as the low density lipoprotein receptor and the insulin receptor. APP is widely expressed in virtually all mammalian cells. In the nervous system, neurons show particularly high expression, but astrocytes, microglia, and endothelial cells also express the precursor. The localization of the APP gene to chromosome 21q is widely believed to explain the observation that patients with trisomy 21 (Down's syndrome) incur β-amyloid deposition as early as late childhood and gradually develop the classical neuropathological features of AD by age 40 or so *(16–18)*.

The primary structure of APP *(10)* shows us that the 40–42 residue Aβ peptide that constitutes the amyloid actually comprises the 28 amino acids immediately outside of the single transmembrane region plus the first 12 or 14 amino acids of that membrane-buried segment (Fig. 1). This topography of the Aβ region led to the assumption that an insult to cell membranes must occur before Aβ could be released intact into the extracellular space of the brain to form amyloid deposits. In turn, this concept seemed consistent with the widely held opinion that tissue amyloid deposits in general were likely to represent secondary byproducts of disease processes rather than serving as an initiating feature which could be linked to the genetic etiology of a disease. However, extensive studies of systemic amyloid diseases as well as AD have shown that this concept is erroneous.

As investigators examined cultured cells that express APP naturally or were transfected with its cDNA to achieve high expression, they found that APP commonly undergoes a proteolytic cleavage just 12 amino acids in front of the membrane-anchoring region, that is, immediately after amino acid 16 of the Aβ region of the precursor *(19, 20)* (Fig. 1). This scission releases the large, soluble ectodomain (referred to as APP$_s$) into the extracellular fluid. The cleavage is caused by an as yet unidentified protease(s) that is referred to as "α-secretase." The APP$_s$ derivative has been found in normal human CSF *(21,22)* and plasma *(23)*. Although a few studies have suggested that its level might be decreased in AD, most studies have found that this change is inconsistent enough as to not be diagnostically useful.

The APP$_s$ that is constitutively secreted by most cells in the body must serve one or several normal functions. Some of these have been suggested by studies in tissue culture. The normal functions of APP$_s$ may include: 1) the inhibition of certain serine proteases (e.g., trypsin, chymotrypsin and factor XIa of the coagulation cascade); 2) the participation in the adhesion of some cell types to the extracellular matrix; and 3) trophic, neuroprotective, and wound-healing properties. In addition, the uncleaved APP holoprotein residing at the cell surface may have its own function, for example, as a molecule that promotes cell-cell interactions or perhaps as a receptor for an as-yet-unknown diffusable ligand.

Although clues to the normal function of APP have emerged from cell culture studies, the use of genetic engineering to entirely delete ("knock out") the APP gene in mice has shown that the gene is not necessary for viability and normal brain development and that the phenotypic consequences are relatively subtle *(24)*. Further study is needed before we can be certain of the functions of APP in the normal nervous system in vivo. Nevertheless, there is no compelling evidence that any putative function of APP is actually lost or diminished in AD subjects. Rather, it appears that the role of APP in AD involves a toxic function imparted by just its Aβ fragment, once it is released from the precursor by proteolysis and begins to aggregate.

A major reinterpretation of our understanding of Aβ came from the discovery in 1992 that APP can be alternatively metabolized in a way that avoids α-secretase cleavage within the Aβ region and instead produces cleavages at the beginning of the Aβ region [by a protease(s) dubbed "β-secretase"] and at the end of this region [by a protease(s) designated "γ-secretase"] *(25–27)* (Fig. 1). In other words, it was found that Aβ is constitutively released from a subset of APP molecules during normal cellular metabolism, without any requirement for preexisting membrane injury or another form of cell damage. Indeed, it was found that intact 40- and 42-residue Aβ peptides were normally present in extracellular fluids such as plasma and CSF *(26,27)*. Moreover, APP-expressing cells cultured in the laboratory (neurons, astrocytes, fibroblasts, and kidney cells, to name a few) all normally secreted Aβ into the culture medium *(25–28)*. These unanticipated findings brought the β-amyloidosis of AD in line with a number of known human amyloid deposition diseases outside of the brain, such as familial amyloidotic polyneuropathy (due to transthyretin amyloidosis) and secondary amyloid deposits (derived from the acute-phase protein, serum amyloid A), that arise in several inflammatory disorders. In virtually all of the amyloidotic diseases of humans, a circulating protein or protein fragment that is normally present in extracellular fluids undergoes progressive polymerization into amyloid fibrils, which form multiple tissue deposits capable of exerting local cytotoxicity *(29)*.

There are at least three major implications of the discovery of normal Aβ secretion for the study of AD *(30)*. First, any genes that are implicated in the etiology of AD can be studied as to their effect on Aβ production, both in transfected cells and transgenic mice bearing a mutant gene and in the CSF and plasma of patients carrying the mutation. Second, the levels of $A\beta_{40}$ and $A\beta_{42}$ can be directly assayed in plasma and CSF to determine whether they were altered in amount and thus are diagnostically useful in subjects with AD. Third, and perhaps most important, cell lines expressing normal or mutant APP and thus secreting Aβ can serve as an in vitro screening system to identify compounds which specifically lower Aβ production without damaging the cells. "Hits" in this assay can then be tested in animals (e.g., normal or transgenic mice) to determine whether they lower Aβ production in vivo. As we will see, all of these principal implications of the discovery of soluble Aβ production have now been realized.

Identification of Genes That Cause or Predispose to Alzheimer's Disease

At the same time that studies of the Aβ peptides of amyloid plaques and the tau protein of neurofibrillary tangles were proceeding, molecular geneticists combined forces with many physicians in searching for loci in the human genome that might contain defective genes underlying the well-recognized autosomal dominant cases of AD (FAD). Geneticists needed a compelling clue as to where in the enormous human genome to begin their search for a faulty gene. This clue came with the recognition that patients with trisomy 21 invariably developed a neuropathological phenotype indistinguishable from that of AD and that the APP gene was located on chromosome 21. First, a linkage of some cases of FAD to the long arm of chromosome 21 was suggested by analysis of anonymous DNA markers in a few families *(31)*, and then, 4 years later, a mutation in the coding region of the APP gene was identified in two families as the first specific molecular cause of AD *(32)*. Extensive further studies have revealed only six missense mutations in APP, occurring in a very small number of autosomal dominant cases of the disease. However, the rarity of this initially defined genetic form of AD does not detract from its mechanistic importance for understanding AD pathogenesis in general. This is because all of the APP missense mutations cluster within or immediately flanking the Aβ region of APP. Indeed, the mutations are found at or near the α-secretase, β-secretase, or γ-secretase cleavage sites for APP proteolysis.

All of the known APP missense mutations linked to familial AD have now been modeled in cultured cells or in transgenic mice, and some of them have also been analyzed directly in the plasma and CSF of mutation-bearing patients. In each case, the APP mutations have been shown to increase the secretion of Aβ into the extracellular fluid, particularly that of the $A\beta_{42}$ form (reviewed in *33*). There is now virtually universal agreement among investigators that the rare APP-linked form of familial AD operates via an amyloid-promoting mechanism. An important corollary of this conclusion is that the neuropathological and clinical phenotypes of the APP-caused cases are highly similar or indistinguishable from those of the other, more common genetic and sporadic forms of the disease.

Apolipoprotein E4 Is a Major Genetic Risk Factor for AD

The next gene to be implicated by genetic studies turned out to be a major risk factor for the common, late-onset form of AD. Biochemical studies searching for CSF proteins capable of binding to Aβ identified apolipoprotein

E as one such protein. Subsequent genetic analyses showed that the naturally occurring ε4 polymorphism of the ApoE gene was substantially overrepresented in AD subjects compared to age-matched controls and thus appeared to represent a major risk factor for the development of the disease *(34)*. There has since been widespread confirmation that inheritance of one or two ApoE ε4 alleles significantly increases the likelihood of developing late-onset AD and decreases its age of onset (e.g., *35*). Conversely, inheritance of the ApoE ε2 allele appears to confer a decreased risk of developing the disorder compared to that seen in humans harboring the common ε3 allele *(36)*.

It remains unclear why the ApoE4 protein (which lacks cysteines) increases the likelihood of AD while ApoE3 and ApoE2 proteins (which contain cysteines) do not. However, a major clue to the mechanism has come from the observation, now confirmed in numerous laboratories, that AD subjects with two ε4 alleles have a significantly higher number and density of Aβ deposits in their brains than subjects with no ε4 alleles, while subjects with one ε4 allele generally fall in between *(37–41)*. In vitro biochemical studies have suggested that ApoE4 may be less effective in retarding the self-aggregation of Aβ into amyloid fibrils than ApoE2 or ApoE3 *(42)*. Alternative hypotheses for the effect of ApoE4 in AD have been proposed. These include the evidence that ApoE4 does not support neurite outgrowth in vitro and is less salutary for normal neuronal structural and function than is ApoE3 *(43)*, and that ApoE4 may permit tau to become dissociated from microtubules and participate in enhanced PHF formation *(44)*. However, the latter hypothesis is inconsistent with the observation that amyloid plaque density, not neurofibrillary tangle density, correlates with ApoE4 gene dosage in AD patients *(37,38)*.

Mutations in the Presenilin Genes Are the Most Common Known Cause of Early-Onset Autosomal Dominant AD

In 1995, linkage analysis and positional cloning led to the identification of a gene on chromosome 14 that is responsible for a sizable fraction of early onset familial AD cases *(45)*. The novel gene, currently called *presenilin 1* (PS-1), encodes a protein that appears to have 6–8 transmembrane domains and thus resembles certain kinds of cell-surface receptors, channel proteins or structural proteins of internal membrane vesicles. Shortly after *presenilin 1* was cloned, a highly homologous second gene, termed *presenilin 2* (PS-2), was identified as the cause of early-onset familial AD in at least two families, one of which was the renowned "Volga German" pedigree that contains many members with presenile AD *(46,47)*. The presenilin gene products are, in turn, highly homologous to a protein called sel12 in the roundworm, *Caenorhabditis elegans,* that appears to function in the recognition of certain cells by other cells during development *(48).*

Based again on the fact that cells that normally secrete Aβ, the PS-1 and PS-2 gene mutations, more than 35 of which have been identified, have been studied in transfected cells and, in some cases, in the plasma and skin fibroblast media of mutation-bearing patients. These analyses demonstrate a reproducible and statistically significant increase in the cellular production of the highly amyloidogenic Aβ$_{42}$ peptides *(49–52).* Recent work *(52a)* has indicated that PS-1 may be a critical co-factor for γ-secretase activity or is γ-secretase itself. As noted earlier, γ-secretase is involved in the final step in the process of generating Aβ from the APP. This research provides a direct link between PS-1 mutations and the increase in Aβ proteins observed in the brains of such patients. Moreover, direct analysis of the brain tissue from several patients bearing a particular PS-1 missense mutation show that there are many more Aβ$_{42}$-immunoreactive amyloid plaques in the brains of these subjects than in sporadic AD subjects with comparable overall neuropathological severity *(53).* The elevation of Aβ$_{42}$ has also been confirmed in the brains of transgenic mice harboring PS-1 mutations *(50,51,54).* Because Aβ$_{42}$ peptide have been shown to be the initially deposited species during β-amyloidosis in Down's syndrome (DS) and conventional AD *(17,18,55),* it is highly likely that the PS-1 and PS-2 mutant genes confer the AD phenotype by selectively enhancing Aβ$_{42}$ production throughout life.

Aβ Deposition Appears To Be a Necessary but Not Sufficient Factor for the Genesis of AD

To summarize at this juncture, four genes that are unequivocally associated with the development of AD have been identified to date, and linkage analyses of other families make it clear that additional genes can be responsible (Table 1). Three of the known genes, APP on chromosome 21, PS-1 on chromosome 14, and PS-2 on chromosome 1, can be said to be causative of AD in the respective families in which mutations in these genes occur. In each of these three cases, there is now compelling evidence that the mechanism of disease involves altered APP catabolism to generate increased amounts of Aβ peptides, particularly the highly amyloid-prone 42 residue form (Table 1). In the case of the ApoE gene on chromosome 19, its ε4 allele is a major genetic risk factor for the development of AD, perhaps contributing to the development of the disorder in some 30–40% or more of all AD patients. However, ApoE4 is not causative, per se, because some patients with one or two ApoE4

Table 1
Genetic Factors Predisposing to Alzheimer's Disease:
Relationships to the β-Amyloid Phenotype

Chromosome	Gene Defect	Age of Onset	Aβ Phenotype
21	βAPP mutations	50s	↑ Production of total Aβ peptides or of $A\beta_{42}$ peptides
19	ApoE4 polymorphism	60s and older	↑ Density of Aβ plaques and vascular deposits
14	Presenilin 1 mutations	40s and 50s	↑ Production of $A\beta_{42}$ peptides
1	Presenilin 2 mutations	50s	↑ Production of $A\beta_{42}$ peptides

Additional chromosomal loci exist but are not yet specifically identified.

alleles show no signs of the clinical disease even late in life, and, conversely, half or more of all AD patients do not bear an ε4 allele. The pathogenetic mechanism of ApoE4 remains to be elucidated but appears to involve enhanced aggregation and deposition of $A\beta_{40}$ peptides (56).

Our discussion thus far has emphasized the possible role of βAPP metabolism and the gradual accumulation of insoluble Aβ deposits in the pathogenesis of the disease. However, many other biochemical and structural abnormalities have also been observed in the brains of AD patients. Although at this moment it is impossible to arrange the heterogeneous molecular and cellular changes found at the end of the disease into a precise temporal sequence of progression, the outlines of a pathogenetic cascade are emerging. Insights into the temporal course of the disorder in its preclinical phase derive primarily from three sources:

1. The study of the accrual of AD-type brain changes in patients with trisomy 21 who have died of other causes at various ages from early childhood to late adulthood
2. Similar analyses of the development of AD-type lesions during the normal aging process in humans and other primates
3. Studies of small animal models of AD, in particular, transgenic mice that overexpresses mutant forms of APP that causes early-onset AD in humans (57,58)

Analyses of DS brains have provided perhaps the most relevant information about how AD may progress. Numerous investigators have reported that the earliest AD-like morphological change found in very young (e.g., 12- to 15-year-old) DS brains is the accrual of amorphous, largely nonfibrillar forms of Aβ deposits referred to as "diffuse plaques." Some or many such deposits are found in limbic and association cortices (and often in striatum, cerebellum, and elsewhere) in trisomic individuals dying after age 12 or so (e.g., 16). Importantly, many such diffuse plaques are also found in the brains of late middle-aged ($\geq$ 60) or older people with normal cognition who have died of other causes. Recent work by Morris and colleagues (*58a*) has shown that clinically silent individuals and those with mild cognitive impairment also show diffuse amyloid deposits when brought to autopsy. Diffuse plaques are also abundantly present in typical AD brains at the end of the patients' lives.

Light- and electron-microscopic studies of diffuse plaques in AD and in DS demonstrate very little or no structural alteration of axons, dendrites, astrocytes, and microglia within and immediately surrounding these amorphous Aβ deposits. This lack of cytopathology appears to correlate with a relative dearth of fibrillar amyloid in the diffuse deposits. As the brains of patients of increasing age with DS are examined, fibrillar plaques with surrounding neuritic and glial dystrophy are detected increasingly after approximately age 30 (e.g., *16,18*). At about the same time, neurofibrillary tangles also begin to appear. Although such temporal correlation is imprecise in the relatively limited number of patients with DS reported to date, a consensus has emerged that diffuse Aβ plaques precede the other AD-type changes that occur in DS. The early accumulation of diffuse plaques is assumed to be caused by the elevated βAPP gene dosage and the documented increase in βAPP expression and Aβ levels found in these patients (e.g., *59*).

APP transgenic mice experience high brain expression of APP from birth and are thus analogous in part to patients with DS. However, the mice reported to date have the additional influence of an FAD-linked missense mutation flanking the Aβ region of APP (*57,58*). Although such animals have high neuronal expression of the APP transgene as well as high levels of soluble Aβ within their brains from birth, they develop diffuse and compacted Aβ plaques resembling those of AD beginning around 5–7 months (mice normally live to about 2–3 years). During the next several months, the transgenic mice show increasing numbers of Aβ deposits, many of which are now Congo red-positive (suggesting that they contain fibrillar amyloid), and electron microscopy clearly reveals filamentous amyloid cores (*60*). Moreover, after Aβ plaques develop, the mice show morphologically and immunocytochemically abnormal neurites intimately associated with the amyloid plaques (*57,58,60*). Cytoskeletal proteins such as the microtubule associated protein 2 (MAP 2), the neurofilament protein, and even the tau protein can show abnormal immunoreactive patterns in these dystrophic neurites and in some nearby neuronal cell bodies (*57,58,60,61*), although full-blown neurofibrillary tangle formation has not been reported to date. A brisk reactive astrocytosis occurs within and around the Aβ plaques, and activated microglial cells occur near the centers of many of the plaques *(60,61)*. Confocal microscopy of the mouse plaques and immunostaining for synaptic proteins indicate that degeneration and loss of synapses is occurring, particularly in the vicinity of the plaques *(57)*. To what extent the progressive amyloidotic, neuritic, astrocytic, and microglial pathology observed in the transgenic mice leads to reproducible behavioral impairment is not yet clear *(57,58,61a)*, but the degree of neuropathological lesions makes this likely.

Although the rather rapid acquisition of AD-like lesions in the mice resulting from high expression of βAPP from birth cannot be considered an ideal model of AD, these transgenic mice clearly provide a highly useful and manipulable experimental model of the Alzheimer process. Additional morphological and neurochemical analyses of various transgenic mice of increasing age will further establish how closely the animals' disease resembles the AD pathological process and in which ways it differs. Several mammalian models of the aging brain also have shown that fibrillar Aβ is toxic to neurons *(60a)*.

Assuming that studies of disease progression in DS and in the transgenic mice are relevant to the mechanism of AD, one may postulate that the gradual accrual of amyloidogenic Aβ peptides in the form of first diffuse and then fibrillar plaques may result in local cellular effects that include reactive astrocytosis, activation of microglial cells, and alterations of nearby axons and dendrites (Fig. 2). The extent to which these cytotoxic events derive from properties of the aggregated Aβ protein itself or from the numerous β-amyloid-associated proteins that have been detected in plaques is yet unclear. These associated polypeptides, some of which have been referred to as "pathological chaperones" because of their putative role in enhancing the aggregation, deposition, and toxicity of Aβ, include the normally secreted proteins, α_1-antichymotrypsin *(62)*, ApoE *(63)*, serum amyloid P component *(64)*, basement membrane-associated heparan sulfate proteoglycan *(65)*, and various components of the classical complement pathway *(66,67)*. Activated microglia, which become associated with maturing plaques, are capable of releasing a number of well-characterized cytokines that can, in turn, stimulate local astrocytes to release yet other proteins, including α_1-antichymotrypsin and ApoE. The serum amyloid P protein, which is associated with all forms of central and peripheral amyloid deposits, is not expressed in the brain and thus must come to the plaque via passage across the blood–brain barrier *(64)*. To what extent other circulating molecules (including Aβ itself) breach the barrier to contribute to the pathological changes is unclear.

It can be concluded that many proteins potentially capable of exerting biological activity on surrounding neurons and glia accumulate within the amyloid plaque. We thus face an embarrassment of riches in terms of potential

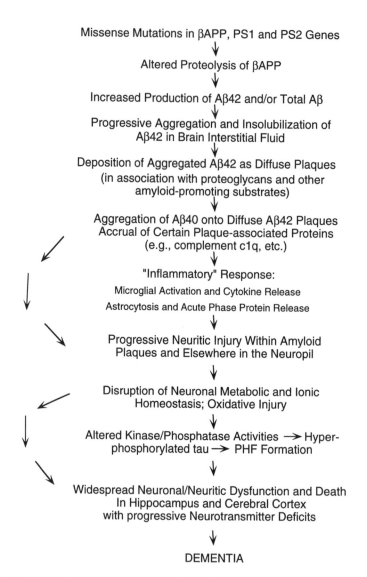

Fig. 2. A hypothetical sequence of the molecular pathogenesis of familial forms of Alzheimer's disease.

effectors of AD cytopathology. At exactly which point axons and dendrites in the vicinity, as well as their cell bodies of origin, undergo an activation of kinases, deactivation of phosphatases, or both, that result in the hyperphosphorylation of tau proteins underlying tangle formation is difficult to say *(68,69)*. In all probability, the multiple molecular and cellular alterations found in AD cortex develop at varying rates but in reasonable proximity to each other. Biochemical and morphological changes can presumably occur in cortical and subcortical neurons and their processes, which are not intimately associated with amyloid deposits. Subcortical neurons in regions such as the cholinergic nucleus basalis of Meynert, the noradrenergic locus ceruleus, and the serotinergic median raphe nuclei, whose axons all project into plaque-rich cortical areas, often show shrinkage, neurofibrillary tangle formation, and cell loss. The complex array of plaque-associated and non-plaque-associated cytopathology one observes by the end stage of AD may ultimately be very difficult to order into a precise sequence of temporal evolution.

The fact that neurofibrillary tangles arise in a variety of etiologically unrelated diseases in the absence of Aβ deposits suggests that they represent a response of neurons to a range of insults and are not specific for the amyloidotic process. The same may also be true of the tau-positive neuropil threads in the cortex, which can also occur in some degenerative diseases bearing tangles but lacking amyloid. On the other hand, the neuritic plaque, with its severe astrocytic and microglial cytopathology, is far more specific for AD and DS. The observation that abundant Aβ deposits can be found in some cognitively normal elderly subjects, theoretically arguing against an important role for amyloid deposition, can be countered by pointing out that the vast majority of these deposits are of the diffuse type, lacking neuritic and glial alteration. This fact presumably explains why they are not associated with clinical dysfunction. A rough analogy could be made to clinically silent fatty streaks of cholesterol in the vasculature; as presumed precursors to clinically important atherosclerotic lesions, their abundance alone does not correlate precisely with disease symptoms, as is the case for diffuse plaques. On the other hand, the total number and density of diffuse and neuritic plaques are usually far higher in AD patients than in age-matched normal subjects (e.g., *70),* just as the extent of cholesterol-rich plaques of all types is often higher in patients with symptomatic atherosclerotic cardiovascular disease than those free of symptoms.

The multiple neurotransmitter alterations in AD brain tissues that began to be uncovered in the late 1970s are now known to include several monoaminergic and neuropeptide deficiencies beyond the loss of cholinergic function that was first described. In the context of the complex, multicellular pathological cascade discussed above, it comes as no surprise that AD does not affect a single neurotransmitter system. Indeed, morphological studies have demonstrated that any one amyloid-bearing neuritic plaque may contain altered neurites derived from neurons of multiple neurotransmitter specificities. These considerations provide one explanation for the general lack of robust symptomatic improvement in patients given cholinergic replacement therapy such as acetylcholinesterase inhibitors. Based on this reasoning, one can provide a flow chart that describes a hypothetical sequence of changes underlying the development of clinical de-

mentia in familial forms of AD (Fig. 2). Clearly, this kind of scheme is specu-
lative, but a number of the elements of the temporal sequence can be justified
on the basis of the published information reviewed above. Whether there are
forms of AD in which the cerebral accumulation of Aβ and the gradual formation of particulate Aβ deposits (diffuse plaques) followed by filamentous amyloid deposits (neuritic plaques) are merely late secondary or tertiary events
remains to be seen. No compelling evidence for such a scenario has arisen.

Molecular Elucidation of Alzheimer's Disease
Predicts Novel and Effective Therapies

A truism of biomedical science is that the development of therapies expected
to slow or arrest the progression of a disease requires as detailed an understanding of the molecular pathogenesis as possible. The tools for screening a wide
array of compounds for efficacy in AD are already in hand and include cell culture systems and the transgenic mouse models, and there is an array of rational
therapeutic targets *(70a)*. Among these potential targets, the inhibition of Aβ secretion from neuronal and nonneuronal cells is being actively pursued. One way
this can be accomplished is by designing specific inhibitors of the β- and γ-se-
cretases, once these proteases are definitively identified and cloned. Screening on
cells that continuously secrete Aβ is well under way and should lead to the identification of compounds that act by a variety of mechanisms. However, there may
be other ways of lowering Aβ production that do not involve direct inhibition of
these enzymes. In any event, screening on cells that continuously secrete Aβ is
well under way and should lead to the identification of compounds that act by a
variety of mechanisms. One specific question regarding this approach relates to
whether chronic treatment with cholinergic agonists will result in increased processing of βAPP molecules by the α-secretase pathway and thus significantly diminished production of Aβ *(71,72)*. Such a possibility can initially be examined
in transgenic mice, in which both cerebral and CSF Aβ levels can be measured,
but it must then be confirmed in treated patients by measuring CSF Aβ levels. A
variety of other first messengers may turn out to be at least as effective as cholinergic agonists in shifting βAPP processing from the β- to the α-secretase pathway. Recent work by Elan scientists *(70b)* suggests yet another approach. They
were able to demonstrate that immunization with Aβ both prevented deposition
of Aβ and to some extent cleared Aβ deposits from the brains of PDAPP transgenic mice. These intriguing results raise the possibility of immunization that
might prevent and reverse the pathological cascade of the disease.

A therapeutic approach that seems particularly attractive is to attempt to slow
the aggregation of the secreted Aβ peptide into its fibrillar, putatively cytotoxic
form. In vitro studies indicate that certain small molecules, including the amy-

loid-binding dye Congo red, can retard the aggregation of synthetic Aβ peptides into high molecular weight aggregates. Compounds that interfere with Aβ assembly into amyloid fibrils could act in the extracellular space of the brain and thus avoid interference with the metabolism of βAPP and other molecules inside cells. Full-length βAPP and its various metabolites, including APP$_s$ and perhaps even Aβ, have normal functions, whereas the aggregated forms of Aβ that plaques are composed of are believed to represent solely pathological moieties. Thus, interfering with Aβ aggregation, if it can be done in a selective fashion, would avoid effects on the metabolism of βAPP and other molecules. The transgenic mouse models, which have fibrillar amyloid plaques, should be a reasonable system in which to evaluate the efficacy and safety of such compounds.

Yet another therapeutic approach based on the growing understanding of presymptomatic events in AD is the use of anti-inflammatory drugs that could interfere in part with the microglial activation, cytokine release, and acute phase response that occur in maturing amyloid plaques. Epidemiological evidence suggests that individuals who have been on nonsteroidal anti-inflammatory drugs may have a lower likelihood of developing the pathological and clinical features of AD. One may assume that the inflammatory process that appears around amyloid plaques is sufficiently distinct from peripheral forms of inflammation that it will require specialized anti-inflammatory compounds, which could again be identified and characterized in transgenic mice.

The devastating impairment of higher cortical functions that characterizes AD must ultimately be attributed to profound neuronal dysfunction and degeneration. Therefore, a variety of neuroprotective strategies can be envisioned in this disorder. One relatively specific approach would be to attempt to design compounds that interfere with any altered signal transduction pathways that are proven in the future to mediate the effects of extracellular amyloid filaments and their closely associated molecules on neuronal homeostasis. However, no single cell-surface receptor for Aβ in its monomeric or aggregated form has yet been found to fully mediate the toxicity. Instead, present evidence predicts that aggregated Aβ, by chronically altering the milieu of the neuronal surface, may trigger dysfunction of several or many cell-surface molecules and subsequent inappropriate activation of more than one second messenger system. Agents that could hypothetically interfere with such a process could include compounds that coat the amyloid aggregates in a way that makes them "invisible" to the cell or molecules that inhibit a downstream effector pathway inside the neuron.

In addition to such approaches directed at the specific neurotoxic cascade putatively induced by amyloid, therapies could be applied that might be equally applicable to AD and other neurodegenerative disorders. Such strategies might include the use of inhibitors of excitotoxicity, agents that block calcium entry, free radical scavengers and other antioxidant treatments. Evidence is mounting from in vitro studies that aggregated Aβ induces multiple features of oxidative injury in cultured neurons (e.g., *73)*. Another general approach to retarding neurodegeneration that might also be applicable to AD would be neurotrophic therapy. However, besides the considerable technical hurdles that must be overcome to chronically deliver neurotrophic peptides to the appropriate sites in the brains of elderly subjects, at least two theoretical concerns arise. First, some indirect evidence from tissue culture studies suggest that nerve growth factor treatment can potentially augment βAPP expression and perhaps its turnover into Aβ, something which would presumably not be desirable on a long-term basis in AD patients. Second, evidence exists that an apparent trophic or sprouting response already occurs in many cortical and limbic neurons (e.g., *74)*. This observation suggests that upregulation of trophic influences may actually be contributing in part to neuronal dysfunction in the disease.

It has been assumed that it will still take a long time to develop compounds that affect any of the therapeutic targets summarized above. But the rate of progress in elucidating the fundamental mechanism of the disease and, in particular, the pathogenic role of Aβ deposition, is sufficiently high to expect more refined therapeutic targets to emerge in the next 2 to 4 years. It may be, for example, that β- and γ-secretase enzymes will be identified, and cloned and then characterized as to possible mechanisms of inhibition. Moreover, prototype inhibitors of the cellular production of Aβ or its subsequent fibrillogenesis could emerge in just the next few years. In any event, a number of therapies advocated for neurodegenerative diseases in general, such as antioxidants and neuronal calcium channel blockers, are already advancing in clinical trials in AD patients soon.

The combined power of genetics, molecular biology, and biochemistry have produced remarkable advances in our understanding of the causes and mechanisms of AD. Given the great prevalence of the disease, the personal tragedy it represents for the patients and their families, and the enormous societal costs, estimated at upwards of $100 billion in the United States alone, one can safely predict that even more intensive effort on the part of academic and pharmaceutical laboratories will be brought to bear on the problem in the months and years ahead. The outcome could be that AD becomes one of the early examples of the amelioration or even prevention of a major, fatal brain disorder based on a thorough understanding of its molecular mechanism.

REFERENCES

1. Nukina N, Ihara Y. One of the antigenic determinants of paired helical filaments is related to tau protein. *J. Biochem.* 1986;99:1541–1544.

2. Kosik KS, Joachim CL, Selkoe DJ. Microtubule-associated protein, tau, is a major antigenic component of paired helical filaments in Alzheimer's disease. *Proc. Natl. Acad. Sci. U.S.A.* 1986;83:4044–4048.

3. Grundke-Iqbal I, Iqbal K, Tung Y-C, Quinlan M, Wisniewski HM, Binder LI. Abnormal phosphorylation of the microtubule-associated protein τ (tau) in Alzheimer cytoskeletal pathology. *Proc. Natl. Acad. Sci. U.S.A.* 1986;83:4913–4917.

4. Kondo J, Honda T, Mori H, Hamada Y, Miura R, Ogawara M, Ihara Y. The carboxyl third of tau is tightly bound to paired helical filaments. *Neuron* 1988;1:827–834.

5. Wischik CM, Novak M, Thogersen HC, Edwards PC, Runswick MJ, Jakes R, Walker JE, Milstein C, Rother M, Klug A. Isolation of a fragment of tau derived from the core of the paired helical filament of Alzheimer's disease. *Proc. Natl. Acad. Sci. U.S.A.* 1988;85:4506–4510.

6. Lee VM-Y, Balin BJ, Otvos L, Trojanowski JQ. A68. A major subunit of paired helical filaments and derivatized forms of normal tau. *Science* 1991;251:675–678.

7. Glenner GG, Wong CW. Alzheimer's disease: initial report of the purification and characterization of a novel cerebrovascular amyloid protein. *Biochem. Biophys. Res. Commun.* 1984;120:885–890.

8. Masters CL, Simms G, Weinman NA, Multhaup G, McDonald BL, Beyreuther K. Amyloid plaque core protein in Alzheimer disease and Down syndrome. *Proc. Natl. Acad. Sci. U.S.A.* 1985;82:4245–4249.

9. Selkoe DJ, Abraham CR, Podlisny MB, Duffy LK. Isolation of low-molecular-weight proteins from amyloid plaque fibers in Alzheimer's disease. *J. Neurochem.* 1986;146:1820–1834.

10. Kang J, Lemaire H-G, Unterbeck A, Salbaum JM, Masters CL, Grzeschik K-H, Multhaup G, Beyreuther K, Muller-Hill B. The precursor of Alzheimer's disease amyloid A4 protein resembles a cell-surface receptor. *Nature* 1987;325:733–736.

11. Kirschner DA, Inouye Y, Duffy LK, Sinclair A, Selkoe DJ. Synthetic β-peptide of Alzheimer disease forms amyloid-like fibrils in vitro. *Proc. Natl. Acad. Sci. U.S.A.* 1987;84:6953–6957.

12. Castano EM, Ghiso J, Prelli F, Gorevic PD, Migheli A, Frangione B. *In vitro* formation of amyloid fibrils from two synthetic peptides of different lengths homologous to Alzheimer's disease β-protein. *Biochem. Biophys. Res. Commun.* 1986;141:782–789.

13. Hilbich C, Kisters-Woike B, Reed J, Masters CL, Beyreuther K. Aggregation and secondary structure of synthetic amyloid βA4 peptides of Alzheimer's disease. *J. Mol. Biol.* 1991;218:149–163.

14. Barrow CJ, Yasuda A, Kenny PTM, Zagorski MG. Solution conformations and aggregational properties of synthetic amyloid β-peptides of Alzheimer's disease. *Mol. Biol.* 1992;225:1075–1093.

15. Jarrett JT, Berger EP, Lansbury Jr, PT. The carboxy terminus of the beta amyloid protein is critical for the seeding of amyloid formation: implications for the pathogenesis of Alzheimer's disease. *Biochemistry* 1993;32:4693–4697.

16. Mann DMA. Cerebral amyloidosis, aging and Alzheimer's disease: a contribution from studies on Down's syndrome. *Neurobiol. Aging* 1989;10:397–399.

17. Iwatsubo T, Mann DM, Odaka A, Suzuki N, Ihara Y. Amyloid β protein (Aβ) deposition: Aβ42(43) precedes Aβ40 in Down syndrome. *Ann. Neurol.* 1995;37:294–299.

18. Lemere CA, Blustzjan JK, Yamaguchi H, Wisniewski T, Saido TC, Selkoe DJ. Sequence of deposition of heterogeneous amyloid β-peptides and Apo E in Down syndrome: implications for initial events in amyloid plaque formation. *Neurobiol. Dis.* 1996;3:16–32.
19. Esch FS, Keim PS, Beattie EC, Blacher RW, Culwell AR, Oltersdorf T, McClure D, Ward PJ. Cleavage of amyloid β-peptide during constitutive processing of its precursor. *Science* 1990;248:1122–1124.
20. Sisodia SS, Koo EH, Beyreuther K, Unterbeck A, Price DL. Evidence that β-amyloid protein in Alzheimer's disease is not derived by normal processing. *Science* 1990;248:492–495.
21. Weidemann A, Konig G, Bunke D, Fischer P, Salbaum JM, Masters CL, Beyreuther K. Identification, biogenesis and localization of precursors of Alzheimer's disease A4 amyloid protein. *Cell* 1989;57:115–126.
22. Palmert MR, Podlisny MB, Witker DS, Oltersdorf T, Younkin LH, Selkoe DJ, Younkin SG. The β-amyloid precursor protein of Alzheimer disease has soluble derivatives found in human brain and cerebrospinal fluid. *Proc. Natl. Acad. Sci. U.S.A.* 1989;86:6338–6342.
23. Podlisny MB, Mamen AL, Schlossmacher MG, Palmert MR, Younkin SG, Selkoe DJ. Detection of soluble forms of the β-amyloid precursor protein in human plasma. *Biochem. Biophys. Res. Commun.* 1990;167:1094–1101.
24. Zheng H, Jiang M, Trumbauer ME, Sirinathsinghji DJS, Hopkins R, Smith DW, Heavesn RP, Dawson GR, Boyce S, Conner MW, Stevens KA, Slunt HH, Sisodia SS, Chen HY, Van der Ploeg LHT. β-Amyloid precursor protein-deficient mice show reactive gliosis and decreased locomotor activity. *Cell* 1995;81:525–531.
25. Haass C, Schlossmacher MG, Hung AY, Vigo-Pelfrey C, Mellon A, Ostaszewski BL, Lieberburg I, Koo EH, Schenk D, Teplow DB, Selkoe DJ. Amyloid β-peptide is produced by cultured cells during normal metabolism. *Nature* 1992;359:322–325.
26. Seubert P, Vigo-Pelfrey C, Esch F, Lee M, Dovey H, Davis D, Sinha S, Schlossmacher MG, Whaley J, Swindlehurst C, McCormack R, Wolfert R, Selkoe DJ, Lieberburg I, Schenk D. Isolation and quantitation of soluble Alzheimer's β-peptide from biological fluids. *Nature* 1992;359:325–327.
27. Shoji M, Golde TE, Ghiso J, Cheung TT, Estus S, Shaffer LM, Cai X, McKay DM, Tintner R, Frangione B, Younkin SG. Production of the Alzheimer amyloid β protein by normal proteolytic processing. *Science* 1992;258:126–129.
28. Busciglio J, Gabuzda DH, Matsudaira P, Yankner BA. Generation of β-amyloid in the secretory pathway in neuronal and nonneuronal cells. *Proc. Natl. Acad. Sci. U.S.A.* 1993;90:2092–2096.
29. Kisilevsky R, Benson MD, Frangione B, Gauldie J, Muckle TJ, Young, ID. Amyloid and Amyloidosis 1993. In: Proceedings of the VIIth International Symposium on Amyloidosis, July 11–15, 1993, Kingston, Ontario, Canada (New York, London: Parthenon Publishing).
30. Selkoe DJ. Physiological production of the amyloid β-protein and the mechanism of Alzheimer's disease. *Trends Neurosci.* 1993;16:403–409.
31. St. George-Hyslop PH, Tanzi RE, Polinsky RJ, Haines JL, Nee L, Watkins PC, Myers RH, Feldman RG, Pollen D, Drachman D, Growdon J, Bruni A, Foncin J-F, Salmon D, Frommelt P, Amaducci L, Sorbi S, Piacentini S, Stewart GC, Hobbs WJ,

Conneally P, Gusella JF. The genetic defect causing familial Alzheimer's disease maps to chromosome 21. *Science* 1987;235:885–889.

32. Goate A, Chartier-Harlin M-C, Mullan M, Brown J, Crawford F, Fidani L, Giuffra L, Haynes A, Irving N, James L, Mant R, Newton P, Rooke K, Roques P, Talbot C, Pericak-Vance M, Roses A, Williamson R, Rossor M, Owen M, Hardy J. Segregation of a missense mutation in the amyloid precursor protein gene with familial Alzheimer's disease. *Nature* 1991;349:704–706.

33. Selkoe DJ. Alzheimer's disease: genotypes, phenotype, and treatments. *Science* 1997;275:630–631.

34. Strittmatter WJ, Saunders AM, Schmechel D, Pericak-Vance M, Enghild J, Salvesen GS, Roses AD. Apolipoprotein E: high-avidity binding to β-amyloid and increased frequency of type 4 allele in late-onset familial Alzheimer disease. *Proc. Natl. Acad. Sci. U.S.A.* 1993;90:1977–1981.

35. Saunders AM, Strittmatter WJ, Schmechel D, George-Hyslop PH, Pericak-Vance MA, Joo SH, Rosi BL, Gusella JF, Crapper-MachLachlan DR, Alberts MJ, Hulette C, Crain B, Goldgaber D, Roses AD. Association of apolipoprotein E allele epsilon 4 with late-onset familial and sporadic Alzheimer's disease. *Neurology* 1993;43:1467–1472.

36. Corder EH, Saunders AM, Risch NJ, Strittmatter WJ, Schmechel DE, Gaskell Jr., PC, Rimmler JB, Locke PA, Conneally PM, Schmader KE, Small GW, Roses AD, Haines JL, Pericak-Vance MA. Protective effect of apolipoprotein E type 2 allele for late onset Alzheimer's disease. *Nature Genet.* 1994;7:180–184.

37. Schmechel DE, Saunders AM, Strittmatter WJ, Crain BJ, Hulette CM, Joo SH, Pericak-Vance MA, Goldgaber D, Roses AD. Increased amyloid β-peptide deposition in cerebral cortex as a consequence of apolipoprotein E gentoype in late-onset Alzheimer disease. *Proc. Natl. Acad. Sci. U.S.A.* 1993;90:9649–9653.

38. Rebeck GW, Reiter JS, Strickland DK, Hyman BT. Apolipoprotein E in sporadic Alzheimer's disease: allelic variation and receptor interactions. *Neuron* 1993;11:575–580.

39. Hyman BT, West HL, Rebeck GW, Buldyrev SV, Mantegna RN, Ukleja M, Havlin S, Stanley HE. Quantitative analysis of senile plaques in Alzheimer's disease: observation of log-normal size distribution and molecular epidemiology of differences associated with apolipoprotein E genotype and trisomy 21 (Down syndrome). *Proc. Natl. Acad. Sci. U.S.A.* 1995;92:3586–3590.

40. Polvikoski T, Sulkava R, Haltia M, Kainulainen K, Vuorio A, Verkkoniemi A, Niinisto L, Halonen P, Kontula K. Apolipoprotein E, dementia, and cortical deposition of β-amyloid protein. *N. Engl. J. Med.* 1995;333:1242–1247.

41. Greenberg SM, Rebeck GW, Vonsattel JPG, Gomez-Isla T, Hyman BT. Apolipoprotein E ϵ4 and cerebral hemorrhage associated with amyloid angiopathy. *Ann. Neurol.* 1995;38:254–259.

42. Evans KC, Berger EP, Cho C-G, Weisgraber KH, Lansbury Jr, PT. Apolipoprotein E is a kinetic but not a thermodynamic inhibitor of amyloid formation: implications for the pathogenesis and treatment of Alzheimer disease. *Proc. Natl. Acad. Sci. U.S.A.* 1995;92:763–767.

43. Nathan BP, Bellosta S, Sanan DA, Weisgraber KH, Mahley RW, Pitas RE. Differential effects of apoliprotein E3 and E4 on neuronal growth in vitro. *Science* 1994;264:850–852.

44. Roses AD, Einstein G, Gilbert J, Goedert M, Han SH, Huang D, Hulette C, Masliah
     E, Pericak-Vance MA, Saunders AM, Schmechel DE, Strittmatter WJ, Weisgraber
     KH, Xi PT. Morphological, biochemical and genetic support for an apolipoprotein
     E effect on microtubular metabolism. *Ann. N.Y. Acad. Sci.* 1996;777:146–157.
45. Sherrington R, Rogaev EI, Liang Y, Rogaeva EA, Levesque G, Ikeda M, Chi H, Lin
     C, Li G, Holman K, Tsuda T, Mar L, Foncin J-F, Bruni AC, Montesi MP, Sorbi S,
     Rainero I, Pinessi L, Nee L, Chumakov I, Pollen DA, Roses AD, Fraser PE,
     Rommens JM, St. George-Hyslop PH. Cloning of a novel gene bearing missense
     mutations in early onset familial Alzheimer disease. *Nature* 1995;375:754–760.
46. Levy-Lahad E, Wasco W, Poorkaj P, Romano DM, Oshima J, Pettingell H, Yu C,
     Jondro PD, Schmidt SD, Wang K, Crowley AC, Fu Y-H, Guenette SY, Galas D,
     Nemens E, Wijsman EM, Bird TD, Schellenberg GD, Tanzi RE. Candidate gene for
     the chromosome 1 familial Alzheimer's disease locus. *Science* 1995;269:973–977.
47. Rogaev EI, Sherrington R, Rogaeva EA, Levesque G, Ikeda M, Liang Y, Chi H,
     Lin C, Holamn K, Tsuda T, Mar L, Sorbi S, Nacmias B, Piacentini S, Amaducci
     L, Chumakov I, Cohen D, Lannfelt L, Fraser PE, Rommens JM, St. George-
     Hyslop PH. Familial Alzheimer's disease in kindreds with missense mutations in
     a gene on chromosome 1 related to the Alzheimer's disease type 3 gene. *Nature*
     1995;376:775–778.
48. Levitan D, Greenwald I. Facilitation of *lin-12*-mediated signalling by *sel-12,* a
     Caenorhabditis elegans S182 Alzheimer's disease gene. *Nature* 1995;377:351–354.
49. Scheuner D, Eckman C, Jensen M, Song X, Citron M, Suzuki N, Bird TD, Hardy
     J, Hutton M, Kukull W, Larson E, Levy-Lahad E, Viitanen M, Peskind E, Poorkaj
     P, Schellenberg G, Tanzi R, Wasco W, Lannfelt L, Selkoe D, Younkin S. Secreted
     amyloid β-protein similar to that in the senile plaques of Alzheimer's disease is in-
     creased *in vivo* by the presenilin 1 and 2 and APP mutations linked to familial
     Alzheimer's disease. *Nature Med.* 1996;2:864–870.
50. Borchelt DR, Thinakaran G, Eckman CB, Lee MK, Davenport F, Ratovitsky T,
     Prada C-M, Kim G, Seekins S, Yager D, Slunt HH, Wang R, Seeger M, Levey AI,
     Gandy SE, Copeland NG, Jenkins NA, Price DL, Younkin SG, Sisodia SS. Familial
     Alzheimer's disease-linked presenilin 1 variants elevate Aβ1-42/1-40 ratio in vitro
     and in vivo. *Neuron* 1996;17:1005–1013.
51. Citron M, Westaway D, Xia W, Carlson G, Diehl T, Levesque G, Johnson-Wood K,
     Lee M, Seubert P, Davis A, Kholodenka D, Motter R, Sherrington R, Perry B, Yao
     H, Strome R, Lieberburg I, Rommens J, Kim S, Schenk D, Fraser P, St George-
     Hyslop P, Selkoe DJ. Mutant presenilins of Alzheimer's disease increase production
     of 42-residue amyloid β-protein in both transfected cells and transgenic mice.
     Nature Med. 1997;3:67–72.
52. Xia W, Zhang J, Kholodenko D, Citron M, Podlisny MB, Teplow DB, Haass C,
     Seubert P, Koo EH, Selkoe DJ. Enhanced production and oligomerization of the 42-
     residue amyloid β-protein by Chinese hamster ovary cells stably expressing mutant
     presenilins. *J. Biol. Chem.* 1997;272:7977–7982.
52a. Wolfe MS, Xia W, Ostaszewski BH, Diehl TS, Kimberly WT, Selkoe DJ. Two
     transmembrane aspartates in presenilin-1 required for presenilin endoproteolysis
     and γ-secretase activity. *Nature* 1999;398:513–517.
53. Lemere CA, Lopera F, Kosik KS, Lendon CL, Ossa J, Saido TC, Yamaguchi H,

Ruiz A, Martinez A, Madrigal L, Hincapie L, Arango L, PC, Anthony DC, Koo EH, Goate AM, Selkoe DJ, Arango V, JC. The E280A presenilin 1 Alzheimer mutation produces increased Aβ42 deposition and severe cerebellar pathology. *Nature Med.* 1996;2:1146–1150.

54. Duff K, Eckman C, Zehr C, Yu X, Prada C-M, Perez-tur J, Hutton M, Buee L, Hairgaya Y, Morgan D, Gordon MN, Holcomb L, Refolo L, Zenk B, Hardy J, Younkin S. Increased amyloid Aβ42(43) in brains of mice expressing mutant presenilin 1. *Nature* 1996;383:710–713.

55. Iwatsubo T, Odaka A, Suzuki N, Mizusawa H, Nukina H, Ihara Y. Visualization of A beta 42(43) and A beta 40 in senile plaques with end-specific A beta monoclonals: evidence that an initially deposited species is A beta 42(43). *Neuron* 1994;13:45–53.

56. Gearing M, Mori H, Mirra SS. Aβ-peptide length and apolipoprotein E genotype in Alzheimer's disease. *Ann. Neurol.* 1996;39:395–399.

57. Games D, Adams D, Alessandrini R, Barbour R, Berthelette P, Blackwell C, Carr T, Clemens J, Donaldson T, Gillespie F, Guido T, Hagopian S, Johnson-Wood K, Khan K, Lee M, Leibowitz P, Lieberburg I, Little S, Masliah E, McConlogue L, Montoya-Zavala M, Mucke L, Paganini L, Penniman E, Power M, Schenk D, Seubert P, Snyder B, Soriano F, Tan H, Vitale J, Wadsworth S, Wolozin B, Zhao J. Alzheimer-type neuropathology in transgenic mice overexpressing V717F β-amyloid precursor protein. *Nature* 1995;373:523–527.

58. Hsiao K, Chapman P, Nilsen S, Ekman C, Harigaya Y, Younkin S, Yang F, Cole G. Correlative memory deficits, Aβ elevation, and amyloid plaques in transgenic mice. *Science* 1996;274:99–102.

58a. Morris JC, Storandt M, McKeel Jr DW, Rubin EH, Price JL, Grant EA, Berg L. Cerebral amyloid deposition and diffuse plaques in "normal" aging: evidence for presymptomatic and very mild Alzheimer's disease. *Neurology* 1996;46:707–719.

59. Querfurth HW, Wijsman EM, St. George-Hyslop PH, Selkoe DJ. βAPP mRNA transcription is increased in cultured fibroblasts from the familial Alzheimer's disease-1 family. *Mol. Brain Res.* 1995;28:319–337.

60. Masliah E, Sisk A, Mallory M, Mucke L, Schenk D, Games D. Comparison of neurodegenerative pathology in transgenic mice overexpressing V717F β-amyloid precursor protein and Alzheimer's disease. *J. Neurosci.* 1996;16:5795–5811.

60a. Geula C, Wu C-k, Saroff D, Lorenzo A, Yuan M, Yankner BA. Aging renders the brain vulnerable to amyloid β-protein neurotoxicity. *Nature Med.* 1998;4(7):827–831.

61. Games D, Carr T, Guido T, Khan K, Soriano F, Tan H, McConlogue L, Lieberburg I, Schenk D, Masliah E. Progression of Alzheimer-type neuropathology in PDAPP$_{717V \rightarrow F}$ transgenic mice. *Soc. Neurosci. Abstr.* 1995;21:258.

61a. Moechars D, Dewachter I, Lorent K, Reverse D, Baekelandt V, Naidu A, Tesseur I, Spittaels K, Haute CV, Checler F, Godaux E, Cordell B, Van Leuven F. Early phenotypic changes in transgenic mice that overexpress different mutants of amyloid precursor protein in brain. *J. Biol. Chem.* 1999;274(10):6483–6492.

62. Abraham CR, Selkoe DJ, Potter H. Immunochemical identification of the serine protease inhibitor, α_1-antichymotrypsin in the brain amyloid deposits of Alzheimer's disease. *Cell* 1988;52:487–501.

63. Namba Y, Tomonaga M, Kawasaki H, Otomo E, Ikeda K. Apolipoprotein E immunoreactivity in cerebral deposits and neurofibrillary tangles in Alzheimer's

disease and kuru plaque amyloid in Creutzfeldt-Jacob disease. *Brain Res.* 1991;541:163–166.

64. Kalaria RN. Serum amyloid P and related molecules associated with the acute-phase response in Alzheimer's disease. *Res. Immunol.* 1992;143:637–641.

65. Snow AD, Mar H, Nochlin D, Kimata K, Kato M, Suzuki S, Hassell J, Wight TN. The presence of heparan sulfate proteoglycans in the neuritic plaques and congophilic angiopathy in Alzheimer's disease. *Am. J. Pathol.* 1988;133:456–463.

66. Eikelenboom P, Stam FC. Immunoglobulins and complement factors in senile plaques: an immunoperoxidase study. *Acta Neuropathol.* 1982;57:239–242.

67. Rogers J, Cooper NR, Websger S, Schultz J, McGeer PL, Styren SD, Civin WH, Brachova L, Bradt B, Ward P, Lieberburg I. Complement activation by β-amyloid in Alzheimer disease. *Proc. Natl. Acad. Sci. U.S.A.* 1992;89:10016–10020.

68. Goedert M, Trojanowski JQ, Lee VM-Y. (1996). The neurofibrillary pathology of Alzheimer's disease. In: *The Molecular and Genetic Basis of Neurological Disease,* 2nd Edition, R.N. Rosenberg, S.B. Prusiner, S. DiMauro and R.L. Barchi, eds. (Boston: Butterworth-Heinemann Publishers), 1996;pp.613–627.

69. Lee VM-Y. Disruption of the cytoskeleton in Alzheimer's disease. *Curr. Opin. Neurobiol.* 1995;5:663–668.

70. Cummings BJ, Cotman CW. Image analysis of β-amyloid load in Alzheimer's disease and relation to dementia severity. *Lancet* 1995;346:1524–1528.

70a. Selkoe DJ. Translating cell biology into therapeutic advances in Alzheimer's disease. *Nature* 1999;399(Suppl.24):A23–A31.

70b. Schenk D, Barbour R, Dunn W, Gordon G, Grajeda H, Guido T, Hu K, Huang J, Johnson-Wood K, Khan K, Kholodenko D, Lee M, Liao Z, Lieberberg I, Motter R, Mutter L, Soriano F, Shopp G, Vasquez N, Vandevert C, Walker S, Wogulis M, Yednock T, Games D, Seubert P. Immunization with amyloid-β attenuates Alzheimer-disease-like pathology in the PDAPP mouse. *Nature* 1999;400:173–177.

71. Nitsch RM, Slack BE, Wurtman RJ, Growdon JH. Release of Alzheimer amyloid precursor derivatives stimulated by activation of muscarinic acetylcholine receptors. *Science* 1992;258:304–307.

72. Hung AY, Haass C, Nitsch RM, Qiu WQ, Citron M, Wurtman RJ, Growdon JH, Selkoe DJ. Activation of protein kinase C inhibits cellular production of the amyloid β-protein. *J. Biol. Chem.* 1993;268:22959–22962.

73. Behl C, Davis JB, Lesley R, Schubert D. Hydrogen peroxide mediates amyloid β protein toxicity. *Cell* 1994;77:817–827.

74. Ihara Y. Massive somatodendritic sprouting of cortical neurons in Alzheimer's disease. *Brain Res.* 1988;459:138–144.

5

Genetic Testing in the Early Diagnosis of Alzheimer's Disease

Deborah Blacker and Rudolph E. Tanzi

INTRODUCTION

Given the clear role of genetic factors in the development of Alzheimer's disease (AD), and the identification of several genes involved in the disease, genetic testing presents some interesting possibilities for the early diagnosis of AD. However, genetic tests for AD are complicated because of the genetic complexity of the disease, which limits the predictive value of genetic tests. Genetic testing for early diagnosis is further complicated because it lies between genetic testing for *diagnosis* of patients who clearly have a dementia consistent with AD, and genetic testing for *prediction* of AD onset in currently asymptomatic individuals.

More critically, genetic tests for AD, whether used for diagnosis or for prediction, carry the risk of invasion of privacy and discrimination in insurance, employment, and other settings *(1–5)*. These types of ethical concerns may be more serious for genetic testing because genetic tests may *appear* more definitive, and because they have implications for other family members. These social and ethical concerns are discussed more fully in Chapter 12.

This chapter focuses on current knowledge of AD genetics and diagnostic and predictive genetic testing, and reviews: 1) what is known about the role of genes in AD onset; 2) available data regarding genetic information in the diagnosis of AD, in the progression from questionable impairment to AD, and in the prediction of AD; 3) available genetic tests for AD and formal recommendations regarding their use; and 4) the implications of all of this information for the role of genetic testing in the early diagnosis of AD. In each case,

From: *Early Diagnosis of Alzheimer's Disease*
Edited by L. F. M. Scinto & K. R. Daffner © Humana Press, Inc., Totowa, NJ

the issues are discussed separately for early-onset AD (conventionally defined as before age 60), and late-onset AD (onset at 60 and beyond), since the genetic data differ for each group.

Genetics of Alzheimer's Disease

AD is a genetically complex and heterogeneous disorder. Roughly 5% of AD occurs under age 60 and is designated early-onset AD. Early-onset AD often displays autosomal dominant inheritance with virtually 100% penetrance *(6–8)*. Three gene defects are known to cause early-onset AD in families: presenilin 1 (PS-1) on chromosome 14 *(9,10)*, presenilin 2 (PS-2) on chromosome 1 *(11,12)*, and the amyloid-β protein precursor (APP) on chromosome 21 *(13,14)*. Late-onset AD has been associated with "public polymorphisms" in genes (i.e., common variations) that serve as genetic risk factors for the disease. While familial clustering is also found in late-onset AD, censoring due to the death of some family members from other age-related illnesses makes it difficult to assess the mode of inheritance. The apolipoprotein E gene (ApoE) on chromosome 19 is associated primarily with late-onset AD *(15,16)*, and appears to act as a risk factor and modifier of age of onset. Several other public polymorphisms have been associated with late-onset AD, but none of these has been definitively established.

Genetics of Early-Onset AD

Initial efforts to understand the role of genetics in AD in the early 1980s focused on extremely rare, large, multigenerational early-onset AD families. The first gene to be genetically linked with this form of AD was *APP (13,14)*, which has been shown to contain six different pathogenic mutations *(6)*, all of which are missense mutations lying within or close to the domain encoding the Aβ peptide, the major component of β-amyloid in AD. However, mutations in APP account for only two to three percent of early-onset AD pedigrees *(6)*. The age of onset of AD reported for individuals with mutations in APP ranges from 39 to 67. Of note, transgenic mice expressing AD mutations in APP produce numerous β-amyloid deposits in the form of classical senile plaques but do not exhibit significant neurofibrillary tangles or neuronal and synaptic loss *(17,18)*.

PS-1 on chromosome 14 was identified in 1995 by a positional cloning strategy *(9,10)*. The PS-2 gene on chromosome 1 was isolated in a group of related families of German descent from the Volga River region in Russia (the "Volga Germans") based on its extensive genetic sequence homology to PS-1 *(11,12)*. PS-1 has been reported to harbor over 50 different AD mutations in over 80 families of various ethnic origins. These mutations account for roughly 30% to 40% of early-onset AD and the vast majority occurring under age 50 *(6,19)*. By contrast, PS-2 has been found to contain only two different familial AD mutations and one apparently "sporadic" AD mutation *(19)*. The reason for the large difference in the number of AD mutations in PS-1 and PS-2 is not obvious, although mutation analysis of PS-1 may have outpaced that of PS-2.

All except two PS mutations are missense mutations that result in single amino acid substitutions. The exceptions are a mutation that deletes exon 9 from PS-1 in three different AD kindreds *(20)* and a splice-donor deletion in intron 4 of PS-1, which leads to truncation following intron 4 *(21)*. Two major clusters of mutations are observed in PS-1 in exons 5 (13 mutations) and 8 (13 mutations), which harbor more than 50% of the known PS-1 mutations.

While the mean age of onset in PS-1-linked AD pedigrees is approximately 45 years (range: 28–64 years), in the Volga German families carrying the N141I mutation in PS-2, it is 52 years, but with a broader range (40–85 years). Thus, it may be necessary to look for PS-2 mutations in AD kindreds with later onset than those that have been traditionally used to search for mutations in early-onset AD genes. The mutations in PS-1 appear to be fully penetrant, with one reported exception *(22)*. Studies to date suggest that ApoE genotype has no effect on the age of onset or phenotype of AD in patients with PS-1 mutations *(23)*. In contrast, ApoE genotype has been reported to affect the age of onset and degree of amyloid burden in patients with APP mutations *(24)*.

Genetics of Late-Onset AD

Late-onset AD is considerably more genetically complex than the early-onset forms of AD. Several lines of genetic and epidemiological evidence from population, family, twin, and segregation studies indicate that genes play a major role in its etiology *(25–30)*. In addition, few other risk factors aside from age itself are clearly established *(31)*. Thus, genetic studies are a principal means of learning about this devastating disease. Several factors must be considered in the search for genes involved in late-onset AD *(7)*. First, the base rate of the disorder is high, and rises steeply with age [10% of individuals over age 65, and as many as 50% of individuals over 85 *(32)*]. Thus, some clustering in families may be due to chance alone. For the same reason, it is also somewhat likely that one family will include multiple sources of disease. Second, late-onset AD occurs very near the end of the life span, so that many individuals do not survive the age of risk. This makes it difficult to assess the mode of inheritance, or even to derive an accurate estimate of the increase in the risk of AD in relatives of AD cases. Third, elderly patients have a greater risk for developing other causes of cognitive decline (e.g., stroke) than younger individuals, making the risk of false positive diagnosis (from the genetic point of view, phenocopies) somewhat higher in this age group. Efforts to avoid false positive diagnosis inevitably lead to diagnostic insensitivity, and thus some AD cases are missed within potentially informative families, further complicating efforts to understand the genetics of late-onset AD.

The only confirmed late-onset AD gene is ApoE-4. ApoE was the second AD-associated gene to be identified and acts as a major risk factor for late-onset AD *(15,16)*. ApoE is the major serum protein involved with cholesterol storage, transport, and metabolism. ApoE has three alleles, designated 2, 3, and 4. In mixed Caucasian populations in the United States and Europe, approximate ApoE allele frequencies are as follows: ApoE-2, 8%; ApoE-3, 80%; and ApoE-4, 12% *(33,34)*. The ApoE-4 allele is associated with increased risk for AD, while the ApoE-2 allele is associated with decreased risk *(7,8,35)*. Investigators first noted that the ApoE-4 allele was overrepresented in early- and late-onset familial and sporadic cases, and this association has been confirmed in numerous studies *(8,35,36)*. The ApoE-2 protective effect *(37)* has been observed less consistently, in part due to a decrease in statistical power to detect this effect associated with lower baseline frequency, but it was clearly confirmed in a large metaanalysis *(35)*. Instead of acting "deterministically," ApoE-4 acts as a risk factor and ApoE-2 as a protective factor for the disease. Although many ApoE-4 homozygotes develop AD, many do not *(36,38,39)*. For example, one population-based study showed that 85% of elderly individuals (average age 81) with the ApoE-4/4 genotype had normal performance on a mental status screening test *(38),* and one family-based study noted that there were 15 individuals who were cognitively intact despite having both the ApoE-4/4 genotype and two younger siblings with AD *(36)*.

Current research suggests that ApoE may act primarily as a modifier of age of onset. For instance, Meyer and coworkers *(40)* found in a population-based study of 4932 elderly individuals that onset occurred earliest in individuals with the ApoE-4/4 genotype, than in those with one copy of ApoE-4, and than in those with none, and that each group showed a plateau beyond which onsets were not observed. This dose-dependent effect of the ApoE-4 allele has been observed in many studies, with earliest onset seen fairly consistently in individuals with two copies of ApoE-4 *(41,42)*. However, some studies find that having only one copy of ApoE-4 has little effect on age of onset *(36)*. The peak effect of ApoE-4 appears to occur in the 60s *(35,36)*. While ApoE-4 has been confirmed as a strong risk factor for AD, it is clearly not necessary for the development of AD at any age: in fact, some 35 to 60 percent of AD cases do not carry the ApoE-4 allele, and only 12 to 15 percent are homozygous for ApoE-4 *(7,43,44)*.

Another group of recent studies have suggested that the observed association of ApoE-4 with AD may be due to linkage disequilibrium (i.e., genetically associated, due to close proximity on the chromosome) with polymorphisms in the promoter for ApoE. These polymorphisms have been found to be associated with both inheritance of ApoE-4 and increased risk for AD *(45,46)*. Thus, it is conceivable that the ApoE-4 genotype is actually in linkage disequilibrium with genetic alterations in the ApoE promoter, which modify age of onset. It will be important to determine whether these or other polymorphisms in the ApoE promoter significantly alter the transcription of the ApoE gene in brain: transcription of ApoE-4 in the brains of *affected* individuals with the ApoE-3/4 genotype has been reported to be 1.5-fold higher than in elderly control subjects with the same genotype *(47)*. In the absence of ApoE, transgenic mice expressing an AD mutant form of human APP displayed dramatically reduced β-amyloid deposition compared to the same mice in the presence of ApoE *(48)*. Thus, increased levels of ApoE protein in brain owing to promoter alterations could conceivably be directly linked to the promotion of AD neuropathology.

Recently, the α_2-macroglobulin (A2M) gene on chromosome 12p12-p13 has been reported to be associated with AD *(49)*. Evidence for association was strong in family-based association tests, with an estimated 3.5-fold increase in risk for the A2M-2 allele tested. The association is biologically plausible, since α_2-macroglobulin is known to attenuate Aβ fibril formation, to affect Aβ degradation, and to interact with the low density lipoprotein receptor, which is an ApoE receptor and has been associated with AD *(50–55)*. However, unlike ApoE-4, the A2M-2 allele had no impact on age of onset, and there was little evidence of a difference in allele frequency between affected family members and the general population. This may be because A2m-2's effect on AD risk depends on the presence of other familial factors, either genetic or environmental. In addition, there was no evidence that the A2M association accounted for the prior report of genetic linkage of AD to the centromeric portion of chromosome 12 *(56)*.

A number of other genes have been reported to be associated with AD. As noted above, the low density lipoprotein receptor-related protein (LRP) gene, which encodes the neuronal receptor for ApoE and resides on the long arm of chromosome 12, has been reported by several groups to be genetically associated with AD *(53,57,58)*. The gene encoding another ApoE receptor, the very low density lipoprotein receptor-related protein (VLDL-R), has also been reported to be associated with AD *(59,60)*. The α_1-antichymotrypsin (ACT) gene has also been proposed as a genetic risk factor for AD *(61)*. In addition, the "K variant" of the butyrylcholinesterase gene on chromosome 3 has been reported to be associated with late-onset AD and to be synergistic with ApoE-4 as a risk factor for AD *(62)*, as has the transferrin gene nearby on chromosome 3, particularly in ApoE-4-positive AD patients *(63)*. Other recently proposed candidate AD genes include the HLA-A2 allele, which has been reported to lower the age of onset of AD *(64)*, and bleomycin hydrolase *(65)*, which is interactive with ApoE-4.

With the exception of ApoE-4, none of these genes can be viewed as established AD risk factors, but all deserve further exploration. While some may prove to be false positives, this large number of genetic associations lends further support to the developing picture of a very complex etiopathogenic pathway leading to the development of late-onset AD.

In view of this complex and still evolving picture, inheritance of mutations in genes like those discussed above and others yet to be identified may be necessary to confer initial susceptibility for AD, while ApoE-4 dose modifies age of onset. In any event, these findings suggest that considerable work remains to elucidate the genetics of late-onset AD, including the development of a better understanding of the role of ApoE, reexamining the many other reported genetic associations, identifying additional genetic risk factors, and elucidating the interaction among AD genetic risk factors. Moreover, we know based on identical twins who are discordant for AD, or who have large differences in age of onset, that environmental factors are also involved in AD; a still greater challenge will be elucidating the role of these factors and their interaction with genetic risk factors.

Data on the Predictive Value of Genetic Tests

The utility of genetic tests for AD, like other tests used in medicine, depends on their informativeness *(66)*. For diagnostic testing, the statistics generally reported to quantify this informativeness are *sensitivity*, the ability of a test to pick up true cases, and *specificity*, the ability of a test to correctly identify noncases. *Predictive value positive*, or the fraction of positive tests that are true positives, is also frequently reported. For diagnostic testing in AD, these are generally measured against an autopsy diagnosis of AD by research diagnostic criteria *(67)*. For prediction of AD onset, or of conversion to AD from less clearcut impairment, the standard is generally a clinical diagnosis of AD by research diagnostic criteria *(68)*. Instead of formal assessment of sensitivity and specificity, prediction studies sometimes simply report conversion rates or odds ratios by genotype.

Still more critical than the test's informativeness per se is its *marginal* informativeness, which takes into account the information already available from standard procedures to which the test would be added or for which the test would be substituted. The informativeness of genetic tests for AD differs greatly for the early- and late-onset forms of the disease, which are discussed separately below.

Early-Onset AD

For early-onset AD, the predictive value of genetic tests has not been formally evaluated, but it can be inferred from what is known about the genetics of the disease. Given the three known fully penetrant autosomal dominant AD genes, predictive testing is at least theoretically possible for some individuals. However, even here the scientific issues remain complex for a number of reasons. A great deal more complexity arises when the personal and social issues associated with genetic testing are taken into account, as discussed in Chapter 12.

First, numerous practical issues limit the predictive value of genetic testing for early-onset AD. In particular, the extensive locus and allelic heterogeneity of early-onset AD vastly complicate the ability to make predictions based on genetic tests, even in families with clearcut autosomal dominant inheritance. The difficulty lies in establishing whether one of the three known genes is involved, and, if so, which one, and in identifying the specific mutation segregating. For families with onsets occurring in the 40s, currently available data suggest that a mutation in PS-1 is very likely to be involved. However, because of the prodigious allelic heterogeneity of this gene, genetic testing involves sequencing the gene looking for any mutations. This makes testing both more complicated (and thus more expensive), and less fully predictive. The meaning of a positive result may be unclear because not all mutations are pathological, and the meaning of a negative result may be unclear because some mutations can be missed or the family may be harboring a mutation in a different gene. Careful review of the nature and location of the specific mutation as it relates to the known pathogenic mutations in PS-1 described above may help clarify matters. In addition, the predictive value is improved considerably if one or more affected members are willing to be tested, and still more if a clear "escapee" (unaffected family members well beyond the age of onset in that family) is also willing.

For onset beyond the 40s, the picture is still less clear. PS-2 and the still rarer APP mutations account for a modest fraction of AD with an age of onset between 50 and 60 years old. PS-1 is also sometimes associated with onset in this interval. While tests for fully penetrant mutations in these genes are in theory highly predictive of the development of AD, mutation screening is impracticable outside of a research context because these two genes account for less than half of AD developing in this age range. Thus, in practice, families segregating these mutations are only likely to be identified in research studies, and no tests for these mutations are available outside of academic settings.

In any case, when considering genetic testing for the early diagnosis of early-onset AD, the marginal information offered by even fully informative genetic testing is unclear, and depends to a great extent on the status of the family and the individual. For *clearly symptomatic* individuals in early-onset families with autosomal dominant inheritance, the probability of AD is already very high: the individual is known to have a 50% chance of carrying a pathogenic mutation, and no other cause of memory impairment is likely at this age. Thus, genetic testing may not contribute greatly to diagnostic confidence. For *questionably affected* individuals in similar families, individuals with subtle symptoms such as mild memory loss, seeking an early diagnosis of AD, the probability that these symptoms represent AD remains fairly high, but undue vigilance about their risk may lead them to over-interpret their symptoms. Thus, the information offered by fully informative genetic testing might provide reassurance for some, and confirmation of their fears for others. For currently *asymptomatic* individuals from such families interested in predicting whether AD will occur, the risk of developing AD at a young age is 50% in those without testing, and could shift to either the population risk (which for early-onset AD is extremely low; their risk for late-onset AD is unaffected) or 100% with fully informative testing. Of course, as described in detail above, genetic testing for early-onset AD is often considerably less than fully informative. More critically, of course, the information offered has risks as well as potential benefits. Fully informed consent for genetic testing must take into account both its informativeness and the consequences of having the information, and given the potential consequences, this process requires formal genetic counseling.

Late-Onset AD

The only clearly confirmed gene involved in late-onset AD is ApoE-4. Other genes involved are altogether unconfirmed or too poorly characterized to be considered for predictive or diagnostic use. In addition, only ApoE-4 shows the significant differences in allele and genotype frequencies between affected and unaffected individuals that would appear necessary for diagnosis or prediction. Thus, the focus of this section is on ApoE.

The role of ApoE testing in early diagnosis, generally in the face of a few mild or non-definitive symptoms, is unclear, since this problem straddles the boundary between diagnosis and prediction. We review here three general classes of studies that may inform decisions about ApoE testing in early diagnosis: 1) studies to date on ApoE-4 and the diagnosis of AD, 2) studies of ApoE's impact on the progression to AD in subjects with mild memory impairment, and 3) studies of ApoE and the development of AD in cognitively intact elderly individuals.

ApoE Genotype

DIAGNOSIS OF AD

Most of the data concerning the role of ApoE testing in the diagnosis of AD address the specificity, sensitivity, and predictive value of ApoE-4 (usually but not always defined as the presence of one or more ApoE-4 alleles) for an autopsy diagnosis of AD, often in the context of its relationship to clinical diagnosis.

Initial reports in well characterized samples with a large proportion of AD cases suggested high sensitivity, specificity, and predictive value. Saunders and colleagues *(69)* studied 67 patients with a clinical diagnosis of AD without a significant family history of the disease. Of these, 85% proved to have AD on autopsy by research diagnostic criteria. All patients who were ApoE-4-positive had positive autopsies, indicating a specificity of 100% in this sample, while 25% of those who were ApoE-4-negative had an AD diagnosis at autopsy, indicating a sensitivity of 75%. Kakulas and associates *(70)* replicated a high specificity in a study of 66 cases of whom 82% met autopsy criteria for AD, but they observed a sensitivity of only 46%.

Later reports with larger samples also suggested that an ApoE test might contribute to the differential diagnosis of AD. Welsh-Bohmer and colleagues *(71)* studied a sample of 162 patients with a clinical diagnosis of AD in a sample collected under the auspices of the Consortium to Establish a Registry for Alzheimer's Disease (CERAD). In this study, 86% proved to have AD on autopsy. ApoE-4 carrier status had a sensitivity of 83% and a specificity of 83% for a later pathological diagnosis of AD. Given the high base rates of disorder, this corresponded to a predictive value positive of 97%, and a predictive value negative of 44%.

More recent studies have taken a broader perspective, and included patients with and without a clinical diagnosis of AD, a more realistic situation from the clinician's point of view. In perhaps the most definitive study to date, Mayeux and colleagues *(72)* studied 2188 patients evaluated for dementia in AD research centers around the United States. Of these, 1833 received a clinical diagnosis of AD, of whom 1643 (87%) also received a pathological diagnosis. Because this study obtained autopsies on patients with and without a clinical diagnosis of AD, Mayeux and colleagues *(72)* were able to estimate the sensitivity and specificity of clinical diagnosis alone, ApoE-4 carrier status alone, and a stepwise process including both. Judged against the pathological gold standard, clinical diagnosis alone had a sensitivity of 93% and a specificity of 55%. ApoE-4 carrier status alone had a sensitivity of 65% and a specificity of 68%. However, if ApoE-4 testing was used only in patients meeting clinical criteria for AD, the sensitivity was 61% and the specificity was 84%. These figures are consistent with earlier studies, but somewhat more stably estimated because of the larger sample sizes. In addition, these more complete data allow one to examine the marginal benefit—and cost—of adding ApoE testing to clinical diagnosis.

CONVERSION TO AD IN INDIVIDUALS WITH MILD SYMPTOMS

Studies of the prediction of conversion to full-blown AD in populations of individuals with questionable status, denoted variously as minimal or mild cognitive impairment or questionable dementia [e.g., a rating of 0.5 on the Clinical Dementia Rating (CDR) scale *(73)*] are most applicable to decision-making about early diagnosis of AD. Several such studies are underway, but only two are currently available in the literature.

Petersen and colleagues *(74)* studied 66 patients with mild cognitive impairment over a period of 4 to 5 years. During this period, 55% converted to frank dementia. ApoE-4 carrier status was a strong predictor of conversion, with a relative risk of approximately fourfold estimated in a survival model based on time to conversion. However, many ApoE-4 positive individuals did not convert, and many ApoE-4 negative individuals did.

Tierney and coworkers *(75)* studied 107 memory impaired patients over a two year period during which 29 developed AD. Of these, 16 (55%) had an ApoE-4 allele while the remaining 13 did not. In the nonconverting 78 patients, 26 (33%) were ApoE-4 positive, while 52 (67%) were not. A set of neuropsychological tests were strongly predictive of outcome, and the combination of these tests and ApoE genotype performed best of all. Again, many ApoE-4 positive individuals did not convert, and many ApoE-4 negative individuals did.

PREDICTION OF AD

Two classes of studies are most relevant to the understanding of ApoE for predictive use. First, there are a large number of population-based studies of the prevalence of AD by ApoE-dose, sometimes including information about age. These studies virtually all show that ApoE-4 carrier status, and especially the ApoE-4/4 genotype, is strongly associated with AD *(7,8,34)*. However, because these include prevalent cases, they have less relevance for early diagnosis.

A small number of studies have looked at the incident cases of AD in a general elderly population. Kukull and associates *(76)* replicated the diagnostic studies using incident cases in a large well-defined population from a large health maintenance organization, comparing 234 AD cases with 304 controls, and showing that ApoE-4 carrier status greatly increased risk for AD: a three-fold increase was noted for carrying one copy of ApoE-4, and a 34-fold increase for two copies. Predicting onset based on carrying one copy of ApoE-4 would have yielded a sensitivity of 52% and a specificity of 74%; using two copies yielded a sensitivity of 23% and a specificity of 99%.

A more relevant design follows a population for the onset of AD as a function of genotype. Payami and collaborators *(25)* followed 114 cognitively intact individuals over age 75 for approximately 4 years, during which time 13 experienced the development of dementia, and an additional 28 developed mild cognitive impairment insufficient to meet diagnostic criteria. They found a strong effect of ApoE-4 status and an independent effect of family history on the risk of developing either outcome.

In another prospective population-based study, Hyman and colleagues *(38)* followed 1899 individuals aged 65 and over and had them repeat a delayed recall task over a 4- to 7-year period. ApoE-2 carriers had decreased risk of developing cognitive decline (odds ratio = 0.53), and ApoE-4 carriers had increased risk of developing such decline (odds ratio = 1.37). However, as noted above, 85% of the elderly ApoE-4 homozygotes in this sample (average age 81) were unimpaired on the mental status test used. In another population-based prospective study, Evans and colleagues *(39)* followed 578 individuals aged 65 years and higher, and found that ApoE-4-positive individuals had a 2.27-fold increased risk of developing AD as compared to persons with the most common genotype, ApoE-3/3. This study also concluded that if ApoE-4 was removed as a risk factor for AD, the incidence of AD would decrease by only 13.7%.

Currently Available Genetic Tests for AD and Formal Recommendations for Their Use

Despite the complexities in genetic testing for AD, the desire for improved diagnostic certainty and the prediction of disease onset is keen. Thus, marketing of tests for AD has recently begun, and is expected to expand with time. Described here are what is currently available, and formal recommendations about how it might be used.

Genetic Tests for Early-Onset AD

For early-onset AD with apparent Mendelian inheritance, there is now a PS-1-based test aimed at individuals with a family history of AD developing before age 50. Because 70 percent of PS-1 mutations are genetically private, the test is based on sequencing the gene for mutations. This test is marketed as a symptomatic or presymptomatic test by Athena Neuroscience, with a recent price list indicating a charge of $895. The actual cost may be higher, however, because better predictive value is obtained when an affected family member and potentially an "escapee" are tested as well, as described above.

For AD developing in the 50s and early 60s with apparent autosomal dominant inheritance, genetic testing is generally not available. It is occasionally possible to screen for mutations in PS-1, PS-2, or APP if the family is thought to be segregating such a mutation based on results obtained in a research project.

Formal panels that have reviewed the possibility of genetic testing for early-onset AD *(77–79)* generally agree that such testing might proceed, whether for diagnosis or prediction, but only in the context of fully informed consent, pre- and postgenetic counseling, and careful protection of confidentiality. Genetic counselling would have to include information about the uncertainties described above, along with the personal and social risks described in Chapter 12. The informed consent process for genetic testing in the diagnosis of AD must consider the patient's competence to understand these very complex issues, and may require input from a surrogate decision-maker *(78,80)*.

ApoE Testing for Late-Onset AD

For late-onset AD, the only genetic test currently available is an ApoE-4 test, which is marketed primarily as an adjunct to clinical diagnosis. ApoE testing was listed on a recent price list at $225 by Athena Neuroscience. The test is also offered by clinical laboratories in many institutions. Given the population at risk for AD, the potential market is enormous. Athena Neuroscience also markets ApoE testing as a package with other tests based on the current understanding of AD pathophysiology. These too are meant to serve as diagnostic adjuncts, and in preliminary studies have high predictive value in selected samples, but have not been subjected to rigorous evaluation.

While ApoE-4's involvement in AD is indisputable, its potential use in the diagnosis and prediction of AD has been marked by considerable controversy. Because it is a risk factor gene and is neither necessary nor sufficient for the development of AD at any age, genetic testing poses problems beyond those encountered in tests for Mendelian diseases, including the Mendelian forms of AD.

Although marketing for diagnostic purposes has been permitted, there is no consensus on whether such use is appropriate *(43,44,77–79,81–83)*. Available data, as detailed above, suggest that positive tests may add confidence in the differential diagnosis of dementia. However, most clinicians and investigators agree that a thorough evaluation for treatable conditions is still required, and thus there is some doubt as to the marginal value of ApoE testing. In addition, most of the data collected to date concern patients who were thoroughly characterized clinically, including evaluation by expert clinicians (e.g., at CERAD sites or AD Research Centers) and complete laboratory and neuroimaging evaluation, and thus may not apply to patients without such an evaluation. Given the potential personal and social implications, then, any additional diagnostic confidence may not be worth the cost. If such testing is undertaken, it should include fully informed consent, pre- and posttest genetic counselling, and careful attention to confidentiality. In addition, clinicians must give careful consideration to the patient's competence to make such a complex decision *(78,80)*, and may need to involve a surrogate in the informed consent and counselling process.

The recommendations for predictive testing using ApoE genotype are clear. Several national panels *(43,44,77–79)* have strongly recommended against using ApoE genotyping to predict future risk for AD, and marketing for this purpose is not allowed. There is a strong consensus that the level of prediction offered by ApoE testing is too low for testing to be appropriate *(84,85)*. However, both patients and physicians sometimes mistake ApoE genotyping for a predictive test, fueled by articles in the press and understandable worry about the disease. Moreover, many individuals have already been tested for ApoE-4 as part of a cardiovascular work up, presenting dilemmas for them and their physicians. Genetic counseling may be useful in helping individuals who already have this information understand its implications. In some cases, individuals with a strong desire to undergo ApoE genotyping for predictive purposes may be referred for genetic counselling to discuss their risk for AD and the limitations of the ApoE test in clarifying that risk. Physicians' understanding of the facts about ApoE and genetic risk factors in general is limited, so educational efforts will be required to enable them to address their patients' concerns in this area *(84,85)*.

Implications for the Early Diagnosis of AD

Formal recommendations such as those described above do not generally address the issue of early diagnosis. Thus, decision-making must use available data to extend the extant recommendations into uncharted territory.

For early-onset AD, testing for early diagnosis is certainly consistent with the available guidelines. However, patients and their families must decide for themselves whether the information gained from such testing is worth the associated emotional and social risks. Those who have preliminary interest in such testing should be referred for formal genetic counseling. Even for individuals with only questionable symptomatology, the patient's ability to participate in the informed consent process and truly understand the scientific data and personal implications should be considered. Most individuals with these very mild symptoms are competent to make their own decisions, but genetic counselling may need to attend to their deficits in memory or executive function, and they may benefit from the participation of a companion.

For late-onset, ApoE testing poses particular challenges. Extrapolating the results from standard diagnosis to early diagnosis, where the symptomatology is insufficient to make a clinical diagnosis, is clearly inappropriate. Studies of conversion from questionable to clear symptoms are better, but generally too small to provide reliable estimates; in any case, they suggest that, although risk is increased, the predictive value is limited. Nonetheless, the personal and social risks remain large. ApoE testing for early diagnosis may in this regard be more similar to predictive testing, but as yet no consensus has emerged. If such testing is considered, fully informed consent, pre- and posttest counseling, and attention to confidentiality are critical. Again, the patient's capacities to understand both the predictive value and the emotional and social risks must be taken into account.

As we anticipate the development of early interventions or preventive strategies for AD, there is considerable pressure to develop the means to recognize the disease very early in its course, almost before it starts. As specific early interventions become available, and as our understanding of genetic testing develops, the cost-benefit ratio of genetic tests will need to be reevaluated. For instance, if a moderately toxic but definitively efficacious intervention is developed, even a test with only modest predictive value might be helpful in decision-making. Another possible scenario is that the value of such an intervention might vary by genotype, for instance, as part of a pharmacogenomic approach.

Meanwhile, it is important to seek additional knowledge that may improve our understanding of AD genetics, to more fully explore the predictive value of genetic tests in a variety of populations, to develop means to communicate that understanding to primary care clinicians and their patients, and to limit the social risks wherever possible. If we anticipate these needs now, we may have safe, sensitive, and specific methods to achieve early diagnosis at our disposal when we are ready to implement therapies aimed at preventing the full manifestation of this devastating disease.

Acknowledgments

We thank Dr. Marilyn Albert for suggestions regarding this chapter. This work was supported by K21 MH01118 (Dr. Blacker) and U01 MH51066 (Dr. Albert).

References

1. Council on Ethical and Judicial Affairs, American Medical Association. Use of genetic testing by employers. *JAMA* 1991;266:1827–1830.
2. Silverman P. Commerce and genetic diagnostics. *Hastings Cent. Rep. Spec. Suppl.* 1995;May–June: S15–S17.
3. Hudson K, Rothenberg K, Andrews L, Kahn M, Collins F. Genetic discrimination and health insurance: an urgent need for reform. *Science* 1995;270:391–393.
4. Geller L, Alper J, Billings P, Barash C, Beckwith J, Natowicz M. Individual, family, and societal dimensions of genetic discrimination: a case study analysis. *Sci. Eng. Ethics* 1996;2:71–87.
5. Hubbard R, Lewontin RC. Pitfalls of genetic testing. *N. Engl. J. Med.* 1995;334: 1192–1194.
6. Tanzi RE, Kovacs DM, Kim T-W, Moir RD, Guenette SY, Wasco W. The gene defects responsible for familial Alzheimer's disease. *Neurobiol. Dis.* 1996;3:159–168
7. Schellenberg GD. Genetic dissection of Alzheimer disease, a heterogeneous disorder. *Proc. Natl. Acad. Sci. U.S.A.* 1995;92:8552–8559.
8. Blacker D, Tanzi RE. The genetics of Alzheimer's disease: current status and future prospects. *Arch. Neurol.* 1998;55:294–296.
9. Schellenberg GD, Bird TD, Wijsman EM, Orr HT, Anderson L, Nemens E, White JA, Bonnycastle L, Weber JL, Alonso ME, Potter H, Heston LL, Martin J. Genetic linkage evidence for a familial Alzheimer's disease locus on chromosome 14. *Science* 1992;258:668–671.
10. Sherrington R, Rogaev EI, Liang Y, Rogaeva EA, Levesque G, Ikeda M, Chi H, Lin C, Li G, Holman K, Tsuda T, Mar L, Foncin J-F, Bruni AC, Montesi MP, Sorbi S, Rainero I, Pinessi L, Nee L, Chumakov Y, Pollen D, Wasco W, Hainus JL, Da Silva R, Pericak-Vance M, Tanzi RE, Roses AD, Fraser PE, Rommens JM, St. George-Hyslop PH. Cloning of a novel gene bearing missense mutations in early onset familial Alzheimer disease. *Nature* 1995;375:754–760.
11. Levy-Lahad E, Wasco W, Poorkaj P, Romano DM, Oshima JM, Pettingell WH, Yu C, Jondro PD, Schmidt SD, Wang K, Crowley AC, Fu Y-H, Guenette SY, Galas D, Nemens E, Wijsman EM, Bird TD, Schellenberg GD, Tanzi RE. Candidate gene for the chromosome 1 familial Alzheimer's disease locus. *Science* 1995;269:973–977.
12. Rogaev EI, Sherrington R, Rogaeva EA, Levesque G, Ikeda M, Liang Y, Chi H, Lin C, Holman K, Tsuda T, Mar L, Sorbi S, Nacmias B, Piacentini S, Amaducci L, Chumakov I, Cohen D, Lannfelt L, Fraser PE, Rommens JM. Familial Alzheimer's disease in kindreds with missense mutation in a gene on chromosome 1 related to the Alzheimer's disease type 3 gene. *Nature* 1995;376:775–778.
13. Tanzi RE, Gusella JF, Watkins PC, Bruns GA, St George-Hyslop P, Van Keuren ML, Patterson D, Pagan S, Kurnit DM, Neve RL. Amyloid β protein gene: cDNA, mRNA distribution and genetic linkage near the Alzheimer locus. *Science* 1987;235:880–884
14. Goate A, Chartier-Harlin M, Mullan M, Brown J, Crawford F, Fidani L, Giuffra L, Haynes A, Irving N, James L, Mant R, Newton P, Rooke K, Roques P, Talbot C, Pericak-Vance M, Roses A, Williamson R, Rossor M, Owen M, Hardy J. Segregation of a missense mutation in the amyloid precursor protein gene with familial Alzheimer's disease. *Nature* 1991;349:704–706.

15. Strittmatter WJ, Saunders AM, Schmechel D, Pericak-Vance M, Enghild J, Salvesen GS, Roses AD. Apolipoprotein E: high avidity binding to β-amyloid and increased frequency of type 4 allele in late-onset familial Alzheimer disease. *Proc. Natl. Acad. Sci. U.S.A.* 1993;90:1977–1981.

16. Saunders AM, Strittmatter WJ, Schmechel D, George-Hyslop PH, Perikak-Vance MA, Joo SH, Rosi B, Gusella JF, Crapper-MacLachlan DR, Alberts MJ, Hulette C, Crain B, Goldgaber D, Roses AD. Association of apolipoprotein E allele e4 with late-onset familial and sporadic Alzheimer's disease. *Neurology* 1993;43:1467–1472.

17. Games D, Adams D, Alessandrini R, Barbour R, Berthelette P, Blackwell C, Carr T, Clemens J, Donaldson T, Gillespie F, Guido T, Hagopian S, Johnson-Wood K, Khan K, Lee M, Leibowitz P, Lieberburg I, Little S, Masliah E, McConlogue L, Montoya-Zavala M, Mucke L, Paganini L, Penniman E, Power M, Schenk D, Seubert P, Snyder B, Soriano F, Tan H, Vitale J, Wadsworth S, Wolozin B, Zhao J. Alzheimer-type neuropathology in transgenic mice overexpressing V717F β-amyloid precursor protein. *Nature* 1995;373:523–527.

18. Hsiao K, Chapman P, Nilsen S, Eckman C, Harigaya Y, Younkin S, Yang F, Cole G. Correlative memory deficits, Aβ elevation and amyloid plaques in transgenic mice. *Science* 1996;274:99–102.

19. Cruts MM, van Duijn CM, Backhovens H, Van den Broeck M, Wehnert A, Serneels S, Sherrington R, Hutton M, Hardy J, St George-Hyslop PH, Hofman A, Van Broeckhoven C. Estimation of the genetic contribution of presenilin 1 and 2 mutations in a population-based study of presenilin Alzheimer disease. *Hum. Mol. Genet.* 1998;7:43–51.

20. Hardy J. Amyloid, the presenilins and Alzheimer's disease. *Trends Neurosci.* 1997;20:154–159.

21. Tysoe C, Whittaker J, Xuereb J, Cairns NJ, Cruts M, Van Broeckhoven C, Wilcock G, Rubinsztein DC. A presenilin-1 truncated mutation in two cases with autopsy-confirmed early-onset Alzheimer's disease. *Am. J. Hum. Genet.* 1998;1:70–76.

22. Rossor MN, Fox NC, Beck J, Campbell TC, Collinge J. Incomplete penetrance of familial Alzheimer's disease in a pedigree with a novel presenilin-1 gene mutation. *Lancet* 1996;347:1560.

23. Van Broeckhoven C, Backhovens H, Cruts M, Martin J, Crook R, Houlden H, Hardy J. APOE genotype does not modulate age of onset in families with chromosome 14 encoded Alzheimer's disease. *Neurosci. Lett.* 1994;169:179–180.

24. Sorbi S, Nacmias B, Forleo P, Piancentini S, Latorraca S, Amaducci L. Epistatic effect of APP717 mutation and apolipoprotein E genotype in familial Alzheimer's disease. *Ann. Neurol.* 1993;38:124–127.

25. Payami H, Grimslid H, Oken B, Camicioli R, Sexton G, Dame A, Howieson D, Kaye J. A prospective study of cognitive health in the elderly (Oregon Brain Aging Study): effects of family history and apolipoprotein E genotype. *Am. J. Hum. Genet.* 1997;60:948–956.

26. Farrer LA, O'Sullivan D, Cupples LA, Growdon JH, Myers RH. Assessment of genetic risk for Alzheimer's disease among first-degree relatives. *Ann. Neurol.* 1989;25:485–493.

27. Farrer LA, Myers RH, Cupples LA, St. George-Hyslop PH, Bird TD, Rossor MN, Mullan MJ, Polinsky R, Nee L, Heston L, et al. Transmission and age-at-onset pat-

terns in familial Alzheimer's disease: evidence for heterogeneity. *Neurology* 1990; 40:395–403.

28. Breitner JC, Silverman JM, Mohs RC, Davis KL. Familial aggregation in Alzheimer's disease: comparison of risk among relatives of early- and late-onset cases, and among male and female relatives in successive generations. *Neurology* 1988;38:207–212.

29. Bergem AL, Engedal K, Kringlen EL. The role of heredity in late-onset Alzheimer disease and vascular dementia: a twin study. *Arch. Gen. Psychiatry* 1997;54:264–270.

30. Lautenschlager NT, Cupples LA, Rao VS, Auerbach SA, Becker R, Burke J, Chui H, Duara R, Foley EJ, Glatt SL, Green RC, Jones R, Karlinsky H, Kukull WA, Kurz A, Larson EB, Martelli K, Sadovnick AD, Volicer L, Waring SC, Growdon JH, Farrer L. Risk of dementia among relatives of Alzheimer's disease patients in the MIRAGE study: what is in store for the oldest old? *Neurology* 1996;46:641–650.

31. Katzman R, Kawas C. The epidemiology of dementia and Alzheimer's disease. In Katzman R, Bick K, editors. *Alzheimer Disease.* New York: Raven Press, 1997:105–121.

32. Evans DA, Funkenstein HH, Albert MS, Scherr PA, Cook NR, Chown MJ, Hebert LE, Hennekens CH, Taylor JO. Prevalence of Alzheimer's disease in a community population of older persons: higher than previously reported. *JAMA* 1989;262: 2551–2556.

33. Wilson PWF, Myers RH, Larson MG, Ordovas JM, Wolf PA, Schaefer EJ. Apolipoprotein E alleles, dyslipidemia, and coronary heart disease. *JAMA* 1994;272:1666–1671.

34. Myers RH, Schaefer EJ, Wilson PWF, D'Agostino R, Ordovas JM, Espino A, Au R, White RF, Knoefel JE, Cobb JL, McNulty KA, Beiser A, Wolf PA. Apolipoprotein E e4 association with dementia in a population-based study: the Framingham Study. *Neurology* 1996;46:673–677

35. Farrer LA, Cupples LA, Haines JL, Hyman B, Kukull WA, Mayeux R, Myers RH, Pericak-Vance MA, Risch N, van Duijn CM. Effects of age, sex, and ethnicity on the association between Apolipoprotein E genotype and Alzheimer disease: a meta-analysis. APOE and Alzheimer Disease Meta Analysis Consortium. *JAMA* 1997;278:1349–1356.

36. Blacker D, Haines JL, Rodes L, Terwedow H, Go RCP, Harrell LE, Perry RT, Bassett SS, Chase G, Meyers D, Albert MS, Tanzi R. APOE-4 and age-at-onset of Alzheimer's disease: the NIMH Genetics Initiative. *Neurology* 1997;48:139–147

37. Corder EH, Saunders AM, Risch NJ, Strittmatter WJ, Schmechel DE, Gaskell PC Jr., Rimmler JB, Locke PA, Conneally PM, Schmader KE, et al. Protective effect of apolipoprotein E type 2 allele for late onset Alzheimer disease. *Nature Genet.* 1994;7:180–184.

38. Hyman BT, Gomez-Isla T, Brigg M, Briggs M, Chung H, Nichols S, Kohout F, Wallace R. Apolipoprotein E and cognitive change in an elderly population. *Ann. Neurol.* 1996;40:55–60.

39. Evans DA, Beckett LA, Field TS, Feng L, Albert MS, Bennett DA, Tycko B, Mayeux R. Apolipoprotein E e4 and incidence of Alzheimer disease in a community population of older persons. *JAMA* 1997;822–827.

40. Meyer MR, Tschanz JT, Norton MC, Welsh-Bohmer KA, Steffens DC, Wyse BW, Breitner JCS. APOE genotype predicts when—not whether—one is predisposed to develop Alzheimer disease. *Nature Genet.* 1998;19:321–322.

41. Corder EH, Saunders AM, Strittmatter WJ, Schmechel DE, Gaskell PC, Small GW, Roses AD, Haines JL, Pericak-Vance MA. Gene dose of apolipoprotein E type 4 allele and the risk of Alzheimer's disease in late onset families. *Science* 1993;261:921–923.

42. Locke P, Conneally PM, Tanzi RE, Gusella JF, Haines JL. APOE and Alzheimer disease: examination of allelic association and effect on age at onset in both early- and late-onset cases. *Genet. Epidemiol.* 1995;12:83–92.

43. American College of Medical Genetics/American Society of Human Genetics (ACMG/ASHG) Working Group on ApoE and Alzheimer's Disease. Statement on use of apolipoprotein E testing for Alzheimer's disease. *JAMA* 1995;274:1627–1629

44. National Institute on Aging/Alzheimer's Disease Association Working Group (NIA/ADA). Apolipoprotein E genotyping in Alzheimer's disease position statement. *Lancet* 1996;347:1091–1095

45. Bullido MJ, Artiga MJ, Recuero M, Sastre I, Garcia MA, Aldudo J, Lendon C, Han SW, Morris JC, Frank A, Vazquez J, Goate A, Valdivieso F. A polymorphism in the regulatory region of APOE associated with risk for Alzheimer's dementia. *Nature Genet.* 1998;18:69–71.

46. Lambert J-C, Pasquier F, Cottel D, Frigard B, Amouyel P, Chartier-Harlin MC. A new polymorphism in the APOE promoter associated with risk of developing Alzheimer's disease. *Hum. Mol. Genet.* 1998;7:533–540.

47. Lambert J-C, Perez-Tur J, Dupire MJ, Galasko D, Mann D, Amouel P, Hardy J, Delacourte A, Chartier-Harlin MC. Distortion of allelic expression of apolipoprotein E in Alzheimer's disease. *Hum. Mol. Genet.* 1997; 6:2151–2154.

48. Bales KR, Verina T, Dodel RC, Du Y, Altstiel L, Bender M, Hyslop P, Johnstone EM, Little SP, Cummins DJ, Piccardo P, Ghetti B, Paul SM. Lack of apolipoprotein E dramatically reduces amyloid β-peptide deposition. *Nature Genet.* 1997;17: 263–264

49. Blacker D, Wilcox MA, Laird NM, Rodes L, Horvath S, Go RCP, Perry R, Bassett SS, McInnis M, Albert MS, Hyman BT, Tanzi RE. Alpha-2 macroglobulin is genetically associated with Alzheimer's disease. *Nature Genet.* 1998;19:357–360.

50. Hughes SR, Khorkova O, Goyal S, Knaeblein J, Heroux J, Riedel NG, Sahasrabudhe S. Alpha-2-macroglobulin associates with β-amyloid peptide and prevents fibril formation. *Proc. Natl. Acad. Sci. U.S.A.* 1998;95:3275–3280.

51. Du Y, Bales KR, Dodel RC, Liu X, Glinn MA, Horn JW, Little SP, Paul SM. Alpha-2-macroglobulin attenuates β-amyloid peptide 1-40 fibril formation and associated neurotoxicity of cultured fetal rat cortical neurons. *J. Neurochem.* 1998;70:1182–1188.

52. Qiu WQ, Borth W, Ye Z, Haass C, Teplow DB, Selkoe DJ. Degradation of amyloid β protein by a serine proteinase alpha-2-macroglobulin complex. *J. Biol. Chem.* 1996;271:8443–8451.

53. Kang DE, Saitoh T, Chen X, Xia Y, Masliah E, Hansen LA, Thomas RG, Thal LJ, Katzman R. Genetic association of the low density lipoprotein receptor-related protein gene (LRP), an apolipoprotein E receptor, with late-onset Alzheimer's disease. *Neurology* 1997;49:56–61.

54. Kounnas MZ, Moir RD, Rebeck GW, Bush AI, Argaves WS, Hyman BT, Tanzi RE,

Strickland DK. LDL receptor-related protein, a multifunctional apolipoprotein E receptor, binds secreted β-amyloid precursor protein and mediates its degradation. *Cell* 1995;82:331–340.

55. Narita M, Holtzman DM, Schwartz AL, Bu G. Alpha-2-macroglobulin complexes with and mediates the endocytosis of β-amyloid peptide via cell surface low-density lipoprotein receptor-related protein. *J. Neurochem.* 1997;69:1904–1911.

56. Pericak-Vance MA, Bass MP, Yamaoka LH, Gaskell PC, Scott WK, Terwedow HA, Menold MM, Conneally PM, Small GW, Vance JM, Saunders AM, Roses AD, Haines JL. Complete genomic screen in late-onset familial Alzheimer disease: evidence for a new locus on chromosome 12. *JAMA* 1997;278:1237–1241.

57. Wavrant-DeVrieze F, Perez-Turs, Lambert J-C, Frigard B, Pasquier F, Delacorte A, Amouyel P, Hardy J, Chartier-Harlin, MC. Association between the low density lipoprotein receptor-related protein (LRP) and Alzheimer's disease. *Neurosci. Lett.* 1997;227:68–70.

58. Hollenbach E, Ackermann S, Hyman BT, Rebeck GW. Confirmation of an association between a polymorphism in exon 3 of LRP and Alzheimer's disease. *Neurology* 1998;50:1905–1907.

59. Okuizumi K, Onodera O, Namba Y, Ikeda K, Yamamoto T, Seki K, Ueki A, Nanko S, Tanaka H, Takahashi H, et al. Genetic association of the very low density lipoprotein (VLDL) receptor gene with sporadic Alzheimer's disease. *Nature Genet.* 1995;11:207–209.

60. Helbecque N, Richard F, Cottel, Neuman E, Guez D, Arnovel P. The very low density lipoprotein (VLDL) receptor is a genetic susceptibility factor for Alzheimer's disease in a European Caucasian population. *Alzheimer Dis. Assoc. Disord.* 1998;13:368–371.

61. Kamboh MI, Sanghera DK, Ferrell RE, DeKosky ST. APOE4-associated Alzheimer's disease risk is modified by alpha 1-antichymotrypsin polymorphism. *Nature Genet* 1995;10:486–488.

62. Lehmann DJ, Johnston C, Smith AD. Synergy between the genes for Butyrylcholinesterase K variant and apolipoprotein E4 in late-onset Alzheimer's disease. *Hum. Mol. Genet.* 1997;6:1933–1936.

63. Namekata K, Imagawa M, Terashi A, Onta S, Oyama F, Ihara Y. Association of transferrin C2 allele with late-onset Alzheimer's disease. *Hum. Genet.* 1997;101:126–129.

64. Payami H, Schellenberg GD, Zareparsi S, Kaye J, Sexton GJ, Head MA, Matsuyama SS, Jarvik LS, Miller B, McManus DQ, Bird TD, Katzman R, Heston L, Norman D, Small GW. Evidence for association of HLA-A2 allele with onset age of Alzheimer's disease. *Neurology* 1997;49:512–518

65. Montoya SE, Aston CE, DeKosky ST, Kamboh MI, Lazzo JS, Ferrell RE. Bleomycin hydrolase is associated with risk of sporadic Alzheimer's disease. *Nature Genet.* 1998;18:211–212.

66. Sackett DL, Haynes RB, Guyatt GH, Tugwell P. Clinical epidemiology. *A Basic Science for Clinicians,* 2nd ed. Boston: Little, Brown, 1991.

67. Khachaturian ZS. Diagnosis of Alzheimer's disease. *Arch. Neurol.* 1985;42:1097–1105.

68. McKhann G, Drachman D, Folstein M, Katzman R, Price D, Stadlan EM. Clinical diagnosis of Alzheimer's disease: report of the NINCDS-ADRDA work group under

the auspices of the Department of Health and Human Services Task Force on Alzheimer's disease. *Neurology* 1984;34:939–944.

69. Saunders AM, Hulete C, Welsh-Bohmer KA, Achmechel DE, Crain B, Buke JR, Alberts MJ, Strittmatter WJ, Breitner JCS, Rosenberg C, Scott SV, Gaskell PC, Pericak-Vance MA, Roses AD. Specificity, sensitivity, and predictive value of apolipoprotein-E genotyping for sporadic Alzheimer's disease. *Lancet* 1996;348:90–93.

70. Kakulas BA, Wilton SD, Fabian VA, Jones TM. Apolipoprotein-E genotyping in diagnosis of Alzheimer's disease. *Lancet* 1996;348:483.

71. Welsh-Bohmer KA, Gearing M, Saunders AM, Roses AD, Mirra S. Apolipoprotein E genotypes in a neuropathological series from the Consortium to Establish a Registry for Alzheimer's disease. *Ann. Neurol.* 1997;42:319–325.

72. Mayeux R, Saunders AM, Shea S, Mirra S, Evans D, Roses AD, Hyman BT, Crain B, Tang M-X, Phelps CH. Utility of the apolipoprotein E genotype in the diagnosis of Alzheimer's disease. *N. Engl. J. Med.* 1998;338:506–511.

73. Hughes CP, Berg L, Danziger WL, Coben LA, Martin RL. A clinical scale for the staging of dementia. *Br J Psychiatry* 1982;140:566–572

74. Petersen RC, Smith GE, Ivnik RJ, Tangalos EG, Schaid DJ, Thibodeau SN, Kokman E, Waring SC, Kurland LT. Apolipoprotein E status as a predictor of the development of Alzheimer's disease in memory-impaired individuals. *JAMA* 1995;273:1274–1278.

75. Tierney MC, Szalai JP, Snow WG, Fisher RH, Tsuda T, Chi H, McLachlan DR, St. George-Hyslop, PH. A prospective study of the clinical utility of ApoE genotype in the prediction of outcome in patients with memory impairment. *Neurology* 1996;46:149–154.

76. Kukull WA, Schellenberg GD, Bowen JD, McCormick WC, Yu C-E, Teri L, Thompson JD, O'Meara ES, Larson EB. Apolipoprotein E in Alzheimer's disease risk and case detection: a case-control study. *J. Clin. Epidemiol.* 1996;49:1143–1148.

77. Post SG, Whitehouse PJ, Binstock RH, Bird TD, Eckert SK, Farrer LA, Fleck LM, Gaines AD, Juengst ET, Karlinsky H, Miles S, Murray TH, Quaid KA, Relkin NR, Roses AD, St. George-Hyslop PH, Sachs GA, Steinbock B, Truschke EF, Zinn AB, Post S, Whitehouse P, Binstock R. The clinical introduction of genetic testing for Alzheimer disease: an ethical perspective. *JAMA* 1997;227:832–836.

78. McConnell LM, Koenig LM, Greely HT, Raffin TA, and the Alzheimer Disease Working Group of the Stanford Program in Genomics, Ethics, and Society. Genetic testing and Alzheimer disease: has the time come? *Nature Med.* 1998;4:757–759.

79. Ronald and Nancy Reagan Research Institute of the Alzheimer's Association and National Institute of Aging Working Group (Reagan Institute). Consensus Report of the Working Group on: "Molecular and Biochemical Markers of Alzheimer's Disease." *Neurobiol. Aging* 1998;19:109–116.

80. Karlinsky H, Geiger O, MacDougall A, Bloch M, Sadovnick D, Burgess M. A pilot experience in genetic counseling for Alzheimer's disease. *Ann. N.Y. Acad. Sci.* 1996;802:120–127

81. Bird TD. Apolipoprotein E genotyping in the diagnosis of Alzheimer's disease: a cautionary view. *Ann. Neurol.* 1995;38:2–3.

82. Mayeux R. Evaluation and use of diagnostic tests in Alzheimer's disease. *Neurobiol. Aging* 1998;19:139–143.

83. Roses AD. Apolipoprotein E genotyping in the differential diagnosis, not prediction, of Alzheimer's disease. *Ann. Neurol.* 1995;38:6–14.

84. Seshadri S, Drachman DA, Lippa CF. Apolipoprotein E epsilon 4 allele and the lifetime risk of Alzheimer's disease: what physicians know and what they should know. *Arch. Neurol.* 1995;52:1074–1079.

85. Task Force on Genetic Testing, NIH-DOE Working Group on Ethical, Legal, and Social Implications of Human Genome Research. Promoting Safe and Effect Genetic Testing in the United States:Principles and Recommendations. http://www.med. jhu.edu/tfgelsi/promoting, 1997.

6

Structural Imaging Approaches
to Alzheimer's Disease

Clifford R. Jack, Jr. and Ronald C. Petersen

The clinical diagnosis of probable Alzheimer's disease (AD) is based on a group of signs, symptoms, and test results *(1–7)*. No single diagnostic test has been identified, and a definitive diagnosis therefore requires biopsy or autopsy confirmation. The formal role of imaging in establishing a clinical diagnosis of probable AD is an exclusionary one—that is, to exclude possible causes of dementia other than AD which may be identified through imaging. However, investigators have sought to identify positive diagnostic imaging criteria, which may aid in the clinical diagnosis of AD. A number of different imaging techniques or modalities have been employed to this end. Functional imaging modalities may reveal a characteristic regional bilateral temporal/parietal lobe or posterior cingulate deficit in patients with AD. Functional deficits identified with positron emission tomography (PET) scanning include regional deficits in glucose and oxygen metabolism as well as blood flow *(8–10)*. Single photon emission computed tomography (SPECT) may reveal similar regional deficits in blood flow *(11–13)*. More recently, deficits in regional cerebral blood volume have been identified with magnetic resonance (MR) perfusion techniques *(14)*. Biochemical alterations have been identified with MR spectroscopy. The two metabolites most commonly targeted for in vivo MR spectroscopy studies are hydrogen and phosphorus. To date, the results with ^{31}P MR spectroscopy in the diagnosis of AD have not been overly promising *(15–17)*. Several studies, however, employing ^{1}HMR spectroscopy have identified decreased *N*-acetyl aspartic acid (NAA) as well as increased myoinositol in the brains of patients with AD *(18,19)* compared to appropriate controls. The final category of imaging techniques that has been employed most extensively in the study of AD is structural anatomic imaging.

From: *Early Diagnosis of Alzheimer's Disease*
Edited by L. F. M. Scinto & K. R. Daffner © Humana Press, Inc., Totowa, NJ

Measures of Cerebral Atrophy

Both computed tomography (CT) and magnetic resonance imaging (MRI) have been employed extensively as cross-sectional imaging modalities in the study of AD. Both of these modalities contain two primary types of information—voxel intensity information and information about gross neuroanatomic structure. Pathological changes in the voxel intensity of brain tissue are most commonly associated with the status of tissue hydration. Tissue damage (cerebral edema, demyelination, astrogliosis) will produce an increase in unbound or free tissue water, which in turn manifests itself as increased signal on T2-weighted MR images, decreased signal on T1-weighted MR images, or decreased intensity on CT images. The association between pathological alterations in tissue intensity and forms of brain injury such as infarction, trauma, and demyelination are well established. Although a number of investigators have attempted to link such signal intensity changes to the primary neurodegenerative pathology found in AD, a consensus has not been reached as to the validity of such a link *(20–23)*. On the other hand, the second basic type of information contained in both MR and CT images—depiction of gross neuroanatomy—has been convincingly linked with the primary neurodegenerative pathology of AD in a consistent and universally recognized fashion. Although deposition of amyloid plaques and neurofibrillary tangles in excess of that expected for age are the pathological hallmarks of AD, cerebral atrophy is a widely recognized concomitant of the primary pathology of AD. The ability of cross-sectional imaging techniques (MR and CT) to accurately depict neuroanatomic structure, and thus accurately identify the cerebral atrophy associated with the disease process in AD, has been confirmed in numerous studies *(20)*.

Because the cerebral atrophy that occurs as part of the primary pathology of AD is a negative phenomenon, it must be characterized as a loss of tissue relative to "normal" elderly individuals. A number of different techniques have been employed to accomplish this. Approaches to the characterization of global or hemispheric cerebral atrophy can be divided into those which employ categorization of MR or CT scans by means of visual ranking, and those which employ a continuous quantitative measure of a particular anatomic feature such as sulcal or ventricular size. In its most rigorous implementation the former approach is accomplished by collecting a battery of example cases, which are representative of the various levels of atrophy (sulcal/ventricular enlargement) into which the study scans will be grouped *(24,25)*. For example, each study scan may be assigned to one of four levels of atrophy: none, mild, moderate, or severe. A finer gradation scale with a greater number of categories to which individual study scans are assigned may also be employed. For this type of visual ranking approach, a panel of expert raters is employed to rank the individual study scans. Quality control is assessed by monitoring measures of inter- and intrarater consistency in ranking scans.

The second general approach to evaluating the cerebral atrophy which occurs in AD is quantitative. The rationale for quantitation is that disease related cerebral atrophy exists along a continuum from mild to moderate to severe (Fig. 1). Because cerebral atrophy exists in nature as a continuous variable, it is logical that a continuous radiological descriptor (quantitative measurement) is better suited to characterize this phenomenon than a categorical radiological descriptor (visual ranking into mild, moderate, or severe categories). In addition, cerebral atrophy has also been identified as a feature of "normal" aging. Although this is not universally accepted, a number of studies have clearly established that age-related cerebral atrophy often occurs in nondemented elderly individuals *(26–29)*. The topic of "normal" aging often involves semantic issues *(30)*. One can consider normal as "typical" aging whereby patients may have comorbidities that are felt to be commonly encountered in aging but not felt to affect cognition. This is in contrast to what some refer to as "supernormal" or optimal aging with virtually no comorbidities. The latter individuals are, however, uncommon. A problem that has plagued attempts at using imaging measures of cerebral atrophy as a marker of AD is distinguishing "pathological" atrophy of AD from the atrophy associated with "normal" aging. The pathological cerebral atrophy associated with the disease process of AD itself is modeled as an additional atrophic burden which is superimposed on the cerebral atrophy that occurs as a feature of "normal" aging. Quantitative approaches lend themselves to separating the effects of normal from pathologic aging because quantitative age-specific levels of cerebral atrophy in "typical aging" can be established for comparison with patients. Several quantitative measures have been employed as markers of the hemispheric atrophy which occur in AD. These can be categorized as linear, area, or volume measurements. These quantitative measures of hemispheric cerebral atrophy were initially employed with CT scanning and later adapted to MR. Because the cerebral hemispheres are morphologically complicated three-dimensional structures, one might assume a priori that greater sensitivity and specificity would be found with volumetric as opposed to more simple linear measurements. In general such a hierarchy has been found with volume measurements outperforming area measurements, which in turn outperform linear measurements *(20)*. Examples of linear measurements made from CT are the width of the frontal horns, width of the third ventricle, and widths of various cortical sulci.

| Cognition | normal ——mild impairment——demented |
| Morphology | no atrophy——mild atrophy——severe atrophy |

Fig. 1. Cognitive and morphologic continuum. Like cognition in the elderly, cerebral morphology exists in nature as a continuum, without discrete categorization into mild, moderate, or severe atrophy. Furthermore, both normal aging and AD are associated with cerebral atrophy in a continuous, not a discrete, manner.

Examples of area measurements made from single CT slices are measures of the area of the lateral ventricles, frontal horn, third ventricle, and interhemispheric fissures. Volume measurements of ventricular size and subarachnoid space size have been made as well *(20)*. More recently MR has been employed as the imaging modality of choice from which measures of brain volume, ventricular volume, total CSF volume, and hemispheric gray and white matter volume are made *(31,32)*.

Medial Temporal Lobe Atrophy

Although almost every study in which imaging measures of global or hemispheric atrophy have been employed has identified a statistically significant difference between the mean value found in AD patients and that found in control subjects, invariably substantial overlap exists between individual members of these two populations which in turn limits the clinical utility of this approach for diagnosis in individual patients *(20)*. It is highly likely that this overlap between controls and AD patients is due in part to the manner in which normal aging is defined when selecting subjects to serve as controls. Most studies have employed as controls individuals who would fall into the category of typical aging. The result is that most elderly control populations in imaging studies include subjects with conditions that predispose toward cerebral atrophy such as hypertension, and some may be in the preclinical stages of dementia. Much better separation between AD patient and controls would be expected if the control group was restricted to "supernormal" or "healthy-aging" individuals.

In an attempt to increase the sensitivity of image derived neuroanatomic measures of cerebral atrophy as a diagnostic marker of AD, a number of investigators in recent years have focused on detecting regional brain atrophy in the medial temporal lobe regions. The rationale for this focus on the medial temporal lobe in AD is the following:

1. A decline in declarative memory is a hallmark of AD.
2. The neuroanatomic substrate for declarative memory is the limbic medial tempo-

ral lobe, particularly the hippocampus and anatomically related areas such as the entorhinal cortex *(33)*.

3. Cell loss and atrophy are consistent features of AD and the limbic anteromedial temporal lobe, particularly the entorhinal cortex and the hippocampus, is involved earliest and most severely by the neurofibrillary pathology of AD *(34–38)*(Fig 2).

Several investigators have employed qualitative ranking *(39–41)* or linear measurements *(43,44)* of anteromedial temporal lobe atrophy on CT scans to effectively separate AD patients from elderly controls. More recently a great deal of interest has arisen in employing MR-based measures of anteromedial temporal lobe atrophy in the diagnosis of AD. The rationale for employing MR (as opposed to CT) to evaluate neuroanatomic changes in this region of the brain is: superior soft tissue contrast with MR; MR does not suffer from beam hardening artifacts in this region of the brain as does CT; and the multiplanar capability of MR which permits the optimal anatomic display of this region of the brain in the coronal plane.

As with quantitative measures of hemispheric atrophy, investigators have employed linear, area, and volume measures of anteromedial temporal lobe atrophy. An example of quantitative MR-based linear measurements of medial temporal lobe atrophy is the interuncal distance *(45,46)*. Seab and colleagues *(47)* described area measures of several neuroanatomic structures from a single MR slice, the most effective measurement at separating controls from AD patients was the area of the hippocampus. Finally, in the past several years a number of investigators have reported MR-based measurements of the volume of various anteromedial temporal lobe structures to assess the atrophy associated with AD *(48–57)*. A variety of structures have been measured. The most common has been the hippocampus, but other neuroanatomic structures which have been employed include the parahippocampal gyrus, temporal horn, amygdala, parahippocampal CSF spaces, and the anterior temporal lobe *(48–57)* (Table 1). A number of these initial studies describing MR-based volume measurements of the medial temporal lobe have reported extremely high sensitivity in separating patients with AD from elderly control individuals. Based on these initial studies, MR-based volume measurements of medial temporal lobe structures have been proposed as a clinically useful test for the diagnosis of AD. However, the published literature does not unequivocally validate the utility of MR-based volume measurements of the medial temporal lobe in AD because:

1. The method of image acquisition varied among some of the reported studies, and the earliest studies were performed during a period of rapid technical evolution of MRI with methods that are no longer state-of-the-art.

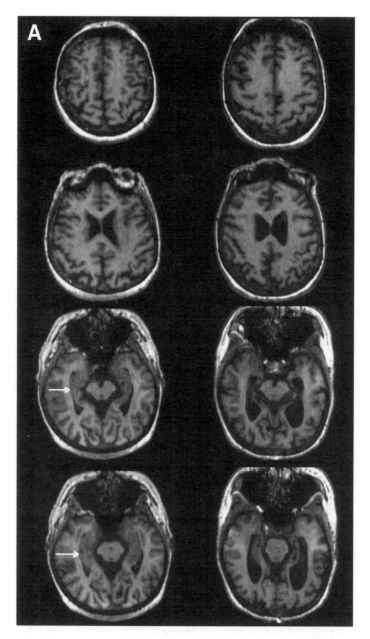

Fig. 2. Selective anteromedial temporal lobe atrophy in AD. **(A)** Axial T1-weighted MR images of two subjects—a 70-year-old woman with probable AD in the column on the right and a 70-year-old cognitively normal woman in the column on the left. From top to bottom the axial images progress from superior to inferior. Note the minimal difference in the appearance of the brain (i.e., presence of cerebral atrophy) between the two subjects in the two more cephalic axial sections through the cerebral hemispheres, and the markedly more striking atrophy particularly of the hippocampus in the patient with AD compared to the control *(arrows)* in the two basal sections through the temporal lobes.

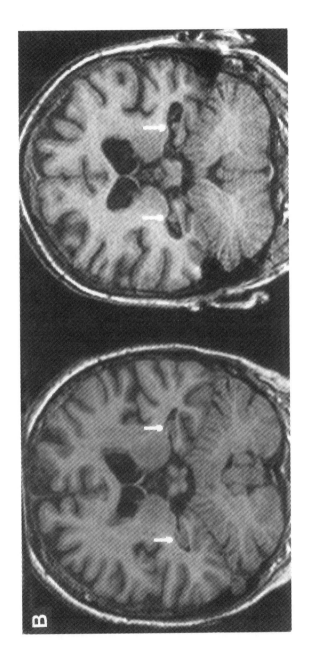

Fig. 2. (*cont.*) (**B**) Coronal T1-weighted MR images of the same two patients in Figure 2A. Note the pronounced atrophy of the hippocampus (*arrows*) in the patient with AD on the right compared to the age- and gender-matched control.

Table 1
Volume Measurements of Medial Temporal Lobe Atrophy in AD

Structure	N	Sens/Spec (Acc)*	Ref.
Hipp/PHG	15	—	49
Hippocampus	44	(85%)	50
Hipp, T Horn	15	100%/100%	56
Amygdala/PHG	31	100%/100%	54
Hipp/CSF	—	(80%)	55
Amygdala	17	—	57
Hipp, amygdala	26	100%/100%	51
Hipp, amygdala	48	(92%)†	52
RT L, T Horn	60	100%/100%	53
Hipp, amygdala, whole brain, fontal lobes, temporal lobes	30	(85%)†	48
Hipp, amygdala, PHG	220	82%/80%‡	58

The neuroanatomic structures measured in each study are indicated: Hipp, hippocampus; PHG, parahippocampal gyrus; T horn, temporal horn; ATL, anterior temporal lobe; CSF, cerebrospinal fluid; N, the total number of subjects in each study.

*The sensitivity and specificity or accuracy (in parentheses) when cited, in discriminating AD patients from controls on the basis of the volume measurements in first column. (Pearlson and colleagues employed SPECT scans in addition to MRI-based volume measurements.)

†Accuracy figure refers to measurements of the right amygdala–hippocampal complex.

‡Sensitivity and specificity figures refer to hippocampal volume measurements.

2. Anatomic boundary criteria for the various medial temporal lobe structures varied significantly among the different studies.
3. Different structures or combinations of medial temporal lobe structures were evaluated in the studies.
4. Most importantly, the studies published before 1997 contain relatively small numbers of subjects. In many cases the control and patient subjects were highly selected, which makes extrapolation of the results to the diagnosis of AD in a general setting problematic.

Medial Temporal Lobe MRI-Based Volume Measurements at Mayo

In order to more thoroughly assess the possible utility of MR-based volume measurements of anteromedial temporal lobe neuroanatomic structures in the diagnosis of AD we undertook a study which employed a large number of control and AD patients, state-of-the-art image acquisition and image-processing techniques, and well-accepted neuroanatomic boundary criteria for the various medial temporal lobe structures that were measured *(58)*. MR-based volume measurements of the hippocampus, parahippocampal gyrus

(PHG), and amygdala were performed in 126 cognitively normal elderly controls and 94 patients with probable AD. These three medial temporal lobe neuroanatomic structures were selected because these areas are involved early in the course of the disease, and are depicted with a high level of anatomic clarity with an appropriately performed MRI study. The clinical characteristics of the 220 study subjects are found in Table 2. The control and AD groups were well matched with respect to gender distribution and education, and fairly well matched with respect to age. AD patients as expected scored substantially lower on cognitive measures. Disease severity in AD patients was assessed by the Clinical Dementia Rating (CDR) scale: very mild, CDR 0.5; mild, CDR 1; moderate, CDR 2 *(59)*. An important distinction is made between establishing a diagnosis of AD and ranking its severity. The former was done according to NINCDS-ADRDA criteria, which emphasize a decline in cognitive performance over time as an important benchmark in establishing a diagnosis of AD. The CDR score was used as a staging instrument to rank disease severity at a specific point in time. It was therefore possible for patients to meet NINCDS-ADRA criteria for AD and also be ranked as only very mildly demented (CDR 0.5).

As mentioned previously, cerebral atrophy is a negative phenomenon that must be assessed by comparing the volumes of the medial temporal lobe structures of interest in affected individuals with a normal reference population. The first aim of this study was therefore to characterize volumetric changes in the hippocampus, amygdala, and PHG in normal aging in both men and women. These volumes were then characterized in patients with AD, and we then assessed the ability of these measures to discriminate between AD and normal aging.

Controls

In the group of 126 cognitively normal controls, the volume of each structure declined with increasing age and did so in parallel for men and women. The mean nonnormalized volumetric decline in cubic millimeters per year of age was 45.63 for hippocampus; 46.65 for the PHG; 20.75 for amygdala. The data in Table 3 indicate that in normal elderly individuals both age and gender affect the volume of the hippocampus, amygdala, and PHG. A third important variable that independently affects the volume of these medial temporal lobe structures is head size. Larger people have larger cranial volumes, and in turn have larger brain volumes including the three medial temporal lobe structures of interest in this study. A method for controlling or normalizing the individual medial temporal lobe structure volumes for interindividual variation in head size was therefore necessary, and this was ac-

Table 2
Characterization of Subjects

	Controls, CDR= 0 (N = 126) Mean ± SD	AD		
Variable		CDR = 0.5 (N = 36) Mean ± SD	CDR = 1 (N = 43) Mean ± SD	CDR = 2 (N = 15) Mean ± SD
Age	79.15 ± 6.73	72.92 ± 8.43	73.47 ± 9.68	75.87 ± 8.71
Education	13.43 ± 2.96	13.33 ± 2.91	12.98 ± 2.69	12.38 ± 2.47
MMSE*	28.60 ± 1.26	21.60 ± 4.36	18.16 ± 4.47	13.93 ± 5.99
DRS*†	135.14 ± 6.95	112.79 ± 13.72	101.33 ± 20.75	89.62 ± 25.58

CDR, Clinical Dementia Rating; MMSE, Mini-Mental State Examination; DRS, Dementia Rating Scale.
*One case in each CDR group with missing values.
†One control, three cases in CDR = 0.5, four cases in CDR = 1, two cases in CDR = 2 with missing values.

complished by dividing the medial temporal lobe structure volume by the measured total intracranial volume of each individual subject *(60,61)*. Mean total intracranial volume in controls was 1393 cm^3(+/-SD 133 mm^3).

Patients With AD

A decline in normalized medial temporal lobe volumes with age was observed among patients with AD, which paralleled the decline seen among control subjects (Table 3 and Fig. 3). Individual volume measurements in control subjects and in patients were affected by the subjects' age and gender in addition total intracranial volume (Table 3). In order to isolate the relationship between disease status (control vs AD) and structure volume, normalized volumetric percentiles in controls specific for age and gender were calculated for each of the three medial temporal lobe structures of interest *(62)*. Age and gender-specific normalized volumetric percentiles among AD patients were then determined and converted to W scores using the inverse of the standard normal distribution (a percentile value of .95 corresponding to a W score of 1.645, for example). Thus, a W of zero indicates that volume is equal to that expected for a normal subject after adjustment for age and gender. A value of −1.96 corresponds to a value which is at the 2.5 percentile of normals. W scores were significantly lower than zero among AD patients ($p < 0.001$) (Table 4). The differences among hippocampus, PHG, and amygdala were significant ($p < 0.001$ ANOVA), and all pairwise comparisons (paired t tests) were also significant (hippocampus vs amygdala, $p < 0.001$;

Table 3.
Relationship Between Normalized Volume, Age, and Gender in Control Subjects and AD patients

Normalized Structure Volume	Controls			AD Patients		
	Intercept	Age	Gender (M = 0, F = 1)	Intercept	Age	Gender (M = 0, F = 1)
	B_0	B_1	B_2	B_0	B_1	B_2
Hippocampus	6.359	−0.0357***	0.263**	5.135	−0.029***	—
Amygdala	2.414	−0.0143*	—	1.790	−0.011***	—
Parahippocampal gyrus	5.458	−0.0371***	0.390***	4.216	−0.025***	0.250*

Values are derived from the following regression equation:

$$V = B_0 + B_1 \text{(age)} + B_2 \text{(gender)}$$

where V = normalized MTL structure volume in mm^3/ccm^3

B_0 = intercept
B_1 = the calculated regression coefficient associated with age
B_2 = the calculated regression coefficient associated with gender

*$p < 0.05$.
**$p < 0.01$.
***$p < 0.001$.

137

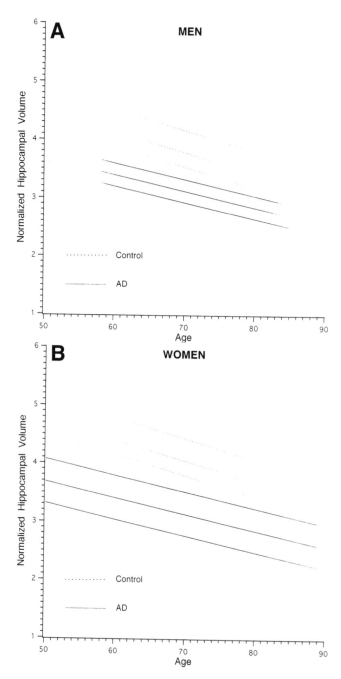

Fig. 3. Normalized hippocampal volume by age in control subjects and patients with AD. Regression of the mean-normalized hippocampal volume by age in male (**A**) and female (**B**) control subjects and patients with AD. The upper and lower limits, dashed lines, represent the 75th and 25th percentile values for each group. Hippocampal volumes of AD patients are smaller than those of age-matched controls. Volumes in both groups decline linearly and in parallel with advancing age. For clinical purposes the position of a memory impaired elderly subject may be plotted and compared to age- and gender-matched controls and AD patients.

Table 4
W Scores* in Patients With Alzheimer's Disease

Variable	CDR = 0.5 (N = 36)		CDR = 1 (N = 43)		CDR = 2 (N = 15)	
	Mean W Value	SD	Mean W Value	SD	Mean W Value	SD
Total hippocampus	−1.752	0.939	−1.989	1.193	−2.225	1.183
Parahippocampal gyrus	−0.874	1.035	−0.996	1.101	−0.512	1.344
Amygdala	−1.026	0.973	−1.337	0.839	−1.355	1.035

The W score is the normal deviate relative to controls, adjusted for age and gender. All mean W scores were significantly different from 0 (the expected value for normal subjects), $p < 0.001$.

139

hippocampus vs PHG, $p < 0.001$, amygdala vs PHG, $p = 0.006$) (Table 4). The mean TIV of AD patients, 1369 cm^3 ($\pm$ SD 138 cm^3), was not significantly different from that of controls.

Discrimination Between Control Subjects and AD Patients of Varying Severity

Using stepwise linear discriminant analysis (including age, gender, and TIV-normalized volumes as independent variables) to predict AD, the only variables that appeared in the final model were hippocampal volume, hippocampal volume squared, and age. Although all these terms were significant at the 0.02 level, the predication equation was dominated by the hippocampal volume term, and the accuracy of the prediction was identical to that obtained using hippocampal W scores alone. The sensitivity of hippocampal volumes to distinguish AD patients from control subjects was assessed by computing the percentage of AD patients with W scores at selected percentiles among control subjects (Table 5). For example, at a fixed specificity of 80%, the sensitivity of hippocampal volumetric measurements in discriminating control subjects from patients was 77.8% for CDR 0.5, 83.7% for CDR 1, and 86.7% for CDR 2. Discrimination between control subjects and AD patients was roughly equivalent among the three AD severity groups at the 50th and 20th percentiles of normal. Discrimination was greater for CDRs 1 and 2 than CDR 0.5 patients at the 10th and 5th percentile of normal. At the first percentile of normal, discrimination improved as the patient's disease severity (CDR score) increased. Hippocampal W values progressively decline (increasing atrophy) with increasing CDR score in Table 4, which suggests that hippocampal volumetric measurements are a sensitive marker of the degenerative neuroanatomic substrate of the progressively more severe memory impairment seen with advancing CDR scores in AD. The most encouraging finding in this study was the ability of hippocampal volumetric measurements to discriminate between control subjects and AD patients with very mild disease. The mean hippocampal volume in very mild (CDR 0.5) AD patients was 1.75 SD below the control mean, and 97.2% of all CDR 0.5 AD patients had hippocampal volumes below the 50th percentile of normal. These data, derived from a large number of subjects, demonstrate that MRI volumetric measurements of hippocampal atrophy are a sensitive marker of the pathology of AD in its most mild form.

The sensitivity and specificity of hippocampal volume measurements in discriminating between controls and AD patients this study is lower than was described in several of the initial studies assessing the efficacy of volume measurements of medial temporal lobe structures in making the diagnosis of AD (48–57). Because of the large number of study subjects involved, the sensitivity

Table 5
Diagnostic Discrimination of Normalized Total Hippocampal Volume Adjusted for Age and Gender*

AD Patients	Indicated Percentile of Normal				
	50%	20%	10%	5%	1%
CDR 0.5 (N = 36)	97.2	77.8	72.2	58.3	36.1
CDR 1 (N = 43)	90.7	83.7	81.4	67.4	53.5
CDR 2 (N = 15)	93.3	86.7	80.0	66.7	66.7
Overall (N = 94)	93.6	81.9	77.7	63.8	48.9

*Percentage of Alzheimer's disease (AD) patients below indicated percentile of normal.
CDR = Clinical Dementia Rating.

and specificity reported here are probably more representative of that which can be expected in a more generalized clinical setting. We believe that this type of MR-based hippocampal volume measurement has sufficient sensitivity and specificity to be a useful clinical adjunct, although it is not 100% accurate and therefore will not be an absolute diagnostic test. A comparison of the normalized hippocampal volume measurements of an individual patient with age and gender specific normal percentiles as illustrated in Table 6 would provide a clinically useful assessment of the presence and severity of hippocampal atrophy. Despite the overlap in hippocampal volume measurements between probable AD patients and elderly controls, a volume assessment of hippocampal atrophy should still be clinically useful in assessing the possibility of AD in individual subjects. For example, given an elderly patient complaining of a memory impairment, if hippocampal volume measurements in that patient fell into the AD range, then a clinical diagnosis of probable AD might be more strongly entertained, whereas if the hippocampal volume measurements fell into the control range, a diagnosis of AD might be considered less likely. There has been growing interest in measuring volumetric changes in individuals wth "mild cognitive impairment" (MCI). Early reports suggest that elders with MCI exhibit diminished hippocampal or medial temporal volumes compared to cognitively healthy normal controls (62a,62b). Elders with MCI may account for some of the observed overlap between nondemented elders and patients with a diagnosis of AD.

The sensitivity and specificity of MRI measures of medial temporal lobe atrophy as a marker of AD generally have been assessed by comparing volume measurements in patients with a clinical diagnosis of probable AD to a matched control population. While estimates of the statistical sensitivity and specificity of the discriminatory power of these measurements may be assessed in this fashion, the "clinical" specificity of MRI measures of medial

Table 6
Age and Gender-Specific Normal Percentiles for Normalized
Hippocampal Volume

Age	Gender	Normal Percentiles				
		1	5	10	25	50
50	M	3.7364	3.9526	4.0593	4.2426	4.4906
	F	3.9998	4.2159	4.3226	4.5059	4.7539
60	M	3.3790	3.5952	3.7019	3.8851	4.1332
	F	3.6424	3.8585	3.9652	4.1485	4.3965
70	M	3.0216	3.2378	3.3445	3.5277	3.7757
	F	3.2850	3.5011	3.6078	3.7911	4.0391
80	M	2.6642	2.8804	2.9871	3.1703	3.4183
	F	2.9275	3.1437	3.2504	3.4337	3.6817
89	M	2.3426	2.5587	2.6654	2.8487	3.0967
	F	2.6059	2.8220	2.9287	3.1120	3.3600

Values in the body of the table represent age and gender-specific mean-normalized hippocampal volume in controls. The units are $mm^3/cm^3 \times 10^3$. The 1st, 5th, 10th, 25th, and 50th percentile values in controls are reported. The presence of hippocampal atrophy in an individual patient can be assessed by comparing the normalized hippocampal volumes of that patient against those of age- and gender-matched controls reported in this table.

temporal lobe atrophy as a marker of AD can only be assessed by comparing these volume measurements among different patient groups; for example, AD vs frontal dementia, or AD vs normal pressure hydrocephalus. Few studies of this type have been done. Hippocampal volume measurements have been shown to discriminate AD patients from patients with dementia due to normal pressure hydrocephalus *(63)*. The clinical specificity of medial temporal volume measurements in discriminating among different conditions that share medial temporal lobe atrophy as a common pathological feature is likely to be low. Medial temporal lobe volume measurements are specific for neuroanatomic degeneration of this region of the brain, but are not disease specific.

Serial Volume Measurements

The purposes of biological markers in AD can broadly be characterized as follows:

1. To diagnose the disease in individual subjects
2. To follow the course of the disease
3. To assess the response to therapeutic intervention in both individuals and in groups (i.e., drug trials)

Most imaging studies in aging and dementia have been cross-sectional in nature and have addressed item 1, that is, identifying imaging criteria that will help to establish the diagnosis of AD in individual subjects. However, items 2 and 3 provide an equally valid rationale for the use of imaging markers in AD. Items 2 and 3, however, necessitate longitudinal as opposed to cross-sectional study design. A particularly attractive use for quantitative MR imaging in AD might center on item 3: to assess the response to therapeutic intervention as an independent marker of the efficacy of a drug in the treatment of AD. The history of imaging markers of hemispheric and regional atrophy in AD has been that significant differences between groups are consistently found, but overlap exists between individual members of the control and the AD populations. While this is a substantial problem if the goal of the imaging marker is to make a clinical diagnosis in individual patients, overlap among individuals becomes less of a problem in the setting of a drug trial where the objective of the study is simply to demonstrate group differences between the treated and the placebo group. In order to effectively perform a longitudinal quantitative imaging study, rigorous attention to the technical details of image acquisition and image processing must be addressed in order to minimize the nonbiological variability in the imaging data. Nonbiological variation in quantitative imaging parameters will tend to obscure changes that are due to biological change. For example, if a multiinstitutional drug trial were instituted with a quantitative MRI measure designated as an independent assessment of drug efficacy, the following items for study quality control would be mandatory. An identical MRI scanning protocol would have to be instituted at each site. While the MRI scanners themselves at the various sites need not be identical, a given patient scanned at two different points in time must be scanned on the same machine. Scanner quality control must be instituted to ensure that instrument drift does not occur over time, and this quality control data should be analyzed at a central site. An initial assessment of the baseline signal to noise ratio, and minimum geometric fidelity criteria should be assessed at each site with a standardized phantom. Monthly measurements of signal to noise and geometric fidelity should be implemented at all sites. The handling, storage, and processing of the MR image data should be performed at a single central site. Essential quality assurance steps for the image processing aspects of the study should include documentation of reproducibility as well as independent cross checking of the numeric output. With this type of rigorous quality control, longitudinal quantitative MRI studies may prove useful in this and other settings in the future.

Several groups have evaluated dementia populations using serial MRI-based volume measurements. Fox and colleagues *(64,65),* evaluated seven members of a family with an amyloid precursor protein 717 Val-Gly pedigree. These individuals were in their 40s and 50s. Three of these individuals deteriorated cognitively over the period of observation, and during this period their hippocampal volumes declined at a more rapid rate than normal controls and unaffected family members. Moreover, right–left hippocampal volumetric asymmetry was present at basline in the affected patients before overt clinical symptoms. At the opposite end of the age spectrum, Kaye and coworkers *(66)* performed serial MRI-based hippocampal and temporal lobe volume measurements as part of a study of the oldest-old. Two groups were identified. A group of cognitively stable persons (mean age: 86.8 years, $n = 18$) and a predementia group (mean age: 90.4 years, $n = 12$). The predemented group declined cognitively over the period of observation and at the time of publication seven were classified as probable AD and five as possible AD. Kaye and coworkers *(66)* found that hippocampal volume declined with age in parallel in the two groups and this measure therefore did not distinguish the normal elderly from predemented subjects. However, the temporal lobe volumes (initially and serially) were atrophic in the predemented group compared to the normal group and this measure separated the two groups. Our own studies *(67)* in serial MRI measurements have focused on subjects who are intermediate in age between the relatively young familial subjects studied by Fox and associates *(64,65)* and the oldest-old studied by Kaye and associates *(66)*. We performed serial MRI-based volume measurements of the hippocampi and temporal horns in 44 subjects. Twenty-two cognitively normal subjects (mean age: 81.5) were individually matched with respect to gender and age ($\pm$ 4 years) with 22 patients with probable AD (mean age: 80.91 years). Each subject underwent an MRI scanning protocol two times, separated by at least 12 months, and the annualized rate of volumetric change for individuals in both of these groups was calculated. The mean annualized rate of hippocampal volume loss among controls was $-1.67\% \pm 1.36\%$ per year and the temporal horns increased in volume by 6.28% $\pm$ 8.03% per year. The mean annualized rate of hippocampal volume loss among AD patients was $-3.84\% \pm 1.93\%$ per year. This rate was significantly greater in cases than in controls, $p < 0.001$. In AD patients, the mean change in temporal horn volume was 13.58% $\pm$ 8.19% per year. This rate was significantly greater among cases than controls, $p = 0.005$. Therefore a statistically significant yearly decline in hippocampal volume and increase in temporal horn volume was identified in normal elderly individuals. The annualized rate of hippocampal atrophy and temporal horn enlargement was approximately two times greater in patients with AD than in individually age and gender matched elderly controls.

Summary

Anatomic imaging measures of cerebral atrophy have been employed in the diagnosis of AD for over a decade. Linear, area, and volume measures of hemispheric and regional atrophy have been assessed with both CT and MRI. Recent attention has focused on MRI-based volume measurements of medial temporal lobe atrophy. Medial temporal volume measurements are a clinically useful marker of functional/anatomic neurodegeneration in this region of the brain, but are not disease specific. Serial MRI-based volume measurements may prove useful in following disease progression in individual patients and as an adjunctive endpoint in AD drug trials.

References

1. American Psychiatric Association, *Diagnostic and Statistical Manual of Mental Disorders.* 3rd ed–Revised. Washington, DC: 1987.
2. Fleming KC, Adams AC, Petersen RC. Dementia: diagnosis and evaluation. *Mayo. Clin. Proc.* 1995;70:1093–1107.
3. Joachim CL, Morris JH, Selkoe DJ. Clinically diagnosed Alzheimer's disease: autopsy neuropathological results in 150 cases. *Ann. Neurol.* 1988;24:50–56.
4. McKhann G, Drachman D, Folstein M, Katzman R, Price D, Stadlan EM. Clinical diagnosis of Alzheimer's disease: report of the NINCDS-ADRDA work group under the auspices of Department of Health and Human Services Task Force on Alzheimer's disease. *Neurology* 1984;34:939–944.
5. Corey-Bloom J, Thal LJ, Galasko D, Folstein M, Drachman D, Raskind M, et al. Diagnosis and evaluation of dementia. *Neurology* 1995;45:211–218.
6. Wade J, Mirsen T, Hachinski V, Fisman M, Lau C, Merskey H. The clinical diagnosis of Alzheimer disease. *Arch. Neurol.* 1987;44:24–29.
7. Kokmen E, Beard CM, O'Brien PC, Offord KP, et al. Is the incidence of dementing illness changing?: a 25-year-time-trend study in Rochester, MN (1960–1984). *Neurology* 1993;43:1887–1892.
8. Foster NL, Chase TN, Fedio P, et al. Alzheimer's disease: focal cortical changes shown by positron emission tomography. *Neurology* 1983;33:961–965.
9. deLeon MJ, George AE, Ferris SH, et al. Regional correlation of PET and CT in senile dementia of the Alzheimer type. *AJNR* 1983;4:553–556.
10. deLeon MJ, George AE, Marcus DL, Miller JD. Positron emission tomography with the deoxyglucose technique and the diagnosis of Alzheimer's disease. *Neurobio. Aging* 1988;9:88–90.
11. Hellman RS, Tikofsy RS, Collier BD, et al. Alzheimer disease: quantitative analysis of I-123-iodoamphetamine SPECT brain imaging. *Radiology* 1989;172:183–188.
12. Holman BL, Johnson KA, Gerada B, Carvalho PA, Satlin A. The scintigraphic appearance of Alzheimer's disease: a prospective study using technetium-99m-HMPAO SPECT. *J. Nucl. Med.* 1992;33:181–185.
13. Jagust WJ, Friedland RP, Budinger TF. Positron emission tomography with [^{18}F]fluorodeoxyglucose differentiates normal pressure hydrocephalus from Alzheimer-type dementia. *J. Neurol. Neurosurg. Psychiatry* 1985;48:1091–1096.
14. Gonzalez RG, Stern C, Carr C, Guimaraes AR, Rosen BR, Growdon JH. Comparison of functional MR imaging cerebral blood volume maps and PET FDG scans in patients evaluated for Alzheimer disease. *Radiology* 1993;189:481.
15. Bottomley PA, Cousins JP, Pendrey DL, et al. Alzheimer dementia: quantification of energy metabolism and mobile phosphoesters with P-31 NMR spectroscopy. *Radiology* 1992;183:695–699.

16. Pettegrew JW, Panchalingam K, Moossy J, et al. Correlation of phosphorous-31 magnetic resonance spectroscopy and morphologic findings in Alzheimer's disease. *Arch. Neurol.* 1998;45:1093–1096.

17. Brown GG, Levine SR, Gorell JM, et al. In vivo ^{31}PNMR profiles of Alzheimer's disease and multiple subcortical infarct dementia. *Neurology* 1989;1423–1427.

18. Shonk TK, Moats RA, Gifford P, et al. Probable Alzheimer disease: diagnosis with proton MR spectroscopy. *Radiology* 1995;195:65–72.

19. Miller BL, Moat RA, Shonk T, et al. Alzheimer disease: depiction of increase cerebral myo-inositol with proton MR spectroscopy. *Radiology* 1993;187:433–437.

20. DeCarli C, Kaye JA, Horwitz B, Rapoport SI. Critical analysis of the use of computer-assisted transverse axial tomography to study human brain in aging and dementia of the Alzheimer type. *Neurology* 1990;40:872–883.

21. Kozachuk WE, DeCarli C, Schapiro MB, et al. White matter hyperintensities in dementia of Alzheimer's type and in healthy subjects without cerebrovascular risk factors: a magnetic resonance imaging. *Arch. Neurol.* 1990;47:1306–1310.

22. Harrell LE, Duvall E, Folks DG, et al. The relationship of high-intensity signals on magnetic resonance images to cognitive and psychiatric state in Alzheimer's disease. *Arch. Neurol.* 1991;48:1136–1140.

23. Bondareff W, Raval J, Woo B, Hauser DL, Colletti PM. Magnetic resonance imaging and the severity of dementia in older adults. *Arch. Gen. Psychiatry* 1990;47:47–51.

24. Bryan RN, Manolio TA, Schertz LD. A method for using MR to evaluate the effects of cardiovascular disease on the brain: the cardiovascular health study. *AJNR* 1994;15:1625–1633.

25. Davis PC, Gray L, Albert M, et al. The consortium to establish a registry for Alzheimer's disease (CERAD). Part III. Reliability of a standardized MRI evaluation of Alzheimer's disease. *Neurology* 1992;42:1676–1680.

26. Gur RC, Mozley PD, Resnick SM, et al. Gender differences in age effect on brain atrophy measured by magnetic resonance imaging. *Proc. Natl. Acad. Sci. U.S.A.* 1991;88:2845–2849.

27. Coffey CE, Wilkinson WE, Parashos IA, et al. Quantitative cerebral anatomy of the aging human brain: a cross-sectional study using magnetic resonance imaging. *Neurology* 1992;42:527–536.

28. Zatz LM, Jernigan TL, Ahumanda AJ. Changes on computed cranial tomography with aging: intracranial fluid volume. *AJNR* 1982;3:1–11.

29. Kaye JA, DeCarli C, Luxenberg JS, Rapoport SI. The significance of age-related enlargement of the cerebral ventricles in healthy men and women measured by quantitative computed x-ray tomography. *J. Am. Geriatr. Society* 1992;40:225–231.

30. Petersen RC. Normal aging, mild cognitive impairment, and early Alzheimer's disease. *Neurologist* 1995;1:326–344.

31. Tanna NK, Kohn MI, Horwich DN, et al. Analysis of brain and cerebrospinal fluid volumes with MR imaging: impact on PET data correction for atrophy: Part II. Aging and Alzheimer dementia. *Radiology* 1991;178:123.

32. Rusinek H, deLeon MJ, George AE, et al. Alzheimer disease: measuring loss of cerebral gray matter with MR imaging. *Radiology* 1991;178:109.

33. Squire LR. Memory and the hippocampus: a synthesis from findings with rats, monkeys, and humans. *Psychol. Rev.* 1992;99:195–231.

34. Ball MJ, Hachinski V, Fox A, Kirshen AJ, Fishman M, Blume W, Kral VA, et al. A new definition of Alzheimer's disease: a hippocampal dementia. *Lancet* 1985;1:14–16.

35. Hooper MW, Vogel FS. The limbic system in Alzheimer's disease: a neuropathologic investigation. *Am. J. Pathol.* 1976;85:1–19.

36. Hyman BT, Van Hoesen GW, Damasio AR, Barnes CL. Alzheimer's disease: cell-specific pathology isolates the hippocampal formation. *Science* 1984;225:1168–1170.

37. Wilcock GK, Esiri MM. Plaques, tangles, and dementia: a quantitative study. *J. Neurol. Sci.* 1982;56:343–356.

38. Tomlinson BE, Blessed G, Roth M. Observations on the brains of demented old people. *J. Neurol. Sci.* 1970;11:205–242.

39. LeMay M. CT changes in dementing diseases: a review. *Am. J. Radiology* 1986;147: 963–975.

40. Sandor T, Albert M, Stafford J, Harpely S. Use of computerized CT analysis to discriminate between Alzheimer patients and normal control subjects. *AJNR* 1988;9:1181–1187.

41. Kido DK, Caine ED, LeMay M, Ekholm S, et al. Temporal lobe atrophy in patients with Alzheimer's disease: a CT study. *AJNR* 1989;10:551–555.

42. George AE, deLeon MJ, Stylopoulos LA, Miller J, et al. CT diagnostic features of Alzheimer disease: importance of the choroida/hippocampal fissure complex. *AJNR* 1990;11:101–107.

43. Jobst KA, Smith AD, Barker CS, et al. Association of atrophy of the medial temporal lobe with reduced blood flow in the posterior parietotemporal cortex in patients with a clinical and pathological diagnosis of Alzheimer's disease. *J. Neurol. Neurosurg. Psychiatry* 1992;55:190–194.

44. Jobst KA, Smith AD, Szatmari M, et al. Detection in life of confirmed Alzheimer's disease using a simple measurement of medial temporal lobe atrophy by computed tomography. *Lancet* 1992;340:1179–1183.

45. Doraiswamy, PM, McDonald WM, Patterson, et al. Interuncal distance as a measure of hippocampal atrophy: normative data on axial MR imaging. *AJNR* 1993;14:141–143.

46. Dahlbeck SW, McCluney KW, Yeakley JW, et al. The interuncal distance: a new MR measurement for the hippocampal atrophy of Alzheimer disease. *AJNR* 1991;12:931–932.

47. Seab JP, Jagust WJ, Wong STS, et al. Quantitative NMR measurements of hippocampal atrophy in Alzheimer's disease. *Magn. Reson. Med.* 1988;8:200–208.

48. Pantel J, Schroder J, Schad LR, et al. Quantitative magnetic resonance imaging and neuropsycholoigcal functions in dementia of the Alzheimer type. *Psychol. Med.* 1997;27:221–229.

49. Kesslak JP, Nalcioglu O, Cotman CW. Quantification of magnetic resonance scans for hippocampal and parahippocampal atrophy in Alzheimer's disease. *Neurology* 1991;41:51–54.

50. Jack CR Jr, Petersen RC, O'Brien PC, et al. MR-based hippocampal volumetry in the diagnosis of Alzheimer's disease. *Neurology* 1992;42:183–188.

51. Lehericy S, Baulac M, Chiras J, et al. Amygdalohippocampal MR volume measurements in the early stages of Alzheimer disease. *AJNR* 1994;15:927–937.

52. Laakso MP, Soininen H, Partanen K, Helkala E-L, Hartikainen P, et al. Volumes of

hippocampus, amygdala and frontal lobes in the MRI-based diagnosis of early Alzheimer's disease: correlation with memory functions. *J. Neural Transmission* 1995;9:73–86.

53. DeCarli C, Murphy DGM, McIntosh AR, et al. Discriminant analysis of MRI measures as a method to determine the presence of dementia of the Alzheimer type. *Psychiatry Res.* 1995;57:119–130.

54. Pearlson G, Harris GJ, Powers RE, Barta PE, et al. Quantitative changes in mesial temporal volume, regional cerebral blood flow, and cognition in Alzheimer's disease. *Arch. Gen. Psychiatry* 1992;49:402–408.

55. Convit A, DeLeon MJ, Golomb J, George AE, et al. Hippocampal atrophy in early Alzheimer's disease: anatomic specificity and validation. *Psychiatric Q.* 1993;64:371–387.

56. Killiany RJ, Moss MB, Albert MS, et al. Temporal lobe regions on magnetic resonance imaging identify patients with early Alzheimer's disease. *Arch. Neurol.* 1993;50:949–954.

57. Cuenod CA, Denys A, Michot JL, et al. Amygdala atrophy in Alzheimer's disease: an in vivo magnetic resonance imaging study. *Arch. Neurol.* 1993;50:941–945.

58. Jack CR Jr, Petersen RC, Xu YC, et al. Medial temporal lobe atrophy on MRI in normal aging and very mild Alzheimer's disease. *Neurology* 1997;49:786–794.

59. Morris JC. The Clinical Dementia Rating (CDR): current version and scoring rules. *Neurology* 1993;43:2412–2414.

60. Jack CR Jr, Twomey CK, Zinsmeister AR, et al. Anterior temporal lobes and hippocampal formations: normative volumetric measurements for MR images in young adults. *Radiology* 1989;172:549–554.

61. Jack CR Jr, Trenerry MR, Cascino GD, Sharbrough FW, So EL, O'Brien PC. Bilaterally symmetric hippocampi and surgical outcome. *Neurology* 1995;45:1353–1358.

62. O'Brien PC, Dyck PJ. Procedures for setting normal values. *Neurology* 1995;45:17–23.

62a. Krasuski JS, Alexander GE, Horwitz B, et al., Volumes of medial temporal lobe structures in patients with Alzheimer's disease and mild cognitive impairment (and in healthy controls). *Biol. Psychiatry* 1998;43(1):60–68.

62b. Jack CR Jr, Petersen RC, Xu YC, O'Brien PC, Smith GE, Ivnik RJ, Boeve BF, Waring SC, Tangalos EG. Kokmen E. Prediction of AD with MRI-based hippocampal volume in mild cognitive impairment. *Neurology* 1999;52(7):1397–1403.

63. Golomb J, deLeon MJ, George AE, Kluger A, et al. Hippocampal atrophy correlates with severe cognitive impairment in elderly patients with suspected normal pressure hydrocephalus. *J. Neurol. Neurosurg. Psychiatry* 1994;57:590–593.

64. Fox NC, Freeborough PA, Rossor MN. Visualisation and quantification of rates of atrophy in Alzheimer's disease. *Lancet* 1996;348:94–97.

65. Fox NC, Warrington EK, Freeborough PA, et al. Presymptomatic hippocampal atrophy in Alzheimer's disease: a longitudinal MRI study. *Brain* 1996;119:2001–2007.

66. Kaye JA, Swihart BS, Howieson D, et al. Volume loss of the hippocampus and temporal lobe in healthy elderly persons destined to develop dementia. *Neurology* 1997;48:1297–1304.

67. Jack CR Jr., Petersen RC, Xu Y, et al. Rate of medial temporal lobe atrophy in typical aging and Alzheimer's disease. *Neurology* 1998;51(4):993–999.

7

Functional Imaging in Alzheimer's Disease

Reisa A. Sperling, Thomas A. Sandson, and Keith A. Johnson

The past decade has seen remarkable advances in the antemortem diagnosis of Alzheimer's disease (AD). While clinical history and examination remain the foundation of the diagnostic process, most clinicians rely on structural tomography, X-ray computed tomography (CT), or magnetic resonance imaging (MRI) to rule out other causes of cognitive impairment, such as cerebral infarction or hydrocephalus. More recently, structural image markers that are positive for the diagnosis of AD have been explored. For example, quantitative volumetric techniques permit size measurements of hippocampal substructure, and open a new avenue for the characterization of AD during life. These techniques are reviewed in Chapter 6.

Functional neuroimaging has sought to identify a physiologic "signature" or functional neuroanatomy that corresponds to the clinical phenomenology of dementia and permits a positive identification of AD. Such a signature image feature could be the foundation for rational therapy as well as early differential diagnosis. This chapter reviews recent research in functional imaging in AD. Following a brief description of image acquisition and image analysis methods, major developments will be considered in roughly the order in which they appeared historically:

1. The description of the central phenomena and anatomy encountered in the imaging of cerebral dysfunction in AD
2. The relation of these image features to clinical and pathologic phenomena and to disease severity
3. The relation of these phenomena to underlying structural abnormality and "atrophy correction"
4. The diagnostic classification performance of various functional techniques in research and clinical settings
5. Studies of the change in functional images over time

From: *Early Diagnosis of Alzheimer's Disease*
Edited by L. F. M. Scinto & K. R. Daffner © Humana Press, Inc., Totowa, NJ

6. Studies in which brain function is measured under conditions of selective functional activation
7. Development of functional MRI methods based on the cerebral blood oxygen level, and the application of these methods to AD
8. The relation of genetic risk factors to image abnormalities
9. The use of functional imaging to characterize the preclinical stage of AD.

This chapter concludes with an overview of some practical issues surrounding the clinical utility of imaging in AD.

Imaging Techniques

Since the early 1980s, functional imaging techniques that utilize radioactive markers of cerebral blood flow or metabolism have been used to infer information about neuronal activity. These techniques include positron emission tomography (PET) and single-photon-emission computed tomography (SPECT). A newer technique, functional magnetic resonance imaging (fMRI), in which no radioactive substances are involved, will be described later in the chapter.

PET and SPECT are nuclear medicine techniques in which a small amount of a radiolabeled substance is injected intravenously and brain images are acquired with specially designed cameras. Such images may be considered "maps" of brain function because a radiopharmaceutical tracer is injected, delivered to, and absorbed by the brain in proportion to the metabolic demands of the tissue. This in turn represents, to a first-order approximation, the state of neural activity. PET imaging uses radiotracers that emit positrons, particles which are emitted from the atomic nucleus, migrate for a few millimeters, and then fly apart to form two high-energy photons (511 KeV). The most commonly used tracers are [^{18}F]deoxyglucose (FDG), a glucose analogue labeled with ^{18}F, to measure cerebral glucose metabolism, and ^{15}O-labeled water to measure cerebral blood flow. Because these substances have very short physical half-lives, they must be made on site at a pharmaceutical level of purity.

Spatial resolution, the threshold below which two points in an image cannot be distinguished is, for PET, typically 6–9 mm, depending on the age of the equipment. Temporal resolution of PET ranges from 30 seconds for ^{15}O blood flow measurements to 45 minutes for FDG. This represents the length of time over which the "state" of functional activity is represented in the image.

Most of the pioneering work in functional imaging has been accomplished at PET centers where relationships between radiopharmaceuticals and brain metabolites have been measured and modeled. Although the number of facilities continues slowly to increase, PET remains quite costly and is generally available only in large academic centers, in part because positron-emitting agents must be made on site at a pharmaceutical level of purity.

Positron-emitting compounds release two gamma rays or photons, while a single, lower energy (140 KeV) photon is emitted in SPECT. Commonly used radiotracers in SPECT are technetium-labeled exametazime (HMPAO or Ceretec) or ethylcysteinate dimer (ECD or "Neurolite"). These agents are taken up by the brain in proportion to blood flow, and, once absorbed by the brain, are chemically altered such that they do not readily exit the brain. This permits image acquisition to take place minutes to hours after injection yet provides an image that is essentially a "snapshot" of the cerebral state present during the several minutes during which the tracer was absorbed by the brain. Thus the spatiotemporal resolution of SPECT is 7–9 mm and 4–5 minutes. SPECT produces images that are similar to PET, but costs are generally lower, because gamma cameras are heavily used in nuclear cardiology, and are available in most medical centers.

Both PET and SPECT can be used to assess regional concentration of specific chemical receptor types *(1–3)*, such as the dopamine transporter *(4)*. Imaging of receptor populations is currently an area of active research, particularly in psychiatric and movement disorders. Such methods may in the future prove useful in the characterization of neurodegenerative diseases such as AD, and may provide neurochemically specific information useful in AD patient management.

Image Analysis

Detailed consideration of the complex field of functional image analysis is beyond the scope of this chapter. However, from the standpoint of imaging studies of AD, sufficient common ground exists that a few generalizations may be offered. As indicated above, PET and SPECT images reflect the "state" of the brain observed over a specific period of time and with a specific degree of spatial detail. Within these constraints, the intensity of each picture element or "pixel" depends on the number of radioactive counts detected by the camera at that particular location in the brain. Functional images may be analyzed using a variety of methods, ranging from single rater visual inspection to manually defined "regions of interest" to highly sophisticated, automated, quantitative techniques.

It should be emphasized that global metabolism or perfusion is often abnormally low in AD, and that optimal identification of regional patterns requires that the global effects be taken into account. A number of methods for doing this have been developed and successfully applied to PET and SPECT. The technique of "normalization" divides regional activity by mean activity in another brain region, relatively unaffected in AD, such as cerebellum, primary visual cortex, or pons *(5–7)* or by whole brain activity. Methods to control for global functional effects have been refined by the use of analysis of covariance (ANCOVA) in both activation *(8)* and resting paradigms *(9)*. More recently, neural net methodology and data-driven statistical techniques, including singular value decomposition to principal components, have been successfully applied to image diagnostic classification of AD *(10–13)*. Use of these advanced analysis methods should improve the ability to detect the earliest functional alterations in AD.

Regional Patterns

Since the earliest studies of functional imaging in Alzheimer's disease *(14–18)*, it has been observed that the regions of greatest reduction in functional activity are found in association cortices, primarily in the temporal and parietal lobes. This regional pattern or "functional signature" (Fig. 1) has been replicated by numerous PET, SPECT, and recent fMRI studies *(9,19–21)*. Premotor and prefrontal cortex abnormalities have also been reported in a number of studies *(22,23)*, but others have observed relative sparing of frontal cortex *(15)*. These apparent discrepancies may reflect variations in clinical presentation or disease severity, as most studies have reported temporoparietal abnormalities earlier in the course of dementia, with frontal abnormalities appearing later in the disease. Primary sensory and somatomotor cortices are usually relatively spared, as are deep gray matter structures and cerebellum. It remains somewhat uncertain why the temporoparietal association cortices show the most significant reductions on functional imaging. Although the temporoparietal neocortex may be particularly susceptible to early pathology in AD *(24,25)*, plaques and tangles are certainly not specific to these areas. Other contributing factors may be selective loss of cholinergic terminals in temporal cortex *(26)* or "deafferentation" of these areas secondary to pathology in deep regions such as the hippocampal complex and basal forebrain.

Most studies have also found that the degree of right-left asymmetry of metabolic activity or cerebral perfusion is increased in patients with AD compared to age-matched controls *(27)*. The majority of patients show greater reductions in left hemisphere metabolism than right, but a subgroup show the reverse asymmetry. These asymmetries in blood flow remain stable over time and have been shown to correlate with variations in clinical presentation (see below).

Correlation With Clinical Parameters

Numerous PET and SPECT studies have reported good correlations between the degree of metabolic or perfusion abnormality and dementia severity *(15,16,28,29)*. Most of these studies utilize standard global assessment

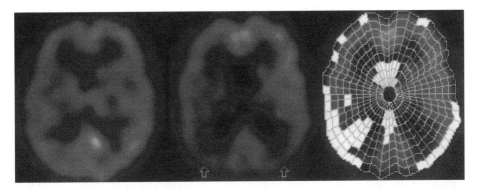

Fig. 1. Brain perfusion SPECT images. **(Left)** Normal control subject. **(Center)** Patient with Alzheimer's disease, showing reduced perfusion is most prominent in the association cortex of the parietal lobes *(arrows).* **(Right)** Quantitative group differences in perfusion are shown superimposed on the AD patient's image. Filled in areas represent those regions significantly reduced in Alzheimer's disease (*n* = 29) compared to age-matched control (*n* = 64; *p* < 0.00l). When parietal perfusion is used to discriminate all subjects (using split-half replication), the accuracy of SPECT is 92%.

tests such as the Mini-Mental State Examination (MMSE), the Blessed Dementia Scale, or the Mattis Dementia Rating Scale *(30).*

Foster and colleagues *(31)* examined a group of patients with moderate-to-severe AD with focal neuropsychological syndromes, and demonstrated hypometabolism in left perisylvian regions in patients with predominate language abnormalities and hypometabolism in right posterior parietal regions in patients with predominant visuospatial deficits. Haxby and colleagues *(22)* also found the lateral asymmetry of cerebral glucose metabolism was associated with relative degree of language and visuospatial impairments in early AD. In another study, Haxby and colleagues *(32)* reported that the parietal/frontal metabolic ratios correlated significantly with neuropsychological deficits in patients with moderate AD. Patients with "disproportionate" parietal hypometabolism showed impairment of verbal comprehension, calculation, and visuospatial functions, while patients with "disproportionate" frontal hypometabolism showed impairment of verbal fluency and attention. These functional imaging findings are consistent with hypotheses about the localization of brain-behavior relationships *(33).*

Variation in functional patterns also may be correlated with the psychiatric and behavioral aspects of AD. Craig and associates *(34)* recently reported that the presence of apathy in patients with AD was correlated with prefrontal and anterior temporal hypoperfusion, and not with posterior temporal or parietal hypoperfusion. Starkstein and coworkers *(35)* used SPECT to study 16 AD patients with delusions and 29 AD patients without delusions. The patients with delusions had significantly lower cerebral blood flow than patients without delusions in left and right temporal regions, but no significant differences between in frontal, parietal, basal ganglionic, or thalamic blood flow.

Recently, several investigators have examined the relationship between cerebral perfusion or metabolism and premorbid abilities. Stern and coworkers *(36)* reported that after controlling for dementia severity, higher level of education in patients with AD was associated with greater reductions in parietotemporal perfusion. Alexander and associates *(37)* found that higher premorbid intellectual ability in individuals, with the same degree of dementia, was associated with lower metabolic rates in several frontal regions and left superior parietal association areas. These studies suggest that a greater burden of pathology may be required to manifest the same level of impairment in individuals with higher education or intellectual capabilities, and support the hypothesis that "cognitive reserve" may affect the clinical expression of dementia. These findings may have significant implications for the "preclinical" diagnosis of AD with functional imaging.

Atrophy Correction

Typical functional maps of the normal brain at rest demonstrate fairly uniform activity in gray matter. When the images indicate an area of abnormal function, a variety of underlying causes should be considered. Diminished metabolism or blood flow is often interpreted as a pure reduction in functional activity, but may actually be due to alterations in underlying structure, such as atrophy or infarction. These defects likely reflect tissue loss rather than tissue dysfunction. One of the primary difficulties in the interpretation of SPECT or PET images in patients with dementia (Fig. 2) is the artifactual underestimate of "function" due to cerebral atrophy *(38)*. Most functional image analysis yields activity in counts per unit volume of space, not in counts/unit volume of brain, a potentially important dimension that more fairly represents functional activity. In diseases associated with aging and neurodegeneration, reduced brain volume is the rule, and any attempt to quantitate a purely functional abnormality would ideally correct for the associated atrophy.

Several groups have applied an "atrophy correction" to their functional imaging studies of AD *(39–41)*. Most of these studies reported a significant increase in "corrected" perfusion or metabolic rates in patients with AD compared to control subjects, although temporoparietal functional abnormalities remained significant after atrophy correction.

Reiman and colleagues *(42)* recently reported that PET scans showed significant metabolic reductions in homozygote apolipoprotein ∈4 carriers before

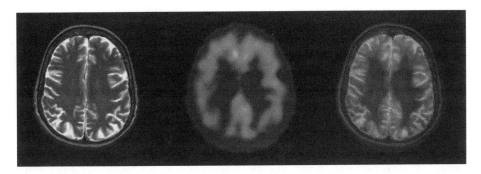

Fig. 2. Axial images from a 73-year-old woman with probable Alzheimer's disease. **(Left)** Structural MRI (T2-weighted) demonstrating posterior parietal atrophy. **(Center)** 99Tc-HMPAO SPECT demonstrating decreased parietal perfusion. **(Right)** Co-registered SPECT and MRI images superimposed showing perfusion deficits corresponding to atrophic parietal regions.

cognitive impairment, but did not find significant hippocampal atrophy in these asymptomatic individuals. These findings suggest that functional and structural alterations may not always occur in parallel, and that functional image abnormalities may precede significant atrophic changes.

Diagnostic Classification

Several studies have attempted to calculate the diagnostic accuracy of PET or SPECT in differentiating AD from normal controls. The studies vary widely in the numbers of subjects, the severity of dementia, and the image analysis methodology. Most of the studies are plagued by lack of a "gold standard," having limited numbers of autopsy-confirmed patients.

A few studies have reported low sensitivity of functional image abnormalities in mild AD. Powers and colleagues *(43)* evaluated the nonquantitative assessment of PET images by blinded reviewers, and reported a low sensitivity (38%) but fairly high specificity (88%). Reed and coworkers *(44)* reported 5/21 probable AD patients with mild memory impairment did not show temporal or parietal perfusion abnormalities.

Most studies, however, have reported sensitivity and specificity in the range of 80–90%. Holman and colleagues *(45)* performed a prospective study of SPECT scans in 132 patients referred for imaging as part of their workup for memory loss or other cognitive abnormalities. Images were evaluated qualitatively by a radiologist blinded to clinical history. The probability of Alzheimer's disease, defined by clinical diagnosis at 1 year follow-up, for patients with bilateral temporoparietal perfusion defects was 82%, but lower for patients with unilateral temporoparietal or frontal perfusion defects. Johnson and associates

(6) reported 88% sensitivity and 87% specificity with a qualitative analysis of IMP-SPECT in probable AD patients compared with age-matched controls. In a subsequent study using quantitative image analysis and HMPAO-SPECT, they reported a sensitivity of 91% and specificity of 86% *(9)*. Bonte and colleagues *(46)* performed SPECT on 54 patients with dementia who had histopathological confirmation of their diagnosis. They found SPECT to have 86% sensitivity, 73% specificity, and 92% positive predictive value.

Combining structural and functional imaging techniques may improve the accuracy of diagnosis (Fig. 2). Pearlson and colleagues *(47)* found combining measures of mesial temporal atrophy on MRI with SPECT measures of temporoparietal perfusion yielded 100% discrimination between a group of 15 patients with AD and 16 normal control subjects. In a larger study of 71 histopathologically confirmed cases of dementia and 84 control subjects, Jobst and associates *(48)* found the combination of medial temporal lobe atrophy as assessed by CT and parietotemporal hypoperfusion on SPECT yielded a sensitivity of 90% with a specificity of 97% for the diagnosis of AD.

Fewer studies have examined the ability of functional imaging to differentiate AD from other dementias. Similar patterns of temporoparietal hypometabolism/hypoperfusion have been reported in Parkinson's disease with dementia (PDD) *(49–51)*. The overlap between AD and PDD may reflect the high incidence of Alzheimer's pathology found in patients with PDD *(52)*. Two recent studies *(53–54)* demonstrated a distinct pattern of reduced occipital glucose metabolism in patients suspected to have dementia with Lewy bodies (DLB) as compared with AD. Parkinson's disease without dementia shows a metabolic pattern similar to normals *(55)*.

The ability to reliably discriminate AD from multiinfarct dementia (MID) remains controversial. Several SPECT studies using qualitative blinded assessments have reported significant differences in the perfusion patterns of AD vs MID *(14,56,57)*, although Duara and coworkers *(19)* did not find a characteristic pattern of metabolic deficits that differentiated AD from MID in a larger PET study. Clearly, combining structural imaging and functional imaging techniques may be helpful in differentiating MID from AD. A substantial subset of patients, however, likely suffer from a mixed dementia with both AD pathology and cerebrovascular disease contributing to the clinical symptomatology, thus making the diagnostic distinction with any methodology extremely difficult.

Functional imaging studies of the frontotemporal dementias caused by Pick's disease and related pathologies show a distinct pattern with frontal and anterior temporal hypometabolism/hypoperfusion and relative sparing of posterior temporal and parietal cortices *(58,59)*. Studies of patients with specific cognitive degenerative syndromes, such as primary progressive aphasia, have demonstrated lateralizing functional abnormalities *(60,61)*. Distinct functional image patterns have also been reported with Jakob-Creutzfeldt disease *(62)* and corticobasal ganglionic degeneration *(63)*.

Several studies have found differences in regional metabolic or perfusion patterns between AD and the " subcortical dementias." Patients with progressive supranuclear palsy (PSP) demonstrate primarily frontal functional abnormalities *(64–66)*. The "pseudodementia" associated with depression has been reported to show prefrontal and limbic system hypoperfusion *(67,68)*. Normal pressure hydrocephalus has been reported to cause more global metabolic reductions without regional abnormalities *(69)*, and the dementia associated with HIV has been associated with widespread multifocal defects *(70,71)*.

Longitudinal Studies

Jagust and colleagues *(20)* studied six AD patients with two PET scans over a mean interval of 15.5 months, and reported a significant decline in parietal metabolic rates as patients worsened clinically. The change over time in the frontal/parietal metabolic ratio correlated with the decline in neuropsychological performance. Left-right metabolic asymmetry was preserved in frontal and occipital regions, but not in parietal regions in this sample. Haxby and coworkers *(27)* reported a longitudinal study of neuropsychological patterns and cerebral metabolic asymmetries. The direction of asymmetry (e.g., left > right) tended to remain constant at follow-up. In addition, the correlation, for either predominately verbal deficits and left hemispheric abnormalities or visuospatial deficits and right hemispheric abnormalities, increased over time.

Activation Studies

While the majority of functional imaging studies in AD have been acquired during a resting condition, several studies have arttempted to study "activation patterns" that are associated with the performance of specific cognitive tasks.

Early cerebral blood flow studies by Ingvar and colleagues *(18)* found that patients with AD had a decrease in the expected flow augmentation when performing mental tasks such as digit span backward and Raven matrices *(30)*. Some of these patients actually showed a decrease from baseline blood flow in association cortices during task activation. More recently, Mentis and colleagues *(72)* performed PET scans on 10 patients with AD and 12 control subjects. They measured cerebral blood flow in response to a visual patterned flash stimulus at varying frequencies. Controls showed a significantly greater increase than AD patients in middle temporal regions and striate cortex, in response to higher frequency stimulation. Becker and associates *(73)* used PET to study verbal memory in patients with Alzheimer's disease and age-matched controls. Patients were asked to repeat or recall word lists of varying lengths during PET acquisition. Paradoxically, the AD patients showed a larger area of activation than controls in regions involved in verbal memory and also showed activation in some cortical areas that did not activate in controls. The authors speculate that this may represent a functional reallocation of brain resources to compensate for dysfunction.

Functional Magnetic Resonance Imaging

A number of functional MRI techniques have recently been developed that can also measure cerebral perfusion. Several studies have been performed with dynamic susceptibility contrast MRI (DSCMRI) in patients with AD. The principle behind this technique is that passage of a concentrated bolus of a paramagnetic contrast agent distorts the local magnetic field sufficiently to cause a transient loss of MR signal on pulse sequences designed to be maximally susceptible to magnetic field inhomogeneities, for example, a T2*-weighted sequence *(74)*. The passage of contrast is imaged over time by sequential rapid scanning of the same slice. The rate of change of signal intensity over time can be calculated and gives a measure that has been shown in animal studies to be directly proportional to cerebral blood volume (CBV).

Gonzalez and collaborators *(75)* studied 10 patients with various types of dementia, including 5 with probable AD, with both PET and DSCMRI. They found a significant correlation between the modalities both quantitatively and qualitatively. Similarly, Johnson and colleagues *(76)* found CBV, as measured by DSCMRI, to correlate well with perfusion by SPECT in 16 patients with AD and 10 age-matched controls. Harris and colleagues *(77)* performed DSCMRI in 13 patients with AD and 13 controls, and found significantly reduced ratios of temporoparietal CBV to cerebellar CBV in the AD group. Three patients with very mild dementia (mean MMSE = 25.0) also had showed reductions in temporoparietal CBVs. Overall, they found that MMSE scores did not correlate well with temporoparietal CBV ratios.

Sandson and colleagues *(21)* performed noninvasive perfusion MRI with the echo-planar imaging and signal targeting with alternation radiofrequency (EPISTAR) technique *(78)* in 11 patients with AD and 8 age- and education-matched controls. The principle of EPISTAR is based on the acquisition of a pair of images, in one of which arterial blood outside of the imaging slice has been magnetically labeled by applying a 180-degree inversion radiofrequency pulse to the protons in the arterial water. Focal areas of hypoperfusion were

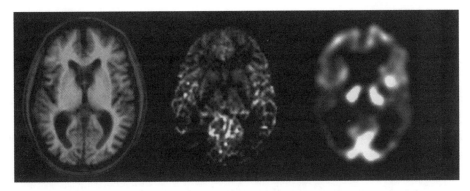

Fig. 3. Axial images from a 53-year old man with biopsy-proven Alzheimer's disease. (**Left**) Structural MRI (T1-weighted). (**Center**) EPISTAR perfusion weighted MRI demonstrating bilateral posterior temporal–occipital perfusion deficits, (**Right**) 99Tc-HMPAO SPECT image demonstrating similar perfusion deficit at same slice plane.

seen in the posterior temporoparietal-occipital region in seven of the patients with AD (Fig. 3). Parietooccipital and temporooccipital to whole-slice signal intensity ratios were significantly lower in the AD patients, and parietooccipital ratios did correlate with dementia severity as measured by the Blessed Dementia Scale-Information-Memory-Concentration subtest *(30)*.

The sensitivity and specificity of the fMRI techniques reported in these preliminary studies are comparable to those reported for PET and SPECT *(6,46,79)*. One advantage of the fMRI techniques over other functional neuroimaging modalities is that the MR structural imaging study can be performed during the same scanning session with the same scan plane, image size (field-of-view), and slice thickness as the functional MR scan. Specific regions of interest (ROI) can therefore be selected with a high degree of certainty on the structural image and directly transferred to the perfusion image at the same anatomical site. Furthermore, there is no exposure to ionizing radiation. EPISTAR offers the advantage of being completely noninvasive. DSCMRI is available as a multislice sequence, while multiple slices can only be acquired sequentially with EPISTAR. Quantification of cerebral blood flow is possible with both DSCMRI and EPISTAR *(80,81)*.

Activational studies with fMRI in Alzheimer's disease are currently ongoing *(82,83)*. These studies utilize another T2*-weighted technique called BOLD *(84)*, which uses changes in the level of oxygenated hemoglobin in capillary beds to visualize areas of regional brain "activation." These preliminary reports have found decreased fMRI activation in hippocampal and prefrontal regions in patients with AD compared with older control subjects *(82,83)*.

Genetic Effects

Several recent reports have suggested that the presence of apolipoprotein E $\epsilon4$ allele may alter the pattern of cerebral metabolism in persons without evidence of clinical dementia. Small and coworkers *(85)* found evidence of parietal hypometabolism and increased parietal asymmetry in nondemented relatives of patients with AD who carried one or two ApoE $\epsilon4$ alleles. Reiman and coworkers *(7)* reported reduced glucose metabolism in posterior cingulate, parietal, temporal, and prefrontal regions in cognitively normal individuals with a family history of AD who were homozygous for the ApoE $\epsilon4$ allele.

In a study of cognitively intact community dwelling elders without a strong family history, and who remained cognitively normal for at least 1 year after SPECT acquisition, we found that the presence of an $\epsilon4$ allele was associated with perfusion abnormalities in temporoparietal cortices, particularly in the hippocampal and parahippocampal areas, as well as orbital frontal regions *(86)*. These findings support the hypothesis that the apolipoprotein E $\epsilon4$ allele may be associated with early pathology in individuals who are still cognitively normal.

The influence of the $\epsilon4$ allele in patients who already have a clinical diagnosis of AD is less clear. Corder and colleagues *(87)* reported no significant difference in cerebral perfusion patterns in patients with AD with or without ApoE $\epsilon4$ alleles, while other studies have suggested that there may be at least some image features that differ in patients with AD with $\epsilon4$ alleles *(86,88,89)*.

Preclinical Diagnosis

Increasing evidence from neuropsychological, neuropathological, structural, and functional imaging studies suggest that the pathophysiological disease process in AD may begin years or even decades prior to the onset of clinical dementia *(90,91)*. It is increasingly imperative to identify individuals in this "preclinical" phase, as emerging pharmacological therapies, such as neuroprotective agents or amyloid precursor secretase inhibitors would likely be most effective in very early stages of the degenerative process.

Even in the absence of genetic risk factors, cerebral perfusion patterns may predict cognitive decline in patients with subtle memory deficits. Johnson and associates *(11)* found a distinct pattern of regional hypoperfusion in 18 subjects with an initial Clinical Dementia Rating scale *(92)* of 0.5, who progressed over 2 years to reach criteria for probable AD (CDR of 1). Perfusion was significantly lower in the posterior cingulate, hippocampal–amygdaloid complex, and other limbic structures of subjects who "converted" to AD within 2 years, compared to 27 subjects who did not show cognitive decline.

Minoshima and coworkers *(93)* also reported posterior cingulate and cinguloparietal hypometabolism in a PET study of eight patients with mild memory impairment who later progressed to probable AD.

Clinical Utility

In this age of shrinking resources for diagnostic workup, the obvious question arises as to the clinical utility of functional imaging in the assessment of dementia. We have found these techniques particularly useful in evaluating patients whose clinical presentation is unusual. Specifically, functional imaging may be useful in patients with prominent behavioral symptoms early in the course of their dementia, when the differential is frontotemporal dementia versus AD. It may also have utility in differentiating the cognitive symptoms associated with mood disorders, such as the "pseudodementia" of depression from abulia associated with early AD. We have also found functional imaging to be helpful diagnostically, in patients who present with a dementing illness at a younger age than typical AD but who demonstrate typical temporoparietal abnormalities. Conversely, the functional imaging can be reassuring in older patients with subjective complaints of memory impairment but who show a normal perfusion pattern. Functional imaging may also be used to provide additional evidence of a correct diagnosis in a patient with a clinical course typical of AD, if family members or loved ones are anxious for further confirmation.

As quantitative methodology becomes more widely used, functional imaging may be very helpful in identifying patients in the earliest stages of dementia for pharmaceutical trials *(94)*. In addition, these techniques may prove useful in identifying image features which may predict response to pharmacological therapy *(95)* and as a physiological marker of response to therapy *(96)*. As potential disease modifying agents become available, the use of functional imaging as a surrogate marker may prove extremely valuable.

References

1. Blin J, Baron JC, Dubois B, Crouzel C, Fiorelli M, Attar-Levy D, Pillon B, Fournier D, Vidailhet M, Agid Y. Loss of brain 5-HT$_2$ receptors in Alzheimer's disease. *Brain* 1993;116:497–510.
2. Kuhl DE, Koeppe RA, Fessler JA, Minoshima S, Ackermann RJ, Carey JE, Gildersleeve DL, Frey KA, Wieland DM. In vivo mapping of cholinergic neurons in the human brain using SPECT and IBVM. *J. Nucl. Med.* 1994;35:405–410.
3. Meyer M, Koeppe RA, Frey KA, Foster NL, Kuhl DE. Positron emission tomography measures of benzodiazepine binding in Alzheimer's disease. *Arch. Neurol.* 1995;52:314–317.
4. Seibyl JP, Marek KL, Quinlan D, Sheff K, Zoghbi S, Zea-Ponce Y, Baldwin RM, Fussell B, Smith EO, Charney DS, et al. Decreased single-photon emission com-

puted tomographic [123I]beta-CIT striatal uptake correlates with symptom severity in Parkinson's disease. *Ann. Neurol.* 1995;38:589–598.

5. Jagust WJ, Johnson KA, Holman BL. SPECT perfusion imaging in the diagnosis of dementia. *J. Neuroimag.* 1995;5:S45–S52

6. Johnson KA, Holman BL, Rosen TJ., Nagel JS, English RJ, Growden JH. Iofetamine I 123 single photon emission computed tomography is accurate in the diagnosis of Alzheimer's disease. *Arch. Intern. Med.* 1990;150:752–756.

7. Reiman EM, Caselli RJ, Yun LS, Chen K, Bandy D, Minoshima S, Thibodeau SN, Osborne D. Preclinical evidence of Alzheimer's disease in persons homozygous for the ε4 allele for apolipoprotein E. *N. Engl. J. Med.* 1996;334:752–758.

8. Friston KJ, Frith CD, Liddle PF, Fr,ackowiak RS. Comparing functional (PET) images: the assessment of significant change. *J. Cereb. Blood Flow Metab.* 1991;11:690–699.

9. Johnson KA, Kijewski MF, Becker JA, Garada B, Satlin A, Holman BL. Quantitative brain SPECT in Alzheinner's disease and normal aging. *J. Nucl. Med.* 1993;34: 2044–2048.

10. Azari NP, Pettigrew MB, Schapiro MB, Haxby JV, Grady CL, Pietrini P, Salerno JA, Heston LL, Rapoport SI, Horwitz B. Early detection of Alzheimer's disease: a statistical approach using positron emission tomographic data. *J. Cereb. Blood Flow Metab.* 1993;13:438–447.

11. Johnson KA, Jones K, Holman BL, Becker JA, Spiers PA, Satlin A, Albert MS. Preclinical prediction of Alzheimer's disease using SPECT. *Neurology* 1998;50(6):1563–1571.

12. Kippenhan JS, Barker WW, Pascal S, Nagel J, Duara R. Evaluation of a neural network classifier for PET scans of normal and Alzheimer's disease subjects. *J. Nucl. Med.* 1992;33:1459–1467.

13. Page MPA, Howard RJ, O'Brien JT, Buxton-Thomas MS, Pickering AD. Use of neural networks in brain SPECT to diagnose Alzheimer's disease. *J. Nucl. Med.* 1996;2:195–200.

14. Benson DF, Kuhl DE, Hawkins RA, Phelps ME, Cummings JL, Tsai SY. The fluorodeoxyglucose ^{18}F scan in Alzheimer's disease and multi-infarct dementia. *Arch. Neurol.* 1983;40:711–714.

15. Foster NL, Chase TN, Mansi L, Brooks R, Fedio P, Patronas NJ, Di Chiro G. Cortical abnormalities in Alzheimer's disease. *Ann. Neurol.* 1984;16:649–654.

16. Frackowiak RSJ, Pozzilli C, Legg NJ, Du Boulay GH, Marshall J, Lenzi GL, Jones T. Regional cerebral oxygen supply and utilization in dementia. *Brain* 1981; 104:753–778.

17. Friedland RP, Budinger TF, Ganz E, Yano Y, Mathis CA, Koss B, Ober BA, Huesman RH, Derenzo SE. Regional cerebral metabolic alterations in dementia of the Alzheimer's type: positron emission tomography with [^{18}F] fluorodeoxyglucose. *J. Comput. Assist. Tomogr.* 1983;7: 590–598.

18. Ingvar DH, Risberg J, Schwartz MS. Evidence of subnormal function of association cortex in presenile dementia. *Neurology* 1975;25:964–974.

19. Duara R, Barker W, Loewenstein D, Pascal S, Bowen B. Sensitivity and specificity of positron emission tomography and magnetic resonance imaging studies in Alzheimer's disease and multi-infarct dementia. *Eur. Neurol.* 1989;29:9–15.

20. Jagust WJ, Friedland RP, Budinger TF, Koss E, Ober B. Longitudinal studies of regional cerebral metabolism in Alzheimer's disease. *Neurology* 1988;38:909–912.

21. Sandson TA, O'Connor M, Sperling RA, Edelman RR, Warach S. Perfusion MRI with EPISTAR in Alzheimer's disease: preliminary results. *Neurology* 1996;47:1339–1342.

22. Haxby JV, Duara R, Cutler NR, Rapoport SI. Relations between neuropsychological and cerebral metabolic asymmetries in early Alzheimer's disease. *J. Cereb. Blood Flow Metab.* 1985;5:193–200.

23. Koss E, Friedland RP, Ober BA, Jagust WJ. Differences in lateral hemispheric asymmetries of glucose utilization between early- and late-onset Alzheimer-type dementia. *Am. J. Psychiatry* 1985;142:638–640.

24. Arriagada PV, Growdon JH, Hedley-Whyte ET, Hyman BT. Neurofibrillary tangles but not senile plaques parallel duration and severity of Alzheimer's disease. *Neurology* 1992;42:631–639.

25. Bierer LM, Hof PR, Purohit DP, Carlin L, Schmeidler J, Davis KL, Perl DP. Neocortical neurofibrillary tangles correlate with dementia severity in Alzheimer's disease. *Arch. Neurol.* 1995;52:81–88.

26. Geula C, Mesulam MM. Systematic regional variations in the loss of cortical cholinergic fibers in Alzheimer's disease. *Cereb. Cortex* 1996;6:165–177.

27. Haxby JV, Grady CL, Koss E, Horwitz B, Heston L, Schapiro M, Friedland RP, Rapoport SI. Longitudinal study of cerebral metabolic asymmetries and associated neuropsychological patterns in early dementia of the Alzheimer type. *Arch. Neurol.* 1990;47:753–760.

28. DeKosky ST, Shih WJ, Schmitt FA, Coupal J, Kirkpatrick C. Assessing utility of single photon emission computed tomography (SPECT) scan in Alzheimer's disease: correlation with cognitive severity. *Alzheimer Dis. Assoc. Discord.* 1990;4:14–23.

29. Waldemar G, Bruhn P, Kristensen M, Johnsen A, Paulson OB, Lassen NA. Heterogeneity of neocortical cerebral blood flow deficits in dementia of the Alzheimer's type: a [^{99m}Tc]-*d,l*-HMPAO SPECT study. *J. Neurol. Neurosurg. Psychiatr.* 1994;57:285–295.

30. Lezak M. *Neuropsychological Assessment.* 3rd ed. New York: Oxford University Press.

31. Foster NL, Chase TN, Fedio P, Patronas NJ, Brooks RA, DiChiro G. Alzheimer's disease: focal cortical changes shown in positron emission tomography. *Neurology* 1983;33:961–965.

32. Haxby JV, Grady CL, Koss E, Horwitz B, Schapiro M, Friedland RP, Rapoport SI. Heterogeneous anterior-posterior metabolic patterns in dementia of the Alzheimer's type. *Neurology* 1988;38:1853–1863.

33. Mesulam MM. Patterns in behavioral neuroanatomy: association areas, the limbic system, and hemispheric specialization. In Mesulam MM, editor. *Principles of Behavioral Neurology.* Philadelphia: FA Davis, 1986;1–70.

34. Craig AH, Cummings JL, Fairbanks L, Itti L, Miller BL, Li J, Mena I. Cerebral blood flow correlates of apathy in Alzheimer's disease. *Arch. Neurol.* 1996;53:1116–1120.

35. Starkstein SE, Vazquez S, Petracca G, Sabe L, Migliorelli R, Teson A, Leiguarda R. A SPECT study of delusions in Alzheimer's disease. *Neurology* 1994;44:2055–2059.

36. Stern Y, Alexander GE, Prohovnik I, Mayeux R. Inverse relationship between edu-

cation and parietotemporal perfusion deficit in Alzheimer's disease. *Ann. Neurol.*
1992;32:371–375.

37. Alexander GE, Furey ML, Grady CL, Pietrini P, Brady DR, Mentis MJ, Schapiro
    MB. Association of premorbid intellectual function with cerebral metabolism in
    Alzheimer's disease: implications for the cognitive reserve hypothesis. *Am. J.
    Psychiatry* 1997;154:165–172.

38. Fazekas F, Alavi A, Chawluk JB, Zimmerman RA, Hackney D, Bilaniuk L, Rosen
    M, Alves WM, Hurtig HI, Jamieson DG. Comparison of CT, MR, and PET in
    Alzheimer's dementia and normal aging. *J. Nucl. Med.* 1989;30:1607–1615.

39. Chawluk JB, Alavi A, Dann R, Hurtig HI, Bais S, Kushner MJ, Zimmerman RA,
    Reivich M. Positron emission tomography in aging and dementia: effect of cerebral
    atrophy. *J. Nucl. Med.* 1987;28:431–437.

40. Meltzer CC, Zubieta JK, Brandt J, Tune LE, Mayberg HS, Frost JJ. Regional hy-
    pometabolism in Alzheimer's disease as measured by positron emission tomography
    after correction for effects of partial volume averaging. *Neurology* 1996;47:
    454–461.

41. Tanna NK, Kohn MI, Horwich DN, Jolles PR, Zimmerman RA, Alves WM, Alavi A.
    Analysis of brain and cerebrospinal fluid volumes with MR imaging: impact on PET
    data correction for atrophy. Part II. Aging and Alzheimer dementia. *Radiology*
    1991;178:123–130.

42. Reiman EM, Uecker A, Caselli RJ, Lewis S, Bandy D, de Leon MJ, De Santi S,
    Convit A, Osborne D, Weaver A, Thibodeau SN. Hippocampal volumes in cogni-
    tively normal persons at genetic risk for Alzheimer's disease. *Ann. Neurol.* 1998;
    44:288–291.

43. Powers WJ, Perlmutter JS, Videen T'O, Herscovitch P, Griffeth LK, Royal HD,
    Siegel BA, Morris JC, Berg L. Blinded clinical evaluation of positron emission to-
    mography for diagnosis of probable Alzheimer's disease. *Neurology*
    1992;42:765–770.

44. Reed BR, Jagust WJ, Seab JP, Ober BA. Memory and regional cerebral blood flow
    in mildly symptomatic Alzheimer's disease. *Neurology* 1989;39:1537–1539.

45. Holman BL, Johnson KA, Garada B, Carvalho PA, Satlin A. The scintigraphic ap-
    pearance of Alzheimer's disease: a prospective study using technetium-99m-
    HMPAO SPECT. *J. Nucl. Med.* 1992;33:181–185.

46. Bonte FJ, Weiner MF, Bigio EH, White CL III. Brain blood flow in the dementias:
    SPECT with histopathologic correlation in 54 patients. *Radiology* 1997;202:
    793–797.

47. Pearlson GD, Harris GJ, Powers RE,, Barta PE, Carmago EE, Chase GA, Noga JT,
    Tune LE. Quantitative changes in mesial temporal volume, regional cerebral blood
    flow, and cognition in Alzheimer's disease. *Arch. Gen. Psychiatry* 1992;49:402–408.

48. Jobst KA, Hindley NJ, King E. The diagnosis of Alzheimer's disease: a question of
    image? *J. Clin. Psychiatry* 1994;11:22–31.

49. Peppard RF, Martin WRW, Clark CM, Carr GD, McGeer PL, Calne DB. Cortical
    glucose metabolism in Parkinson's and Alzheimer's disease. J. Neurosci. Res.
    27:561–568.

50. Sperling RA, Johnson KA, Becker JA, Satlin A, Garada B, Holman BL, Growdon

JH. SPECT cerebral perfusion in neurodegenerative diseases with dementia. *Neurology* 1993;43:956S.

51. Vander Borght T, Minoshima S, Giordani B, Foster NL, Frey KA, Berent S, Albin RL, Koeppe RA, Kuhl DE. Cerebral metabolic differences in Parkinson's and Alzheimer's diseases matched for dementia severity. *J. Nucl. Med.* 1997;38: 797–802.

52. Hakim AM, Mathieson G. Dementia in Parkinson disease: a neuropathologic study. *Neurology* 1979;29:1209–1214.

53. Imamura T, Ishii K, Sasaki M, Kitagaki H, Yamaji S, Hirono N, Shimomura T, Hashimoto M, Tanimukai S, Kazui H, Mori E. Regional cerebral glucose metabolism in dementia with Lewy bodies and Alzheimer's disease: a comparative study using positron emission tomography. *Neurosci. Lett.* 1997;235:49–52.

54. Ishii K, Imamura T, Sasaki M, Yamaji S, Sakamoto S, Kitagaki H, Hashimoto M, Hirono N, Shimomura T, Mori E. Regional cerebral glucose metabolism in dementia with Lewy bodies and Alzheimer's disease. *Neurology* 1998;51:125–130.

55. Sasaki M, Ichiya Y, Hosokawa S, Otsuka M, Kuwabara Y, Fukamura T, Kato M, Goto I, Masuda K. Regional cerebral glucose metabolism in patients with Parkinson's disease with or without dementia. *Ann. Nucl. Med.* 1992;6:241–246.

56. Cohen MB, Graham LS, Lake R, Metter EJ, Fitten J, Kulkarni MK, Sevrin R, Yamada L, Chang CC, Woodruff N, Kling AS. Diagnosis of Alzheimer's disease and multiple infarct dementiar by tomographic imaging of iodine-123 IMP. *J. Nucl. Med.* 1986;27:769–774.

57. Gemmell HG, Sharp PF, Besson JAO, Crawford JR, Ebmeier KP, Davidson J, Smith FW. Differential diagnosis in dementia using the cerebral blood flow agent ^{99m}Tc HM-PAO: a SPECT study. *J. Comput. Assist. Tomogr.* 1987;11:398–402.

58. Miller BL, Ikonte C, Ponton M, Levy M, Boone K, Darby A, Berman N, Mena I, Cummings JL. A study of the Lund-Manchester research criteria for frontotemporal dementia: clinical and single-photon emission CT correlations. *Neurology* 1997;48:937–942.

59. Pickut BA, Saerens J, Marien P, Borggreve F, Goeman J, Vandevivere J, Vervaet A, Dierckx R, De Deyn PP. Discriminative use of SPECT in frontal lobe-type dementia versus (senile) dementia of the Alzheimer's type. *J. Nucl. Med.* 1997;38:929–934.

60. McDaniel KD, Wagner MT, Greenspan BS. The role of brain single photon emission computed tomography in the diagnosis of primary progressive aphasia. *Arch. Neurol.* 1991;48:1257–1260.

61. Turner RS, Kenyon LC, Trojanowski JQ, Gonatas N, Grossman M. Clinical, neuroimaging, and pathologic features of progressive nonfluent aphasia. *Ann. Neurol.* 1996;39:166–173.

62. Benson DF, Mazziotta JC. Positron emission tomographic scanning in the diagnosis of Jakob-Creutzfeldt disease. [Abstract]. *Ann. Neurol.* 1991;30:238.

63. Eidelberg D, Dhawan V, Moeller JR, Sidtis JJ, Ginos JZ, Strother SC, Cederbaum J, Greene P, Fahn S, Powers JM, Rottenberg DA. The metabolic landscape of cortico-basal ganglionic degeneration: regional asymmetries studied with positron emission tomography. *J. Neurol. Neurosurg. Psychiatry* 1991;54:856–862.

64. Blin J, Baron JC, Dubois B, Pillon B, Cambon H, Cambier J, Agid Y. Positron emis-

sion tomographhy study in progressive supranuclear palsy: brain hypometabolic pattern and clinicometabolic correlations. *Arch. Neurol.* 1990;47:747–752.

65. Johnson KA, Sperling RA, Holman BL, Nagel JS, Growdon JH. Cerebral perfusion in progressive supranuclear palsy. *J. Nucl. Med.* 1992;33:704–709.

66. Neary D, Snowden JS, Shields RA, Burjan AWI, Northen B, MacDermott N, Prescott MC, Testa HJ. Single photon emission tomography using ^{99m}Tc-HMPAO in the investigation of dementia. *J. Neurol. Neurosurg. Psychiatry* 1987;50:1101–1109.

67. Ito H, Kawashima R, Awata S, Ono S, Sato K, Goto R, Koyama M, Sato M, Fukuda H. Hypoperfusion in the limbic system and prefrontal cortex in depression: SPECT with anatomic standardization technique. *J. Nucl. Med.* 1996;37:410–414.

68. Mayberg HS. Clinical correlates of PET- and SPECT-identified defects in dementia. *J. Clin. Psychiatry* 1994;55:12–21.

69. Jagust WJ, Friedland RP, Budinger TF. Positron emission tomography with [^{18}F] fluorodeoxyglucose differentiates normal pressure-type hydrocephalus from Alzheimer-type dementia. *J. Neurol. Neurosurg. Psychiaty.* 1985;48:1091–1096.

70. Rottenberg DA, Moeller JR, Strother SC, et al. The metabolic pathology of the AIDS dementia complex. *Ann. Neurol.* 1987;22:700–706.

71. Rottenberg DA, Sidtis JJ, Strother SC, Schaper KA, Anderson JR, Nelson MJ, Price RW. Abnormal cerebral glucose metablism in HIV-1 seropositive subjects with and without dementia. *J. Nucl. Med.* 1996;37:1133–1141.

72. Mentis MJ, Horwitz B, Grady CL, Alexander GE, VanMeter JW, Maisog JMa, Pietrini P, Schapiro MB, Rapoport SI. Visual cortical dysfunction in Alzheimer's disease evaluated with a temporally graded "stress test" during PET. *Am. J. Psychiatry* 1996;153:32–40.

73. Becker JT, Mintun MA, Aleva K, Wiseman MB, Nichols T, DeKosky ST. Compensatory reallocation of brain resources supporting verbal episodic memory in Alzheimer's disease. *Neurology* 1996;46:692–700.

74. Edelman RR, Mattle HP, Atkinson DJ, Hill T, Finn JP, Mayman C, Ronthal M, Hoogewoud HM, Kleefield J. Cerebral blood flow: assessment with dynamic contrast-enhanced T2*-weighted MR imaging at 1.5 T. *Radiology* 1990;176:211–220.

75. Gonzalez RG, Fischman AJ, Guimaraes AR, Carr CA, Stern CE, Halpern EF, Growdon JH, Rosen BR. Functional MR in the evaluation of dementia: correlation of abnormal dynamic cerebral blood volume measurements with changes in cerebral metabolism on positron emission tomography with fludeoxyglucose F 18. *Am. J. Neuroradiol.* 1995;16:1763–1770.

76. Johnson KA, Renshaw JA, Becker A. Comparison of functional MRI and SPECT in Alzheimer's disease [Abstract]. *Neurology* 1995;45:A405–A406.

77. Harris GJ, Lewis RF, Satlin A, English CD, Scott TM, Yurgelum-Todd DA, Renshaw PF. Dynamic susceptibility contrast MRI of regional cerebral blood volume in Alzheimer's disease. *Am. J. Psychiatry* 1996;153:721–724.

78. Edelman RR, Siewert B, Darby DG, Thangaraj V, Nobre AC, Mesulam MM, Warach S. Qualitative mapping of cerebral blood flow and functional localization with echoplanar MR imaging and signal targeting with alternating radio frequency. *Radiology* 1994;192:513–520.

79. Herholz K, Adams R, Kessler J. Criteria for the diagnosis of Alzheimer's disease with positron emission tomography. *Dementia* 1990;1:156–164.

80. Buxton RB, Frank LR, Siewart B. A quantitative model for EPISTAR perfusion imaging. Proceedings of the Society for Magnetic Resonance in Medicine, Berkeley, CA: 1990;132.

81. Rempp KA, Brix G, Wenz F, Becker CR, Guckel F, Lorenz WJ. Quantification of regional cerebral blood flow and volume with dynamic susceptibility contrast-enhanced MR imaging. *Radiology* 1994;193:637–641.

82. Corkin S, Kennedy AM, Bucci J, Moore CI, Locascio JJ, Stern CE, Rosen BR, Gonzalez RG. Relation between recognition performance and fMRI data in Alzheimer's disease older normal subjects. *Neurosci. Abstr.* 1997;193.5.

83. Bates JF, Savage CR, Buckner RL, Schacter DL, Weisskoff R, Rosen B, Whalen PJ, Kennedy DN, Stern CE, Albert MS. Abnormal activiation of the hippocampal formation in mild Alzheimer's disease during visual encoding. *Neurosci. Abstr.* 1997;843.1.

84. Kwong KK, Belliveau JW, Chesler DA, Goldberg IE, Weisskoff RM, Poncelet BP, Kennedy DN, Hoppel BE, Cohen MS, Turner R, et al. Dynamic magnetic resonance imaging of human brain activity during primary sensory stimulation. *Proc. Natl. Acad. Sci. U.S.A.* 1992;89:5675–5679.

85. Small GW, Mazziotta JC, Collins MT, Baxter LR, Phelps ME, Mandelkern MA, Kaplan A, La Rue A, Adamson CF, Chang L, Guze BH, Corder EH, Saunders AM, Haines JL, Pericak-Vance MA, Roses AD. Apolipoprotein E type 4 allele and cerebral glucose metabolism in relatives at risk for familial Alzheimer disease. *JAMA* 1995;273:942–947.

86. Sperling RA, Jones KJ, Rentz DM, Albert MS, Holman BL, Becker JA, Scinto LFM, Daffner KR, Johnson KA. SPECT cerebral perfusion and apolipoprotein E genotype. [Abstract]. *Neurology* 1998;50:A438.

87. Corder EH, Jelic V, Basun H, Lannfelt L, Valind S, Winblad B, Nordberg A. No difference in cerebral glucose metabolism in patients with Alzheimer's disease and differing apolipoprotein E genotypes. *Arch. Neurol.* 1997;54:273–277.

88. Higuchi M, Arai H, Nakagawa T, Higuchi S, Muramatsu T, Matsushita S, Kosaka Y, Itoh M, Sasaki H. Regional cerebral glucose utilization is modulated by the dosage of apolipoprotein E type 4 allele and α_1-antichymotrypsin type A allele in Alzheimer's disease. *NeuroReport* 1997;8:2639–2643.

89. Lehtovirta M, Soininen H, Laasko MP, Partanen K, Helisalmi S, Mannermaa A, Ryynänen M, Kuikka J, Hartikainen P, Riekkinen PJ Sr. SPECT and MRI analysis in Alzheimer's disease: relation to apolipoprotein E ϵ4 allele. *J. Neurol. Neurosurg. Psychiatry* 1996;60:644–649.

90. Morris JC, Storandt M, McKeel DWJr, Rubin EH, Price JL, Grant EA. Cerebral amyloid deposition and diffuse plaques in "normal" aging: evidence for presymptomatic and very mild Alzheimer's disease. *Neurology* 1996;46:707–719.

91. Snowdon DA, Kemper SJ, Mortimer JA, Greiner LH, Wekstein DR, Markesbery WR. Linguistic ability in early life and cognitive function and Alzheimer's disease in late life. Findings from the Nun Study. *JAMA* 1996;275:528–532.

92. Morris JC, Ernesto C, Schafer K, Coats M, Leon S, Sano M, Thal LJ, Woodbury P. Clinical dementia rating training and reliability in multicenter studies: the Alzheimer's Disease Cooperative Study experience. *Neurology* 1997;48:1508–1510.

93. Minoshima S, Giordani B, Berent S, Frey KA, Foster NL, Kuhl DE. Metabolic re-

duction in the posterior cingulate cortex in very early Alzheimer's disease. *Ann. Neurol.* 1997;42:85–94.

94. Foster NL. PET Imaging. In Terry RD, Katzman R, Bick KL, editors. *Alzheimer's Disease* New York: Raven Press, 1994:87–103

95. Mega MS, O'Connor SM, Lee L, Dinov ID, Cummings JL, Toga AW. Orbital frontal and anterior cingulate pretreatment perfusion defects on 99mTc-HMPAO-SPECT are associated with behavioral response to cholinesterase inhibitor therapy in Alzheimer's disease. *Neurology* 1998;50(4):A250.

96. Nakano N, Fukatsu R, Fujii M, Murakami S, Hayashi S, Saito S, Hayashi Y, Fujimori K, Takahata N. Effects of cholinesterase inhibitor, E2020, on the regional cerebral blood flow in Alzheimer's disease as measured by ^{99m}Tc-ECD SPECT. *Neurobiol. Aging* 1998;19:S178.

8

Neuropsychological Detection of Early Probable Alzheimer's Disease

Dorene M. Rentz and Sandra Weintraub

Introduction

Alzheimer's disease is the most common of the degenerative dementias affecting up to 47% of the population over the age of 85 *(1,2)*. As the age distribution shifts over the next quarter century, the increasing prevalence of Alzheimer's disease poses a significant health care crisis and intensifies the need for greater research efforts toward detection, treatment, and cure. While initiatives to develop noninvasive biological tests for Alzheimer's disease are underway [i.e., ApoE *(3)*, CSF amyloid *(4)*, tau *(5)*, Pupil Test *(6)*], to date, cognitive and behavioral deficits remain the earliest, most reliable evidence of disease. Yet, by the time neuropsychological deficits are detected, it is likely that the pathological disease process has been present for many years *(7–9)*. Now that new medicines are on the horizon to slow disease progression, a major challenge lies in identifying affected, but not yet demented, individuals in the earliest phases of illness when treatment can have a more profound impact on functional status and rate of decline.

Since neuropsychological deficits are still the best way to detect early symptoms, the goal would be to identify the cognitive changes that depart from the "usual" course of aging and that specifically predict Alzheimer's disease. This chapter begins with a review of studies that have defined the parameters of age-related cognitive change, or what has been called "normal" or "usual" aging. We then describe the neuropsychological profile of probable Alzheimer's disease (PrAD) and contrast that with the profile of groups characterized as "preclinical" or "at-risk." We will discuss methods for predicting the development of PrAD based on neuropsychological test scores and patterns. Finally, some of the challenges facing early detection are considered.

From: *Early Diagnosis of Alzheimer's Disease*
Edited by L. F. M. Scinto & K. R. Daffner © Humana Press, Inc., Totowa, NJ

"Usual" Age-Related Cognitive Change

Intellectual decline in certain cognitive domains has been described as an inevitable consequence of normal aging but the severity of these changes varies widely among individuals *(10,11)*. The "classic aging" pattern that has been observed using the *Wechsler Adult Intelligence Scale* suggests that the verbal IQ remains relatively stable over time while the performance IQ declines *(12–14)*. The robustness and stability of verbally mediated cognitive processes in the face of aging is especially useful when making distinctions between normal aging and disease states. The downward trend in the performance IQ, however, is not unidimensional nor does it influence all individuals in the same manner. Furthermore, the sensitivity of the performance tests to many factors, including diminished motoric reaction time, makes them less useful for detecting and characterizing changes that might signal dementia.

Several other observations on age-related cognitive change are also pertinent. Results from the Seattle Longitudinal Study *(15)* showed that there is a great degree of overlap in the performance of older and younger cohorts along several cognitive dimensions. On tests of vocabulary, spatial orientation, inductive reasoning, numerical skills, immediate memory, and life planning tasks, there was a 90% overlap in test scores between younger and older subjects up to the age of 67. With the exception of inductive reasoning test scores, which began to show some evidence of decline after that point, the overlap remained stable until the age of 74. On some tasks, overlap was apparent until the late 80's. Prior to the late 70's, the magnitude of age-related cognitive change would not be expected to hamper work performance or activities of daily living *(15)*.

Cross-sectional neuropsychological studies have yielded similar conclusions. In one study, a series of standard neuropsychological tests of attention, memory, and visuospatial skills were administered to individuals from age 60 to 80, and their performance was compared to an index sample made up of individuals between 16 and 60 years of age *(16)*. Different tests showed different rates of change from one group to the next, with memory tests showing the earliest and most significant decline. However, on some of the tests, there was no evidence of significant change with increasing age. Furthermore, when the proportion of individuals in the older groups who failed one or more tests (i.e., scored less than 95% of normal subjects or greater than 1.7–2 SD below the mean) was calculated, one-third of those in the oldest age group did not fail any of the tests. These findings were very important because they demonstrated that 1) not all tests are equally sensitive to decline, and 2) not all individuals experience decline to the same degree.

Similar conclusions were reached in a study using computerized neuropsychological tests to study age-related change in a group of physicians in 6 age cohorts between 28 and 92 years of age *(17)*. For approximately half the subtests (those measuring attention, immediate verbal recognition memory, and visual perceptual skill) performance did not change appreciably until the age of 75. For an additional 25% of subtests (largely delayed recognition memory measures) significant changes were detected after the age of 65. Three subtests measuring visual memory and reasoning showed a significant decrease in scores in the 55–64 age group and all others beyond that age. Finally, one subtest of the ability to compare strings of letters and symbols showed no significant change in scores across all age groups. Thus, it was only by the age of 75 that average test scores in almost all domains were significantly lower than the average scores of individuals in the index group (under the age of 35). This was a highly biased sample with respect to their level of intellectual ability and education so their results may not be easily generalized. However, even in this high-functioning group, it was abundantly clear that, as revealed in the increasing magnitude of the standard deviations, there was considerable variability in the oldest cohorts. This tendency for increased variability in many measures in older individuals introduces significant problems when trying to evaluate the significance of test scores in the individual patient *(18,19)*.

The most consistent finding from both cross-sectional and longitudinal studies is that delayed recall and attention scores are most vulnerable to the effects of aging *(20)*. Since these functions are also central in the symptomatology of Alzheimer's disease, mild declines in memory performance are difficult to discriminate from early Alzheimer's disease. In a study of community dwelling, nondemented elders, Petersen and colleagues *(21)* showed that learning scores (i.e., acquisition) decline uniformly with increasing age and with no relationship to prior level of education. Delayed recall (i.e., rate of forgetting) remained relatively stable across age when adjusted for the amount of material initially learned. In related studies, Petersen and colleagues *(22)* and Branconnier and coworkers *(23)* also demonstrated that recognition memory is relatively unaffected by normal aging but is specifically sensitive to dementia. These results suggest one strategy for deciding if an individual patient's memory is impaired: if learning, delayed recall, or recognition memory scores fall below average levels, then the suspicion of a dementing process increases.

Neuropsychological Deficits Characteristic of Dementia Associated with Alzheimer's Disease

Criteria for the clinical diagnosis of probable or possible Alzheimer's disease (PrAD or PoAD, respectively) were proposed in 1984 and still constitute the standard in most research studies *(24)*. The criteria for PrAD specify the presence of a progressive memory disorder accompanied by deficits in other cognitive domains, including aphasia, visuoperceptual/constructional deficits, and abnormalities of reasoning and personality. The diagnostic criteria have been validated against neuropathological findings at autopsy *(25)* and have been shown to be associated with the plaques and tangles of Alzheimer's disease as specified by diagnostic criteria *(26)* in 85–100% of cases *(9,27–28)*.

Neuropsychological studies of patients with PrAD have provided detailed information about the nature of specific cognitive impairments. The most essential and consistent feature of PrAD is the presence of a defect of explicit learning and memory. In preclinical phases of the illness, as shown in follow-up studies of initially nondemented individuals, some patients show deficits in the initial learning of information while retention is preserved *(29,30)*. A loss of information over a delay interval has also been cited as a differentiating feature between usual aging and PrAD *(31)*. In large cohort studies, declines in delayed recall measures or accelerated forgetting were found to be the best discriminators between patients with a diagnosis of mild Alzheimer's disease and nondemented controls *(32–34)*. As the severity of the disease increases, patients also show a constriction of immediate recall. The early loss of delayed recall makes it difficult to continue to characterize further memory deterioration in these patients if only recall measures are used. Recognition memory can be preserved in moderate stages when patients are incapable of spontaneous recall. Implicit learning, including the acquisition of motor skills *(35),* and some types of priming are commonly spared in PrAD *(36)*.

Next to amnesia, the most common deficits in PrAD occur in the realm of language *(28,37–41)*. Patients may perform poorly on naming tests at a time when there is no other evidence of a language impairment, either in social interaction or by formal testing. There is some discussion as to whether or not a naming impairment reflects dissolution of the semantic system in general or whether it is a true aphasic deficit *(41)*. However, many PrAD patients go on to develop symptoms of fluent aphasias, including anomic, transcortical sensory, and Wernicke's aphasia *(38–40)*. The degree of anomia has been associated with rapidity of disease progression *(42)*. The use of less sophisticated grammatical constructions in writing in early adult development has also been shown to be a strong predictor of the development of Alzheimer's disease in late life *(43)*.

Although less well-characterized than the amnestic and aphasic symptoms, attentional deficits are also observable and often constitute the earliest non-memory symptom observed in PrAD *(28, 44)*. Patients may generally not have reduced forward digit spans in the early stages, which makes the presence of a memory disorder even more striking, but as the disease progresses, span length is reduced *(45)*. Deficits in attentional tasks requiring working memory, persistence, or divided attention, such as the Stroop Test *(46)* and Trail

Making Tests *(47)*, are common in patients with mild to moderate dementia severity *(48,49)*.

Many test batteries for PrAD include constructions as a measure of visuospatial processing since they may deteriorate early in the course of illness. However, constructions are complex tasks requiring not only visuospatial but also executive functions such as planning, sequencing, and organization. Therefore, failure on these tasks can occur for one of several reasons. Performance on more "pure" measures of visual processing such as the Facial Recognition Test *(50)* and the Judgment of Line Orientation Test *(50)* can often be preserved and may be selectively impaired only in that group of patients with progressive visuospatial dysfunction who show Balint's syndrome, visual agnosia, or simultagnosia early in the course of illness, and an unusual distribution of plaques and tangles in the visual association cortex *(51,52)*.

Although individuals in very early stages of dementia may continue to function adequately in daily living activities, the cognitive deficits soon begin to affect, first, complex activities such as performing one's job or traveling, and ultimately, overlearned skills such as dressing or feeding oneself. Several measures are available to assess ADLs, including Instrumental Activities of Daily Living *(53)*, Record of Independent Living *(54)*, the Activities of Daily Living Questionnaire *(31)*, and the Direct Assessment of Functional Status *(55)*, but these are only informative for patients in whom dementia is already obvious.

Mild Cognitive Impairment in the Elderly: "At Risk" or "Preclinical" Dementia

Despite living independently in the community, many elders show some degree of abnormal cognitive decline on standardized testing. When community dwelling elders with "mild cognitive impairments" are studied longitudinally, some go on to develop dementia *(56–59)* while some do not *(60–61)*. The presence of mild cognitive problems, by themselves, in community dwelling elders, is not necessarily predictive of a preclinical stage of Alzheimer's disease but can also be associated with the variability seen in normal aging and a variety of medical, neurological, and psychiatric illnesses *(62–64)*. Therefore, the ability to distinguish age associated cognitive change from symptoms that herald a future dementia is critical in research on aging, particularly for those investigating early markers of Alzheimer's disease. With this in mind, several attempts have been made over the last 10 years to develop operationalized criteria for making these distinctions *(65–67)*.

Historically, memory loss has been shown to be the best discriminator between dementing and nondementing conditions of aging *(31–33)*. As early as

1962, Kral *(68)* introduced the terms "benign" (or malignant) senescent forget-fulness" in recognition of the fact that memory loss could be normal or abnormal. However, these terms were poorly operationalized and insufficiently validated to be useful in research. In 1986, a National Institute of Mental Health Work Group on aging and memory *(65)* proposed diagnostic criteria for "Age-Associated Memory Impairment" (AAMI). Their inclusion criteria included:

- Above age 50
- Gradual onset of subjective memory problems that affect everyday life
- The absence of dementia as indicated by a MMSE score of 24 or higher
- Adequate intellectual function as determined by a scaled score of 9 on the WAIS-R Vocabulary Test
- Proposed cutoff scores of 1 standard deviation below the mean established for young adults on tests of memory [i.e., Benton Visual Retention Test *(49)*, Logical Memory subtest of the WMS *(69)*, and Associate Learning subtest of the WMS *(69)*]

Problems were encountered applying the proposed criteria and a revised and expanded version was introduced, which 1) limited the age range from 50–79; 2) utilized standardized self-report memory questionnaires; and 3) suggested a more comprehensive battery of memory tests *(66)*. With these criteria the identification of two other subtypes were introduced. These included "Age Consistent Memory Impairment" (ACMI), which identifies persons whose memories appear to be aging in accord with normative expectations (i.e., ±1 SD of the mean established for age on 75% or more of the tests administered) and "Late Life Forgetfulness" (LLF), which identifies those persons whose scores are mildly but quite consistently below average on memory tests (i.e., between 1 and 2 SD below the mean established for age on 50% or more of the tests administered). The aim of these revised criteria was to help investigators specify more clearly the variability within normal elderly populations on tests of memory and to allow for more controlled experimentation.

Petersen et al. *(66a)* followed over 4 years a group of community dwelling elders from primary care clinics who were at risk for developing Alzheimer's disease. Based on their findings, elders received a diagnosis of mild cognitive impairment (MCI) if they met the following criteria:

- Complaint of defective memory
- Normal activities of daily living
- Normal general cognitive function
- Abnormal memory function for age (i.e., 1.5 SD below mean for age on standardized tests of memory)
- Absence of dementia

Petersen et al. *(59a)* reported that elders diagnosed with MCI, using the above criteria, converted to a diagnosis of Alzheimer's disease at a rate of 12% per year over 4 years. In contrast to previous definitions of "at risk" populations, Petersen et al.'s diagnosis of MCI may prove valuable as criteria for early treatment and are now being used in several multicenter clinical trials.

The presence of "mild cognitive impairments," particularly on objective tests of memory, has been shown to be a good predictor of subsequent further deterioration in community dwelling elders *(56–59a,66a)* while the absence of "cognitive impairments" seems to predict no further decline *(60,61)*. Thus, many individuals with mild impairments may be in preclinical phases of Alzheimer's disease, although there continues to be debate over this conclusion. Malec and associates *(61)* showed that an elder sample who reported no cognitive problems but were identified as "at risk" for future cognitive decline did not show any further decline in learning or memory over a 3- to 5-year interval. They proposed that group membership in an "at risk" category for nonclinical subjects without cognitive complaints was not a powerful predictor of future cognitive decline.

Conversely, several other studies found that subjective memory complaints without objective evidence on standardized tests of memory were better at predicting the presence of depression in community dwelling elders than differentiating those "at risk" for future dementia *(60,70–73)*. Others found that subjective memory complaints were predictive of future dementia only when accompanied by objective signs of memory deterioration on testing *(60,71,73)*. However, informants' or relatives' ratings of cognitive deficits in "at risk" elders were the best predictors of subsequent decline and also significantly correlated with declines on standardized tests of memory *(70,73)*.

Use of Neuropsychological Tests and Test Batteries for Detecting and Predicting Early Alzheimer's Disease

A number of studies have investigated the utility of neuropsychological measures for differentiating nondemented from mildly demented patients and predicting which normal subjects will progress to a dementia state. These studies range from the use of simple screening measures or single neuropsychological tests for classification and detection of disease to more sophisticated regression formulas for deriving predictions from selected tests with a high degree of sensitivity and specificity for dementia and Alzheimer's disease.

The development of global screening measures such as the Mini Mental State Examination (MMSE) *(74)* or the Blessed Dementia Rating Scale *(75)* were early attempts at discriminating cognitively intact normals from those with dementia. They are still widely used in research for this purpose because of their reported utility in identifying those at high risk for developing Alzheimer's disease *(76)*. However, there are several reports in which these measures have been shown to be insensitive to early dementia and may produce false negative results *(7,77)* or lead to neuropsychological findings in which performances of persons with "questionable" dementia overlap with those of healthy older adults *(9)*. In the "Aging and Alzheimer's Disease" study currently under way at the Brigham and Women's Hospital, we are following 141 community dwelling elders. All subjects underwent a medical/psychiatric history interview and neuropsychological evaluation. The Information, Memory and Concentration subtest (IMC) of the Blessed Dementia Scale was administered as well as a more extensive neuropsychological test battery measuring the domains of attention, memory, language, visuospatial skills, and premorbid IQ. Each domain had one or more tests. Test scores were judged abnormal if they fell beyond 2 standard deviations below the mean, a criterion more generous than that required by the NIMH proposed standards for distinguishing age associated memory loss. Subjects were assigned to one of three categories depending on their test performance: 1) no cognitive impairment; 2) impairment in one cognitive domain; 3) impairments in two or more cognitive domains. We compared IMC scores to their cognitive classification status. We found that 72% of the 109 subjects who scored well within the normal range on the IMC (scores of 0 and 1) had impairments in one or more cognitive domains and 28% had impairments in two or more cognitive domains. The deficits essentially occurred on tests of memory and/or attention. There was no effect of age, education, and IQ on their classification. We then converted the Blessed score into predicted MMSE scores based on the formula of Thal and colleagues *(78)*, since this screening measure is also widely used in aging and dementia research. The results were similar. Of those subjects who obtained conversion scores of greater than 26 on the MMSE, 58% had impairments in one or more cognitive domains, and 18% had impairments in two or more cognitive domains *(79)*. These subjects would have been classified as normal controls if these common screening measures were used.

To address the need for a more reliable, rapidly administered screening test designed to detect elders with PrAD, Solomon et al. *(79a)* developed the 7 Minute Neurocognitive Screening Battery (known as the 7 Minute Screen). Unlike the MMSE and the IMC, this screening tool consists of four brief tests that take advantage of the evolving understanding of the cognitive differences between PrAD and the normal aging process. Purported to take an average of 7 minutes 42 seconds to administer, this screening test demonstrated a high degree of sensitivity (92%) and specificity (96%) in a random sample of elders referred to a

Memory Disorders Clinic. A logistic regression formula is used to determine the likelihood that a patient has signs of PrAD. The test's ability to distinguish between other forms of dementia is unclear. However, the 7 Minute Screen has the potential of being a more reliable test for detecting elders in early stages of PrAD than other screening tests being used by primary care physicians.

Despite the appeal of using a simple screening test for detecting early cognitive decline, there are inherent limitations in utilizing them for determining normal cognitive status. First, the recruitment of elderly subjects based on a common method of self-referral often attracts a large number of persons with subjective memory complaints who may be in preclinical phases of Alzheimer's disease. Second, screening measures are insensitive in detecting cognitive deficits in intellectually superior individuals because of the simplicity of the items. Conversely, they overestimate deficits in intellectually limited individuals who may not have the knowledge to answer even simple questions. This creates both type I and type II research errors in subject classification. However, global screening measures are particularly useful for tracking dementia severity and charting its course over time *(31)*.

If testing time is limited and screening measures are determined to be unreliable in detecting early dementia in the elderly, the researcher can turn to single neuropsychological test scores which have shown some degree of success in predicting dementia. For example, memory recall scores on the Fuld Object Memory Evaluation *(80)* and the Bushke Selective Reminding Test *(81–83)* predicted the development of dementia 1 year before the clinical onset of symptoms.

Performance on the California Verbal Learning Test (CVLT) *(84)* differentiated at-risk control subjects with a positive family history of dementia from those without such a history *(85)*. The addition of a delayed recall measure to a neuropsychological battery increased the predictive accuracy of identifying patients with PrAD to 95.2% *(86)*. Recognition memory on an odor detection test was found to be significantly impaired in subjects with questionable Alzheimer's disease and may be an early predictor of the disease state *(87)*. The degree of anomia on the Boston Naming Test predicted a more rapidly progressive disease course *(42)*. Finally, performance on category fluency measures discriminated patients from normal controls with 100% sensitivity and 92.5% specificity *(88)*.

Earlier we mentioned that the capacity to detect preclinical or very early Alzheimer's disease on the basis of particular neuropsychological measures has also been the focus of several cross-sectional studies. Petersen and colleagues *(22)* examined several aspects of memory function to determine which indices of performance were most sensitive at differentiating early Alzheimer's disease from normal aging. Furthermore, using logistic regression models that included measures of memory, verbal and nonverbal intelligence, attention, and language, they found that an index of learning, especially with semantic cueing, was most sensitive at separating the two groups and appeared to be the best discriminator at detecting very mild Alzheimer's disease. This corresponds with the work of Robinson-Whelen and Storandt *(29)* and Grober and Kawas *(30)*, who found that deficits in the initial learning of information was a better predictor of preclinical Alzheimer's disease than deficits in retention or accelerated rates of forgetting *(31–34)*.

The use of a limited battery of tests to accurately discriminate between patients with early PrAD and normal controls was suggested in 1984 by Storandt and colleagues *(89)*. They found four tests that could successfully identify 98% of the cases as either healthy or mildly demented. These were the Logical Memory and Mental Control subtests of the Wechsler Memory Scale *(69)*, Trail Making Test A *(47)*, and a word fluency task for the letters S and P *(90)*. Following these subjects longitudinally, Storandt and coworkers *(91)* found that those who developed early or preclinical Alzheimer's disease over the next 2.5 years had performed less well initially than those who remained nondemented over the same time period. These results are consistent with other researchers who found that lower test scores on initial examination were predictive of subsequent decline *(57,59)*.

Several important longitudinal studies have identified predictors of dementia, particularly, Alzheimer's disease, in preclinical community dwelling elders. The first of these reports came from the Bronx Aging Study where it was reported that 64 of 317 initially nondemented individuals or 20% of their sample, developed dementia over a 4-year period *(92)*. Four neuropsychological test scores were selected from multiple logistic regression procedures to be the most predictive. These included the delayed recall measure from the Selective Reminding Test *(93,94)*, the recall measure from the Fuld Object Memory Evaluation *(80)*, WAIS Digit Symbol *(95)* and Verbal Fluency *(88)*. They also developed an actuarial equation which could predict group membership on an individual basis. This model was able to correctly identify 32 of 64 individuals who developed dementia yielding a sensitivity of 50% and a positive predictive value of 68%. However, 238 of 253 individuals who did not develop dementia were accurately classified yielding a high specificity of 94%. Several limitations to this study have been pointed out. PrAD was not differentiated from other forms of dementia. Second, the findings could not be generalized to groups with different sociodemographic profiles. Third, the results may have been confounded by the use of the same tests for diagnosis and for prediction. However, the actuarial equation was useful in determining who will not go on to develop dementia, therefore accurately identifying "low-risk" groups.

Tierney and colleagues *(59)* found that two independent neuropsychological tests [i.e., delayed recall from the Rey AVLT *(96)* and Mental Control from the WMS *(69)*] could predict with a high degree of accuracy memory-impaired, but not demented, patients who were at high risk for developing PrAD. Through a logistic regression equation, they found that these two tests alone could accurately classify a subgroup of preclinical individuals who went on to develop PrAD with 89% accuracy, 76% sensitivity and 94% specificity. This sample differed from that used in the Bronx study because subjects were already identified as having memory problems over the previous three months (a Global Dementia Score of 2 or 3) *(97)* and referred by their primary care physician for this reason. They were evaluated thoroughly, including the use of neuropsychological tests, and were classified as having a dementia or not. Only those subjects without dementia (i.e., MMSE ≥24; Dementia Rating Scale ≥123 and failure to meet DSM-III-R criteria) were included for further study. At 2 years later, the diagnostic process was repeated: 29 subjects (24%) met criteria for dementia and for PrAD and 94 did not. Similar to the findings of the Canadian Study of Elby *(62)* the group that went on to receive a diagnosis of dementia had lower scores at entry than the cognitively impaired group. The addition of ApoE genotypes did not increase the predictive value beyond that of the neuropsychological test scores *(98)*. This finding differed from that of Petersen and colleagues *(99)* in which ApoE genotype had an effect on the predictive utility of neuropsychological test scores.

It is clear that the preclinical phases of Alzheimer's disease might be characterized by more than just changes in memory. Examining a cohort of nondemented elders in the North Manhattan Aging Project who subsequently developed dementia one year later, Jacobs and associates *(100)* reported changes in confrontation naming, abstract reasoning and delayed memory recall.

Neuropsychological tests of memory and attention were found in other longitudinal studies of normal elder samples to successfully discriminate between those who continued to decline from those whose cognitive functions remained stable over time. Memory measures that were most discriminating included tests of word list recall, facial recognition memory, percent retained from the recall of stories, object function recall, and Paired Associative Learning. The attention tests included Digit Symbol and Digit Span from the Wechsler Intelligence Scales *(57,101)*.

In summary, memory loss is an early symptom of Alzheimer's disease, and most studies examining the neuropsychological characteristics of "at risk" populations have found impairments on memory tasks to differentiate those subjects who progress to a clinical dementia from those who do not *(82,83,101)*. Table 1 summarizes the studies providing neuropsychological predictors. However, as a number of longitudinal studies suggest, tests of verbal fluency, naming, abstract reasoning and complex attention, in addition to memory measures, may improve the power of prediction in cognitively im-

Table 1
Neuropsychological Studies That Attempted to Establish Test Predictors for Discriminating Between Patients With PrAD From Normal Controls

Author (Ref.)	Distinguish Normal Controls From PrAD	Distinguish Nondemented Elders at Risk for Dementia or PrAD	Distinguish Nondemented but Cognitively Impaired at Baseline Who Developed PrAD	Test
Storandt et al. 1984 (89)	X			Logical Memory (WMS); Mental Control (WMS); Trail Making A: Word Fluency (letters S and P)
Fuld et al. 1990 (81)		X		Free Recall on the Fuld Object Memory Test (FOME)
Morris et al. 1991 (9)	X			Logical Memory (WMS); Hard Paired Associates (WMS); Information (WAIS); Boston Naming Test; Trail Making A
Flicker et al. 1991 (56) and 1993 (57)			X	Shopping List-Test of verbal recall; Misplaced Objects Test-Visuospatial recall; Object Function Recognition Task; and Object Identification Task
Bondi et al. 1994 (85)		X	X	Recall on initial learning trials, Delayed Recall, Intrusion Errors, Heightened Recency Effects on the California Verbal Learning Test (CVLT)

180

Study			Tests
Masur et al. 1994 (92)		X	Delayed Recall-Selective Reminding Test (SRT); *Recall (FOME); Digit Symbol-(WAIS-R)*; Verbal Fluency
Petersen et al. 1994 (21)	X		Free and Cued Recall (Selective Reminding Test); Controlled Oral Word Association Test
Petersen et al. 1999 (59a)		X	Free and Cued Recall (Selective Reminding Test); Controlled Oral Word Association Test
Jacobs, et al. 1995 (100)		X	Boston Naming Test; Immediate Recall on the Selective Reminding Test; and Similarities (WAIS-R)
Locascio et al. 1995 (31)		X	Delayed Recall of a Story & Delayed Recall of a Geometric Figure
Linn et al. 1995 (101)		X	Measures of verbal memory (Logical Memory WMS); and Auditory Digit Span
Tierney et al. 1996 (59)		X	Delayed Recall from the Rey AVLT; Mental Control (WMS)
Grober and Kawas, 1996 (30)		X	Free and Cued Recall (Selective Reminding Test)

PrAD, probable Alzheimer's disease; WMS, Wechsler Memory Scale; WAIS, Wechsler Adult Intelligence Scale; CVLT, California Verbal Learning Test; WAIS-R, Wechsler Adult Intelligence Scale-Revised paired normal elders who go on to develop a frank dementia state *(57,92,100,101)*. Yet, others suggest that the combination of a biologic assay such as ApoE or the Pupil Dilation Test in conjunction with neuropsychological testing may provide for the best prediction of early, preclinical Alzheimer's disease *(6,99,103)*.

Challenges Facing Early Diagnosis

Early detection of cognitive change that heralds Alzheimer's disease poses some challenging obstacles. Early symptoms of dementia are commonly overlooked because they are relatively mild, do not call for immediate medical attention and are commonly discarded as signs of old age, fatigue, poor physical health or depression, even by primary care physicians. When a patient is initially evaluated for dementia with neuropsychological tests, it is exceedingly rare to have preexisting baseline tests for comparison. While most elderly people will have had prior measures of other health indicators (e.g., measures of blood pressure, cardiac function, pulmonary function, blood tests) as a matter of routine heath care, very few individuals will have had prior cognitive testing unless there was a specific problem in the past (including early learning disabilities or prior impairment of cognitive functions). Estimates of prior level of functioning can be derived but these can be quite imprecise especially in patients with limited education. This is especially a problem for evaluating patients with superior levels of intellectual functioning who may obtain test scores in the average range but for whom this level of performance constitutes a decline.

Another challenge to identifying serious cognitive decline is that there are substantial individual differences in the course of cognitive aging *(15,17,18)*. Changes in test scores over time may be normal for one individual but abnormal for another. The lack of screening instruments that are sensitive to mild cognitive symptoms in very early stages poses yet another problem. Early cognitive decline can be very insidious and hard to detect with the instruments available to primary care physicians, such as the Mini Mental State Examination *(74)*, the Blessed Dementia Scale *(75)*, or the 7 Minute Screen *(79a)*. These tests are convenient and do not require special expertise for administration. However, even the most astute general practitioner will fail to detect an incipient dementia in the individual with a very high premorbid level of ability who may be experiencing subjective symptoms of decline but who may obtain a normal score on these screening tests of mental state. Thus, early detection requires careful neuropsychological examination by a professional with the clinical expertise to recognize patterns that depart from normality. Even for the expert neuropsychologist, however, early detection can still pose problems in the patient with low IQ or limited education. Many of the standard instruments have not been adequately normed on older subjects stratified according to levels of education, race, gender, or social and cultural factors although this problem is being addressed *(102,104–106)*.

Finally, even if there existed the ideal cognitive screening test, the presence of dementia may be marked not by cognitive decline but by changes in mood, personality, and comportment (i.e., judgment, decision-making, social inappropriateness), all complex behavioral functions for which we have no suitable tests. Despite these seemingly daunting obstacles, however, this chapter has demonstrated the benefits of neuropsychological assessment for detecting early Probable Alzheimer's Disease.

Acknowledgments

Dr. Rentz has been supported by a grant from Johnson & Johnson Company to Brigham & Women's Hospital. Dr. Weintraub is supported in part by an Alzheimer's Disease Core Center grant (NSIP,30AG-13854-01) from the National Institute on Aging to Northwestern University.

References

1. Evans DA, Funkenstein HH, Albert MS, Scheer PA, Cook NC, Chown MJ, Hebert LE, Hennekens CH, Taylor JO. Prevalence of Alzheimer's disease in a community population of older persons: higher than previously reported. *JAMA* 1989;262: 2551–2556.
2. Herbert LE, Scherr PA, Beckett LA, Albert MS, Pilgrim DM, Chown MJ, Funkenstein HH, Evans DA. Age-specific incidence of Alzheimer's disease in a community population. *JAMA* 1995;273:1354–1359.
3. Saunders AM, Strittmatter WJ, Schmechel D, et al. Association of apolipoprotein E allele E4 with late onset familial and sporadic Alzheimer's disease. *Neurology* 1993;43:1467–1472.
4. Motter R, Vigo-Pelfrey C, Kholodenko D, Barnour R, Johnson-Wood K, Galasko D, Chang L, Miller B, Clark C, Green R, Olson D, Southwick P, Wolfert R, Munroe B, Lieberburg I, Seubert P, Schenk D. Reduction of β-amyloid peptide$_{42}$ in the cerebrospinal fluid of patients with Alzheimer's disease. *Ann. Neurol.* 1995; 38:643–648.
5. Arai H, Terajima M, Miura M, Higuchi S, Muramatsu T, Machida N, Seiki H, Takase S, Clark CM, Lee V, Trojanowski JQ, Sasaki H. Tau in cerebrospinal fluid: a potential diagnostic marker for Alzheimer's disease. *Ann. Neurol.* 1995;38: 649–652.
6. Scinto LFM, Daffner KR, Dressler D, Ransil BJ, Rentz D, Weintraub S, Mesulam M-M, Potter H. A potential noninvasive neurobiological test for Alzheimer's disease. *Science* 1994;226:1051–1054.
7. Katzman R, Terry R, DeTeresa R, Brown T, Davies P, Fuld P, Renbing X, Peck A. Clinical, pathological and neurochemical changes in dementia: a subgroup with preserved mental status and numerous neocortical plaques. *Ann. Neurol.* 1988; 23:138–144.

8. Crystal H, Dickson,D, Fuld P, Masur D, Scott R, Mehler M, Masdeu J, Kawas C, Aronson M, Wolfson L. Clinico-pathologic studies in dementia: nondemented subjects with pathologically confirmed Alzheimer's disease. *Neurology* 1988;38:1682–1687.

9. Morris JC, McKeel DW, Storandt M, Rubin EH, Price L, Grant EA, Ball MJ, Berg L. Very mild Alzheimer's disease: informant-based clinical, psychometric and pathologic distinction from normal aging. *Neurology* 1991;41:469–478.

10. Rinn WE. Mental decline in normal aging: a review. *J. Geriatr Psychiatry Neurol.* 1988;1,144–158.

11. LaRue A. Cognition in normal aging. In Puente AE, Reynolds CR, editors. *Critical Issues in Neuropsychology: Aging and Neuropsychological Assessment..* New York: Plenum, 1992:47–75.

12. Botwinick J. Intellectual abilities. In Birren J, Schaie KW, editors. *Handbook of the Psychology of Aging.* New York: Van Nostrand Reinhold, 1977:580–605.

13. Storandt M. Age, ability level and method of administering and scoring the WAIS. *J. Gerontol.* 1977;32:175–178.

14. Albert MS, Heaton RK. Intelligence testing. In Albert MS, Moss MB, editors. *Geriatric Neuropsychology.* New York: Guilford Press,1988:13–32.

15. Schaie KW. The Seattle Longitudinal Study: a 21 year exploration of psychometric intelligence in adulthood. In Schaie KW, editor. *Longitudinal Studies of Adult Psychological Development.* New York: Guilford Press, 1983.

16. Benton AL, Eslinger PJ, Damasio AR. Normative observations on neuropsychological test performances in old age. *J. Clin. Neuropsychol.* 1981;3:33–4.

17. Weintraub S, Powell DH, Whitla DK. Successful cognitive aging: individual differences among physicians on a computerized test of mental state. *J. Geriatr. Psychiatry* 1994;28:15–34.

18. Nelson EA, Dannefer D. Aged heterogeneity: fact or fiction?—the fate of diversity in gerontological research. *Gerontologist* 1992;32:17–23.

19. Sliwinski M, Lipton RB, Bushke H, Stewart W. The effects of preclinical dementia on estimates of normal cognitive functioning in aging. *J. Gerontol.* 1996;51:218–225.

20. Salthouse TA. *Theoretical Perspectives on Cognitive Aging.* Hillsdale, NJ: Lawrence Earlbaum Associates, 1991.

21. Petersen RC, Smith G, Kokmen E, Ivnik RH, Tangalos EG. Memory function in normal aging. *Neurology* 1992;42:396–401.

22. Peterson RC, Smith GE, Ivnik RJ, Kokmen E, Tangalos EG. Memory function in very early Alzheimer's disease. *Neurology* 1994;44:867–872.

23. Branconnier RJ, Cole JO, Spera KF, De Vitt DR. Recall and recognition as diagnostic indices of malignant memory loss in senile dementia: a Bayesian analysis. *Exp. Aging Res.* 1982;8:189–193.

24. McKhann G, Drachman D, Folstein M, Katzman R, Price D, Stadlan EM. Clinical diagnosis of Alzheimer's disease: report of the NINCDS-ADRDA work group under the auspices of the Department of Health and Human Services Task Force on Alzheimer's Disease. *Neurology* 1984;34:939–944.

25. Boller F, Lopez OL, Moosy J. Diagnosis of dementia: clinicopathological correlations. *Neurology* 1989;29,76–79.

26. Khachaturian ZS. Diagnosis of Alzheimer's disease. *Arch. Neurol.* 1985;42: 1097–1105.

27. Wade JP, Mirsen TR, Hachinski VC, Fisman M, Lau C, Merskey H. The clinical diagnosis of Alzheimer's disease. *Arch. Neurol.* 1987;44:24–29.
28. Price BH, Gurvit H, Weintraub S, Geula C, Leimkuhler E, Mesulam M-M. Neuropsychological patterns and language deficits in twenty consecutive cases of autopsy-confirmed Alzheimer's disease. *Arch. Neurol.* 1993;50:931–937.
29. Robinson-Whelen S, Storandt M. Immediate and delayed prose recall among normal and demented adults. *Arch. Neurol.* 1992;49:32–34.
30. Grober E, Kawas C. Learning and retention in preclinical and early Alzheimer's disease. *J. Int. Neuropsychol. Soc.* 1996;2:12.
31. Locascio JJ, Growden JH, Corkin S. Cognitive test performance in detecting, staging and tracking Alzheimer's disease. *Arch. Neurol.* 1995;52:1087–1099.
32. Welsh KA, Butters N, Hughes J, Mohs R, Heyman A. Detection of abnormal memory decline in mild cases of Alzheimer's disease using CERAD neuropsychological measures. *Arch. Neurol.* 1991;48:278–281.
33. Welsh KA, Butters N, Hughes JP, Mohs RC, Heyman A. Detection and staging of dementia in Alzheimer's disease. *Arch. Neurol.* 1992;49:448–452.
34. Morris JC, Edland S, Clark C, Galasko D, Koss E, Mohs R, van Belle G, Fillenbaum G, Heyman A. The Consortium to Establish a Registry for Alzheimer's Disease (CERAD). Part IV. Rates of cognitive change in the longitudinal assessment of probable Alzheimer's disease. *Neurology* 1993;43: 2457–2465.
35. Eslinger PJ, Damasio AR. Preserved motor learning in Alzheimer's disease: implications for anatomy and behavior. *J. Neurosci.* 1986;6:3006–3009.
36. Moscovitch M. Multiple dissociations of function in amnesia. In Cermak LS, editor. *Human Memory and Amnesia.* Hillsdale, NJ.: Erlbaum, 1982:337–370.
37. Faber-Langendoen K, Morris JC, Knesevich JW, LaBarge E, Miller JP, Berg L. Aphasia in senile dementia of the Alzheimer's type. *Ann. Neurol.* 1988;23:365–370.
38. Cummings JL, Benson DF, Hill MA, Read S. Aphasia in dementia of the Alzheimer type. *Neurology* 1985;35:394–397.
39. Kirshner H, Webb W, Kelly M, Wells CE. The naming disorder of dementia. *Neuropsychologia* 1984;22:23–30.
40. Hier DB, Hagenlocker K, Shindler AG. Language disintegration in dementia: effects of etiology and severity. *Brain Lang.* 1985;25:117–133.
41. Martin A, Fedio P. Word production and comprehension in Alzheimer's disease: the breakdown of semantic knowledge. *Brain Lang.* 1983;19:124–141.
42. Knesevich JW, LaBarge E, Edwards D. Predictive value of the Boston Naming Test in mild senile dementia of the Alzheimer type. *Psychol. Res.*1986;19:155–161.
43. Snowdon DA, Kemper SJ, Mortimer JA, Greiner LH, Wekstein DR, Markesbery WR. Linguistic ability in early life and cognitive function and Alzheimer's disease in late life. *JAMA* 1996;275:528–532.
44. Morris JC, Fulling K. Early Alzheimer's disease. *Arch. Neurol.* 1988;45:345–349.
45. Kaszniak AW, Garron DC, Fox J. Differential effects of age and cerebral atrophy upon span of immediate recall and paired associate learning in older patients with suspected dementia. *Cortex* 1979;15:285–295.
46. Trenerry MR, Crosson B, DeBoe J, Leber WR. *Stroop Neuropsychological Screening Test.* Odessa, FL: Psychological Assessment Resources, 1989.

47. Reitan RM. Validity of the Trail Making Test as an indication of organic brain damage. *Percept. Mot. Skills* 1958;8: 271–276.

48. Grady CL, Haxby JV, Horwitz B, Sundaram G, Berg M, Schapiro M, Freidland RP, Raporport SI. A longitudinal study of the early neuropsychological and cerebral metabolic changes in dementia of the Alzheimer's type. *J. Clin. Exp. Neuropsychol.* 1988;10:576–596.

49. Grady CL, Grimes AM, Patronas N, Sunderland T, Foster NL, Rapoport SI. Divided attention, as measured by dichotic speech performance, in dementia of the Alzheimer type. *Arch. Neurol.* 1989;46:317–320.

50. Benton AL, deS Hamsher K, Varney NR, Spreen O. *Contributions to Neuropsychological Assessment.* New York: Oxford University Press,1983.

51. Weintraub S, Mesulam M-M. Four neuropsychological profiles in dementia. *Handb. Neuropsychol.* 1993;8:253–282.

52. Benson DF, Davis J, Snyder BD. Posterior cortical atrophy. *Arch. Neurol.* 1988;45:789–793.

53. Lawton M, Brody E. Assessment of older people: self-maintaining and instrumental activities of daily living. *Gerontologist* 1969;9:179–186.

54. Weintraub S. The Record of Independent Living: an informant-completed measure of activities of daily living and behavior in elderly patients with cognitive impairment. *Am. J. Alzheimer Care* 1986;1:35–39.

55. Loewenstein DA, Amigo E, Duara R, Guterman A, Hurwitz D, Berkowitz N, Wilkie F, Weinberg G, Black B, Gittelman B, Eisdorfer C. A new scale for the assessment of functional status in Alzheimer's disease and related disorders. *J. Gerontol.* 1989;44:P114–121.

56. Flicker C, Ferris SH, Reisberg B. Mild cognitive impairment in the elderly: predictors of dementia. *Neurology* 1991;41:1006–1009.

57. Flicker C, Ferris SH, Reisberg B. A two-year longitudinal study of cognitive function in normal aging and Alzheimer's disease. *J. Geriatr. Psychiatry Neurol.*1993; 34:294–295.

58. O'Neill D, Surmon DJ, Wilcock GK. Longitudinal diagnosis of memory disorders. *Age Ageing* 1992;21:393–397.

59. Tierney MC, Szalai JP, Snow WG, Fisher RH, Nores A, Nadon G, Dunn E, St. George-Hyslop PH. Prediction of probable Alzheimer's disease in memory-impaired patients: a prospective longitudinal study. *Neurology* 1996;46:661–665.

59a. Petersen RC, Smith GE, Waring SC, Ivnik RJ, Tangalos EG, Kokmen E. Mild cognitive impairment: clinical characterization and outcome. *Arch Neurol.* 1999; 56:303–308.

60. Flicker C, Ferris SH, Reisberg B. A longitudinal study of cognitive function in elderly persons with subjective memory complaints. *J. Am. Geriatr. Soc.* 1993;41: 1029–1032.

61. Malec JF, Smith GE, Ivnik RJ, Petersen RC, Tangalos EG. Clusters of impaired normal elderly do not decline cognitively in 3 to 5 years. *Neuropsychology* 1996;1:66–73.

62. Elby EM, Hogan DB, Parhad IM. Cognitive impairment in the nondemented elderly: results from the Canadian Study of Health and Aging. *Arch. Neurol.* 1995;52:612–619.

63. Gutierrez R, Atkinson JH, Grant I. Mild neurocognitive disorder: needed addition to the nosology of cognitive impairment (organic mental) disorders. *J. Neuropsychol. Clin. Neurosci.* 1993;5:161–177.

64. Elias MF, Wolf PA, D'Agostino RB, Cobb J, White LR. Untreated blood pressure level is inversely related to cognitive functioning: the Framingham study. *Am. J. Epidemiol.* 1993;138:353–364.

65. Crook T, Bartus RT, Ferris SH, Whitehouse P, Cohen GD, Gershon SG. Age-associated memory impairment: proposed diagnostic criteria and measures of clinical change: report of a National Institute of Mental Health Work Group. *Dev. Neuropsychol.* 1986;2:261–276.

66. Blackford RC, LaRue A. Criteria for diagnosing age-associated memory impairment; proposed improvement from the field. *Dev. Neuropsychol.* 1989;5:295–306.

66a. Petersen RC, Smith GE, Waring SC, Ivnik RJ, Kokmen E, Tangalos EG. Aging, memory, and mild cognitive impairment. *Int. Psychogeriatr.* 1997;9:65–69.

67. Zaudig M. A new systematic method of measurement and diagnosis of "mild cognitive impairment" and dementia according to ICD-10 and DSM-III-R criteria. *Int. Psychogeriatr.* 1992;4:203–219.

68. Kral VA. Senescent forgetfulness: benign and malignant. *Can. Med. Assoc. J.* 1962;86:257–260.

69. Wechsler D, Stone CP. *Wechsler Memory Scale.* New York: Psychological Corporation, 1973.

70. McGlone J, Gupta S, Humphrey D, Oppenheimer S, Mirsen T, Evans DR. Screening for early dementia using memory complaints from patients and relatives. *Arch. Neurol.* 1990;47:1189–1193.

71. Schmand B, Jonker C, Hooijer C, Lindeboom J. Subjective memory complaints may announce dementia. *Neurology* 1996;46:121–125.

72. Small GW, LaRue A, Komo S, Kaplan A, Mandelkern MA. Predictors of cognitive change in middle-aged and older adults with memory loss. *Am. J. Psychiatry* 1995;152:1757–1764.

73. Tierney MC, Szalai JP, Snow WG, Fisher RH. The prediction of Alzheimer's disease: the role of patient and informant perceptions of cognitive deficits. *Arch. Neurol.* 1996;53:423–427.

74. Folstein MF, Folstein SE, McHugh PR. Mini-Mental State: a practical method for grading the cognitive state of patients for the clinician. *J. Psychiat. Res.* 1975;12: 189–198.

75. Blessed G, Tomlinson BE, Roth M. The association between quantitative measures of dementia and of senile change in the cerebral grey matter of elderly subjects. *Br. J. Psychiatry* 1968;114:797–811.

76. Katzman R, Aronson MK, Fuld PA. Development of dementing illness in an 80-year-old volunteer cohort. *Ann. Neurol.* 1989;25:317–324.

77. Kokmen E, Smith GE, Petersen RC, Tangalos E, Ivnik RJ. The short test of mental status: correlations with standardized psychometric testing. *Arch. Neurol.* 1991;48:725–728.

78. Thal LJ, Grundman M, Golden R. Alzheimer's disease: a correlational analysis of the Blessed Information-Memory-Concentration Test and the Mini-Mental State Examination. *Neurology* 1986;36:262–264.

79. Rentz DM, Calvo VL, Scinto LFM, Sperling RA, Budson AE, Daffner KR. Detecting early cognitive decline in high functioning elders. *J Geriatr Psych.* In Press.

79a. Solomon PR, Herschoff A, Kelly B, Relin M, Brush M, De Veaux RD, Pendleburg WW. A 7 Minute Neurocognitive Screening Battery Highly Sensitive to Alzheimer's Disease. *Arch Neurol.* 1998;55:349–355.

80. Fuld PA. *The Fuld Object Memory Evaluation.* Chicago, IL: Stoelting Instrument Company, 1981.

81. Fuld PA, Masur DM, Blau AD, Crystal H, Aronson MK. Object memory evaluation for prospective detection of dementia in normal functioning elderly: predictive and normative data. *J. Clin. Exp. Neuropsychol.* 1990;12:520–528.

82. Masur D, Fuld PA, Blau AD, Thal LJ, Levin HS, Aronson MK. Distinguishing normal and demented elderly with the Selective Reminding Test. *J. Clin. Exp. Neuropsychol.* 1989;11:615–630.

83. Masur DM, Fuld PA, Blau AD, Crystal H, Aronson MK. Predicting development of dementia in the elderly with the Selective Reminding Test. *J. Clin. Exp. Neuropsychol.* 1990;12:529–538.

84. Delis DC, Kramer JH, Kaplan E, Ober BA. *The California Verbal Learning Test.* New York: Psychological Corporation, 1987.

85. Bondi M., Monsch AU, Galasko D, Butters N, Salmon DP and Delis DC. Preclinical cognitive markers of dementia of the Alzheimer type. *Neuropsychology* 1994;8:374–384.

86. Knopman DS, Ryberg S. A verbal memory test with high predictive accuracy for dementia of the Alzheimer type. *Arch. Neurol.* 1989;46:131–145.

87. Nordin S, Murphy C. Impaired sensory and cognitive olfactory function in questionable Alzheimer's disease. *Neuropsychology* 1996;10:113–119.

88. Monsch AU, Bondi MW, Butters N, Salmon DP, Katzman R, Thal LJ. Comparisons of verbal fluency tasks in the detection of dementia of the Alzheimer type. *Arch. Neurol.* 1992;49:1253–1258.

89. Storandt M, Botwinick J, Danziger WL, Berg L, Hughes CP. Psychometric differetiation of mild senile dementia of the Alzheimer type. *Arch. Neurol.* 1984;41:497–499.

90. Thurston LL, Thurston TG. *Examiner Manual for the SRA Primary Mental Abilities Test.* Chicago, IL: Science Research Associates, 1949.

91. Storandt M, Botwinick J, Danziger WL. Longitudinal changes: patients with mild SDAT and matched healthy controls. In Poon LW, editor. *Handbook For Clinical Memory Assessment of Older Adults.* Hyattsville, MD: American Psychological Association, 1989:277–284.

92. Masur DM, Sliwinski M, Lipton RB, Blau AD, Crystal HA. Neuropsychological prediction of dementia and the absence of dementia in healthy elderly persons. *Neurology* 1994;44:1427–1432.

93. Bushke H. Selective reminding analysis of memory and learning. *J. Verb. Learn. Behav.* 1973;12:543–550.

94. Bushke H, Fuld PA. Evaluating storage, retention, and retrieval in disordered memory and learning. *Neurology,* 1974;24:1019–1025.

95. Wechsler D. *Manual for the Wechsler Adult Intelligence Scale.* New York: Psychological Corporation, 1955.

96. Lezak M. *Neuropsychological Assessment.* 2nd ed. New York: Oxford University Press, 1982.
97. Reisberg B, Ferris SH, deLeon MJ, Crook T. The Global Deterioration Scale for assessment of primary degenerative dementia. *Am. J. Psychiatry* 1982;139:1136–1139.
98. Tierney MC, Szalai JP, Snow WG, Fisher RH, Tsuda T, Chi H, McLachlan DR, St. George-Hyslop PH. A prospective study of the clinical utility of ApoE genotyping in the prediction of outcome in patients with memory impairment. *Neurology* 1996;46:149–154.
99. Petersen RC, Smith GE, Ivnik RJ, Tangalos EG, Schaid DJ, Thibodeau SN, Kokmen E, Warig SC. Apolipoprotein E status as a predictor of the development of Alzheimer's disease in memory-impaired individuals. *JAMA* 1995;273:1274–1278.
100. Jacobs DM, Sano M, Dooneief G, Marder K, Bell KL, Stern Y. Neuropsychological detection and characterization of preclinical Alzheimer's disease. *Neurology* 1995;45:957–962.
101. Linn RT, Wolf PA, Backman DL, Knoefel JE, Cobb JL, Belanger AJ, Kaplan EF, D'Agostino RB. The "preclinical phase" of probable Alzheimer's disease. *Arch. Neurol.* 1995;52:485–490.
102. Tuokko H, Woodward TS. Development and validation of a demographic correction system for neuropsychological measures used in the Canadian Study on Health and Aging. *J. Clin. Exp. Neuropsychol.* 1996;18:479–616.
103. Smith GE, Ivnik RJ, Malec JF, Thibodeau SN. Mayo Cognitive Factor scale scores and APO-E status in normal controls in probable Alzheimer's patients. *Clin. Neuropsychol.* 1994;8:354.
104. Ivnik RJ, Malec JF, Smith GE, Tangalos EG, Petersen RC, Kokmen E, Kurland LT. Mayo's older Americans normative studies, WAIS-R, Wechsler Memory Scale-Revised and AVLT norms for ages 56 through 97. *Clin. Neuropsychol.* 1992; 6(Suppl):1–104.
105. Ivnik RJ, Malec JF, Smith GE, Tangalos EG, Petersen O. Neuropsychological test norms above age 55: COWAT, BNT, MAE Token, WRAT-R Reading, AMNART, STROOP, TMT and JLO. *Clin. Neuropsychol.* 1996;10:262–278.
106. Richardson ED, Marottoli RA. Education-specific normative data on common neuropsychological indices for individuals older than 75 years. *Clin. Neuropsychol.* 1996;10:375–381.

9

Peripheral Markers of Alzheimer's Disease

Directions From the Alzheimer Pathogenic Pathway

Maire E. Percy, David F. Andrews, and Huntington Potter

INTRODUCTION

The development of tests that will indicate the presence of Alzheimer's disease (AD), or that will identify persons who are at very high risk of developing AD at an early potentially reversible stage, is driven by clinical needs and research interests. There is evidence that brain changes leading to AD may begin more than four decades before the appearance of clinical symptoms *(267,361)*. For this reason, there is optimism that it will be possible to develop tools to detect AD before symptoms have progressed to the point where they meet the criteria for probable AD (symptomatic markers), identify persons at highest risk for developing clinical manifestations of AD (preclinical markers), and to monitor the progression of AD so that treatments to slow down the course of AD (ultimately, to prevent it) can be developed and evaluated. Such tools have the potential for substantial cost-savings at many different levels. Furthermore, they would aid clinical trials of drug treatments by simplifying the selection and subgrouping of study participants and by enabling the effects of drug treatments to be measured objectively. Aside from possible clinical application, efforts to develop earlier tests for AD are increasing our understanding of the aberrant biological processes that result in AD, information that will help with the rational development of treatment.

Biological processes, factors, or chemicals that are expressed aberrantly in a particular disease are referred to as *biomarkers* of the disease. Measurements of a wide variety of biomarkers are currently being evaluated as tools for the earlier diagnosis of AD. In the AD field, some researchers are focusing on biomarkers that are known to reflect the underlying disease process.

From: *Early Diagnosis of Alzheimer's Disease*
Edited by L. F. M. Scinto & K. R. Daffner © Humana Press, Inc., Totowa, NJ

Others are studying phenomenological correlates of AD with the hope that they will be informative. There are several important components in biomarker research. First the biomarker should be connected to the disease in a rational way. They must be evaluated to determine if they are symptomatic or predictive. Second, biomarker studies require the collection of valid and reliable data. Assurance must be provided that measures of biomarkers are not affected by factors purely technical. Finally, biomarker data must be interpreted appropriately. The challenge at hand is to be able to distinguish persons with AD at an incipient stage not only from healthy normal individuals but from others with neurological and nonneurological disorders that can mask as AD at an early stage of development.

This chapter begins with an overview of general considerations in biomarker studies. Risk factors for AD and the pathogenesis of AD have been reviewed to emphasize the complexity of AD and to explain at least in part why AD is expressed systemically as well as in the central nervous system. Biomarkers that may be relatively specific to AD [such as neuronal thread protein, tau, and a specific form of amyloid-β protein (Aβ)], as well as markers that may reflect a relatively nonpecific response to injury in the central nervous system (CNS) (such as certain indicators of the acute phase response and inflammatory markers) and other correlates of AD are discussed and critically assessed. The potential of biomarker testing in AD is compared with the demonstrated potential of clinical dementia test batteries and brain imaging. The chapter concludes with an approach for using different types of information in combination for the earlier diagnosis of definite AD.

General Considerations in Biomarker Studies

Criteria of a Biomarker for AD

A biomarker for AD may have several uses including diagnosis, population screening, predictive testing, monitoring progression or response to treatment, and studying brain-behavior relationships. After an association between a biomarker and AD has been established, the biomarker must be evaluated to determine if it is an indicator and/or a predictor of AD, and if it is useful in all types of AD and at all stages. Ideally, a biomarker for AD should be connected in a known way to AD brain pathology and be able to detect AD early in its course and to distinguish it from other dementias. It should be quick, easy, reliable, inexpensive to perform, and safe and acceptable to the persons being tested as well as to clinicians. It is considered unlikely that a single biomarker will be able to fulfill all of these criteria *(385)*.

Characterization of the Performance of Diagnostic Tests

In order to interpret a biomarker test result, one needs to know what is the probability of definite AD given a positive test result, and what is the probability that the disease is absent if the test is negative, as discussed in Chapter 1. Mayeux *(244)* has summarized the terms that are used to characterize the performance of a diagnostic test. The prior probability is defined as the frequency of the disease in the particular group of patients being investigated. If this group includes all affected individuals in a particular region, then the frequency is equivalent to the prevalence. The terms *sensitivity* and *specificity* describe the accuracy of the test. Sensitivity is defined as the percentage of individuals with the disease whose test results are positive, and specificity refers to the percentage of individuals without the disease whose test results are negative. The predictive values (positive and negative) describe the probability of disease. Positive predictive value (PPV) is the percentage of people with positive test results who actually have the disease. This indicates how likely it is that the disease is present if the test result is positive. Negative predictive value (NPV) is the percentage of people with negative test results who do not have the disease. Mathematical definitions of the terms used to describe the performance of a diagnostic test are given in Table 1. In the section "Tests in Combination for the Earlier Detection of AD," a strategy for calculating the probability that a person with a collection of suspicious symptoms of AD actually has definite AD is presented.

Sources of Variability in Biomarker Tests

Introduction

Biomarkers can be affected by biological and technical factors other than the disease in question. In this section we draw attention to factors that might result in variability of biomarker expression in AD.

Subject Age, Gender, Genetic Risk Factors, Ethnic Background, and Family History

Measures of biological parameters frequently are affected by subject age and gender. Furthermore, age and gender effects can be different in patients and healthy normal individuals used as "controls." Ideally, age and gender effects should be established for healthy control individuals and patients. One way of minimizing age and gender effects is to pair each case with a control individual that is matched with respect to gender and age. If there is reason to believe that ethnic background will affect the biomarker, then this parameter

Table 1
Definitions of Terms Encountered in the Evaluation and Use of Diagnostic Tests

A. Comparison of results of a diagnostic test with the true disease state

	The True Situation	
Test Result	Disease	No Disease
Positive	a: True positive	b: False positive
Negative	c: False negative	d: True negative
Population	Patients	Nonpatients

B. Prior probability, sensitivity and specificity

$$\text{Prior probability} = \frac{\text{true positives} + \text{false negatives}}{\text{total population}}$$

$$\text{Sensitivity} = \frac{\text{true positives } (a)}{\text{true positives } (a) + \text{false negatives } (c)}$$

$$\text{Specificity} = \frac{\text{true negatives } (d)}{\text{true negatives } (d) + \text{false positives } (b)}$$

C. Positive and negative predictive value

$$\text{Positive predictive value (PPV)} = \frac{\text{true positives } (a)}{\text{true positives } (a) + \text{false positives } (b)}$$

$$\text{Negative predictive value (NPV)} = \frac{\text{true negatives } (d)}{\text{true negatives } (d) + \text{false negatives } (c)}$$

After ref. 244.

also should be factored in and controlled for *(181,324)*. In carrier detection studies, family history of a particular disorder has been shown to affect the predictive power of a biological test result *(295)*. In the development of direct tests for AD, subject age and gender and any available genetic information (e.g., family history of AD or lack of it; age at onset of AD), or knowledge of specific genetic markers to which AD is linked or associated—positively or negatively) likewise could be evaluated as explanatory variables *(292)*. (An example of how such information might be used in earlier AD diagnostics is given in the section "Tests in Combination for the Earlier Detection of AD.") It is known that increasing subject age is the strongest risk factor for AD. Compared to males, females have a 2 to 3-fold increased risk of developing AD *(171,345,384)*. A recent longitudinal study of subjects age 75 years and older has shown that a family history of AD increases the rate of cognitive decline independently of the apolipoprotein E ε4 (ApoE 4) allele, which presently is thought to be the most significant genetic risk factor for AD *(292,326–328,333)*.

Inclusion/Exclusion Criteria

The specification of criteria for selecting study participants is of great importance. Ideally, participants should be recruited in a random fashion, and inclusion/exclusion criteria and other relevant characteristics should be described in sufficient detail so that the study population can be replicated by another group. A dilemma in studies of prevalent diseases in which subject age is a risk factor is whether the reference group should consist of relatively young individuals who are likely to be free of disease, or age-matched individuals of whom a significant proportion actually may have the disease in question! Alternatively, persons in the reference population might be screened for signs of disease and excluded from the study. Researchers must be aware of the consequences of the nature of the control group(s) on interpretation of their data.

Environmental Factors

As biological parameters can vary in a diurnal fashion or be affected by season of the year, cases and control individuals should be tested under parallel conditions *(77,132,297)*. The level of recent physical activity or degree of psychological stress sometimes can affect results and should be noted *(423)*. Information about current health status (including medications the participant is taking) should be collected, since these can affect levels of biomarkers *(301)*. Because every test is associated with some degree of intraperson variation, it is necessary to determine whether adequate information can be obtained with one test on each individual, whether repeated independent measurements using the same test are necessary, or whether measures of different independent tests should be combined to increase the sensitivity and/or specificity to the desired level *(299)*. Test results can be interpreted in terms of the results found in a "normal" population. A convenient way of expressing a test result is to convert it into Z scores (i.e., the number of standard deviations away from the mean of the reference population). In longitudinal studies, test values of each individual at the beginning of the study can be used as reference *(306)*.

Technical Factors

AD biomarkers include blood, cerebrospinal fluid (CSF), or urine tests that can be affected by many factors. For example, in the case of blood tests, protocols for collecting, transporting, processing, storing, and assaying samples must be specified and rigorously adhered to for both cases and controls *(295)*.

Factors that can affect measures of biological substances in plasma include the gauge of the needle used to draw the blood (this must be sufficiently large to prevent distortion of blood cells), type of anticoagulant and/or tube used for collection of the blood, nature and duration of sample storage before processing (chilling blood will leach components out of cells and solidify lipids), the *g*-force and duration of centrifugation used for recovery of the plasma, temperature at which the centrifugation is done, the type of pipette used to harvest the plasma (glass pipettes will trigger clotting), the type of vial used for storing sample aliquots, and the conditions for storing the processed sample prior to analysis (i.e., refrigerated, frozen at −20°C or −80°C, duration). The addition of stabilizing buffers and/or a protease inhibitor cocktail to any biological fluid or extract which is at risk of losing its activity or of becoming proteolytically degraded in vitro is strongly recommended. Finally, multiple freeze–thaw cycles are to be avoided.

If a test is based on analysis of cultured cells, important factors that might affect results are characteristics of the cell donor (i.e., gender, age, type/stage of AD), whether the culture is primary or secondary, and the passage number (how many times the cells have been allowed to divide before they are assayed). The number of divisions an untransformed cell culture can undergo before they begin to die is inversely proportional to the age of the cell donor *(133)*. If the cells are transformed, the nature of the transforming agent (e.g., chemical or viral) may be important. For data interpretation, researchers must be aware that cultures can easily become contaminated by droplets containing rapidly growing transformed cells such as HeLa *(280)*. (The HeLa cell line was originally established from a human uterine carcinoma; it contains DNA from human papillomavirus type 18.) Details of the culture conditions (type of culture medium, percentage of fetal calf serum added, internal incubator temperature, the incubator atmosphere, cell concentration, whether replenishment of the culture medium requires disbursement or centrifugation of the cells, the size of the flask, the amount of medium in the flask), and how long the cells were in logarithmic growth before the experiment, are some other important factors that can affect gene expression, growth and physiological properties of cells. For example, it is known that old cell cultures or cells that have been stressed by growth in serum-deficient culture medium will produce excessive amounts of Aβ *(1)*. Researchers must ensure that a potential AD effect on particular properties of cultured cells is not a passage number effect, or an effect of treating AD cells differently than control cells.

It is important to know how reproducible a laboratory screening procedure is. Interassay, intraperson, and interperson coefficients of variation should be determined *(299)*. If interassay coefficients are not reasonable and are not less than the interperson variation, then there may be a problem with the test and/or experimental design which must be investigated *(299)*. Factors known to result in abnormally high interassay coefficients of variation include differences or ranges in ambient temperature or temperature of assay reagents, faulty micropipets, failure to control for the time dependence of an assay (especially in rapid immunoassays in which an antigen–antibody reaction is not allowed to reach equilibrium) *(298)*, the use of "standards," which themselves are not stable or which differ from one laboratory to another, inexperience of the technician conducting the test, or involvement of different technicians in data generation. Preparing reagents with the required degree of accuracy, and working within their limits of stability, also are fundamental to the success of any laboratory assay *(301)*. The validity of a biomarker test (i.e., what exactly is the test measuring) also is of fundamental importance. For example, in immunoassays the specificity of the antibody being used must be demonstrated and appropriate positive and negative standards should be used as reference *(256)*. World Health Organization Standards should be made available for AD testing as they have been for other biomarker assays *(411)*.

Similarly, for neuropsychological, neurobehavioral and other types of testing, the chosen protocols must have documented and adequate test–retest reliability, interrater reliability and validation *(142)*. For any test to work, attention must be paid to quality control.

Statistical Approaches for Data Analysis

Attention to detail in experimental design and analysis is essential. A paired case/control study design and analysis is preferred when a methodological procedure is affected by "environmental factors" *(301)*. For example, because the measurement of superoxide dismutase (SOD) activity in a biological sample is affected by ambient temperature, as well as the oxygen concentration in the lysates and in the assay reagents, the interassay coefficient of variation is large. To minimize such environmental effects, we assayed in parallel red cell extracts from a patient with clinical manifestations of AD and a paired control matched for subject age and gender. To determine if there were an Alzheimer effect on SOD activity, a paired analysis with corrections for gender and age effects was used to test the null hypothesis that the mean difference between pairs of patients and controls was zero *(301)*.

The powerful technique of logistic regression enables populations to be effectively separated on the basis of one or more quantitative, overlapping characteristics. This approach enables multiple independent measurements from one or more tests into a single clinical indicator which then can be combined with family history information to yield the probability that an individual has a particular disease. For example, in order to distinguish female carriers of

Duchenne muscular dystrophy (DMD) on the basis of serum creatine kinase (CK) measurements, we developed a procedure to combine independent serial measurements of CK on individuals into a single index which then was combined with family history information to yield the probability that the individual being tested was a carrier of the DMD gene *(299)*. In order to efficiently distinguish female carriers of hemophilia from healthy normal individuals, logistic coefficients were derived from the ratio of measurements of factor VIII activity (which is defective in hemophilia A) and von Willebrand factor (to which factor VIII binds) into a single index which was combined with family history information to yield the probability that the individual being tested was a carrier of hemophilia A *(300)*.

The construction of receiver operator characteristic (ROC) curves (plots of sensitivity versus corresponding specificity for different cutoff values) enables an observer to see at a glance how different cutoff values affect the sensitivity and specificity of a test, an innovation which is very practical since these two test characteristics are not always equally important in a clinical setting *(67)*.

The application of artificial neural networks (ANNs) may be useful for separating populations on the basis of differing patterns. For example, French and colleagues *(105)* compared the classification abilities of linear discriminant analysis (LDA) using the results of 11 neuropsychological tests as predictors of AD. LDA and ANNs correctly identified 71.9% and 91.1% of cases, respectively. Furthermore, ANNs were more powerful in discriminating severity levels within the dementia population.

Tissues That Should Be Sampled

Biomarker tests should be done on tissues that express the disease in question. In the case of AD, many investigators are evaluating markers in the CSF. CSF is secreted in the brain, primarily by the choroid plexus. Because it exists in steady state with the extracellular fluid surrounding neurons and glia, it is the body fluid most likely to reflect disturbances of the CNS. Although CSF sampling is an invasive procedure that must be done by an experienced clinician, serious side-effects are quite rare. The potential benefits of a CSF test for AD must be balanced against any risks and discomfort associated with the procedure. Some researchers are examining markers in blood, urine, skin, and cell lines derived from blood or skin, although it is not presently clear to what extent changes in the latter tissues reflect disease or metabolic perturbations from predisposing risk factors. Yet others are combining the results of genetic tests with neuropsychological or brain imaging test data *(4,361)*.

Evaluation of a Biomarker

The challenge in AD is to find a biomarker that will distinguish AD from other conditions that mask as AD at the earliest possible stage. The potential of a biomarker for probable AD is initially evaluated from studies of persons with a clinical diagnosis of probable AD and healthy normal individuals. Its positive and negative predictive power based on autopsy diagnosis should then be evaluated. Once a biomarker shows promise in increasing the diagnostic accuracy of probable AD using autopsy diagnosis as a "gold" standard, its value in early or presymptomatic diagnosis should be evaluated in longitudinal studies of individuals with questionable symptoms of AD, and different categories of presymptomatic individuals at high risk for AD. A fundamental problem with such evaluation is that a diagnosis of probable AD in living individuals or of definite AD made on the basis of neuropathological findings alone or in combination with clinical findings, cannot be made with certainty.

Although guidelines exist for the clinical and autopsy diagnosis, both have shortcomings. In as many as 10% to 40% of cases, a clinical diagnosis of AD does not agree with autopsy findings. Part of the problem lies with the clinical diagnosis. Clinical guidelines often do not distinguish between "pure AD" and AD with a mixed pathology that includes vascular dementia and white matter lesions. These guidelines identify two main subgroups of patients: presenile AD with an age of onset <65 years, and senile AD with an age of onset >65 years; the second subgroup can contain a high proportion of "mixed" cases *(402)*. Current clinical guidelines also often do not distinguish between AD and frontotemporal dementia, or Lewy body disease. Furthermore, there is substantial interpathologist disagreement on the interpretation of autopsy findings *(36)*. Thus studies of biomarkers must go hand in hand with improved inclusion/exclusion criteria for study participants and improved guidelines for the clinical and autopsy diagnosis of AD *(164,232)*. The importance of guidelines for the clinical and autopsy diagnosis of AD in biomarker studies cannot be overemphasized.

The Alzheimer Pathogenic Pathway

Risk Factors

Genetic risk factors for AD are discussed in Chapter 5. In the current chapter, genetic and environmental risk factors are summarized in Tables 2 and 3 to emphasize the complex and heterogeneous nature of AD, to remind the reader that some AD biomarkers may be metabolic perturbations resulting from such predisposing risk factors, and to underscore the potential that knowledge of predisposing risk factors for AD might have in its earlier diagnosis.

Table 2
Genetic Markers for Alzheimer Disease

Marker	Uses	Target Population	Accuracy*	Reference
Confirmed Nuclear Genetic Markers				
APP mutations (chromosome 21)	Dx,PREDT	EOFAD	SP: <1 ST: 0.05-0.07	115 270 373
ApoE 4 (chromosome 19)	Dx,PREDT,Rx	LOAD non-PS-1 EOAD		144 245
Clinical diagnosis			SP: 0.55; ST: 0.93	
ApoE 4 alone			SP: 0.68; ST: 0.65	
Clinical diagnosis + ApoE 4			SP: 0.84; ST: 0.61	
PS-1 (or S182) gene mutations (chromosome 14)	Dx,PREDT	EOFAD	SP: 1 ST: 0.70-0.75	11, 270, 350 351
PS-2 (or STM2) gene mutations (chromosome 1)	Dx,PREDT	EOFAD	SP: 1 ST: 0.05-0.20	211 212 322
Nonrandom association between alpha 1-ACT and ApoE loci in women				174, 175
α_2-Macroglobulin deletion (chromosome 12)				23
Transferrin C2 allele (chromosome 3)		LOAD		396
C2 allele frequency is markedly increased in ApoE 4 homozygotes				393 271
Other Reported Nuclear Genetic Markers				
Increased frequency of certain HLA haplotypes and Gm allotypes		EOFAD		408
Association of a rare HLA-linked C4*B2 allele		SDAT		274
Variant chromosome 22p+		one LOFAD kindred		302
HLA DR 1,2,3 variants (protective against AD) (chromosome 6)		LOAD		58

Marker	Disease	Ref.
HLA DR 4,5,6 variants (chromosome 6)	LOAD	58
ApoA-IV-2P variant (chromosome 11)	LOAD	56
LRP genotype (chromosome 12) (involvement is controversial)	LOFAD, LOAD	176,178
Association between butyrylcholinesterase variant K and ApoE 4 variant (controversial)	LOAD	210
HLA-A2 variants (chromosome 6)	EOAD	291
ApoE promoter polymorphism (chromosome 19)	LOAD	201
Tau variants (chromosome 17)	FTDP-17	309 397 148
CYP2D microsatellite polymorphism (chromosome 19)	Lewy body variant of AD	377
Association between PS-1 and α1-ACT genotypes	sporadic AD	405
Unidentified (X chromosome)		426

Possible Mitochondrial DNA Markers

Marker		Ref.
Mitochondrial tRNA 4336G variants:		
Possible association with AD and Parkinson's disease		352
Possible association with AD		83
Somatic mitochondrial 4977 nt deletions (in Alzheimer brains)		147 51
12S mitochondrial rRNA polymophisms		380

201

α_1-ACT, α_1-antichymotrypsin; AD, Alzheimer disease; ApoE, apolipoprotein E; APP, amyloid precursor protein; CYP2D, cytochrome P4502D variant; Dx, diagnostic; EOFAD, early onset familial Alzheimer disease; FTDP-17, frontotemporal dementia and Parkinsonism linked to chromosome 17; G_m allotype, marker on IgG heavy chains; HLA, human leukocyte antigens; LOAD, late onset Alzheimer disease; LOFAD, late onset familial Alzheimer disease; LRP, an apolipoprotein E receptor; PREDT, predictive; PS-1 and PS-2, presenilin 1 and 2; rRNA, ribosomal RNA; Rx, treatment; SDAT, senile dementia of the Alzheimer type; SP, specificity; ST, sensitivity.
*Information about diagnostic accuracy from ref. 321.

Table 3
Other Risk Factors for Alzheimer Disease Including Environmental Risk Factors and Genetic/Environmental Interactions

Category	Likely Relative Risk or Probability That Association of Risk Factor Is Due to Chance	Reference
Old age*	Strongest risk factor	141
Down syndrome*	Not definitely established; possibly as many as 50% of people with Down syndrome may develop clinical manifestations of AD	59
Family history:*		
Positive family history of dementia & family history of Down syndrome	4.2	392
Negative family history of dementia & family history of Down syndrome	2.6	392
Positive family history of dementia & family history of Parkinson disease	3.3	392
Negative family history of dementia & family history of Parkinson disease	2.4	392
ApoE genotype interactions:		
Herpes simplex virus 1 in brain & an ApoE 4 allele	16.8	161
Head injury & an ApoE 4 allele	10	379
Head injury, no ApoE 4 allele	No increase	379
ApoE 4 alone*	2	379
Caucasian & ApoE 4	5.3	379
Hispanic & ApoE 4	3.2	379
African-American & ApoE 4	0.6	379
Female gender*	2-3	171
Maternal vs. paternal inheritance	2.8	82
Magnetic field exposure	2.4/2.7	98
Low head circumference (lowest quintile) for males/females	2.3/2.9	336
History of depression and positive/ negative family history of AD	2.0/2.1	392
Late maternal age and positive/negative family history of AD	1.7/2.0	392
Aluminum in drinking water $\geq$100 μg/l	1.7	251
Association with diabetes/diabetes treated with insulin	1.3/3.2	284

Table 3 *(continued)*

Category	Likely Relative Risk or Probability That Association of Risk Factor Is Due to Chance	Reference
Low socio-economic status (including low level of education)	$p < 0.05$	*93*
Starvation/malnutrition associated with late-onset AD and sporadic AD	$p < 0.05$	*136*
Physical underactivity associated with early-onset AD	$p < 0.05$	*136*
Nervous breakdown more than 10 years before, associated with early-onset AD	$p < 0.05$	*136*
Increased frequency of HLA-BW15 + cytomegalovirus antibodies	$p < 0.05$	*316*
Adult exposure to tuberculosis	$p < 0.05$	*104*
Spirochetes in all brain samples		*258*
No spirochetes in brain		*126*
Association with insulin resistance syndrome	$p < 0.05$	*200*

*Consistently confirmed risk factors for AD. See also refs. 344, 372.

There are considerable data that suggest all genetic and/or environmental risk factors for AD perturb the metabolism of amyloid precursor protein (APP), and result in excessive production of APP derivatives called Aβ which play an important role in the disorder. This view has arisen from the observation that the AD brain is characteristically laden with amyloid deposits that are surrounded by dead neurons. Many researchers believe that these amyloid deposits cause AD. A report that people with mutations in the APP or presenilin (PS-1 and PS-2) genes have more Aβ peptide ending at Aβ 42(43) than normal in their plasma supports the opinion that an increased extracellular concentration of Aβ 42(43) leads to increased deposition of this particular form of Aβ in the brain *(335)*. This concept is also supported by in vitro experiments using transfected cells. For a review of the cell biology of APP and the possible mechanism of AD see Selkoe *(341)* and Chapter 4. See also refs. *143,230,242,243,341,407,418.* Second, while the biological basis for the association of the ApoE 4 allele with AD is not known, the age of onset of AD and Aβ deposition in the brain are correlated with the ApoE 4 allele dosage, suggesting that this risk may also be mediated directly or indirectly through Aβ. Finally, treatment of cells and animals with fibrillar preparations of Aβ in vitro can be cytotoxic *(420)*. However, the excessive production of Aβ may be the manifestation of underlying cellular injury which possibly arises from excessive intracellular oxidation *(42)* and/or ischemic stress *(165)*. Oxidative processes might lead to vascular and/or cellular abnormalities, which result in excessive production of Aβ as a compensatory or repair process. According to this second view the Alzheimer pathogenic process (including the deposition of amyloid) constitutes a defensive reaction to cellular malfunction, injury or stress that results from genetic mutations/variations and/or environmental risk factors, and may reflect the body's attempt to seal and "wall off" leaky cells and vasculature, inactivate faulty neurons, and maintain brain homeostasis in so far as is possible *(247,248)*. In support of the latter hypothesis is the fact that excess Aβ is produced by an injured brain and by normal cells when they become senescent or are severely stressed or injured *(1,111,165)*. Mattson and colleagues *(243)* have pointed out that APP has characteristics of a pleiotrophic cytokine/trophic factor like transforming growth factor-beta (TGF-β) and tumour necrosis factor-alpha (TNF-α). These interact with one another and mediate a variety of injury-related changes and molecular interactions. It has been suggested that amyloid deposition is a primitive mechanisms of wound healing that takes place in the absence of immunoglobulins *(99)*. Researchers are urged to keep an open mind about the biological function of amyloid deposition in AD in the development of treatments for AD *(103)*. A fundamental question is whether treatment for AD should focus on prevention of injury to neurons and blood vessels or on reduction of amyloid production, which might exacerbate the condition if its deposition is a response to injury.

It is suggested that the following processes are involved in the pathogenesis of AD: metabolic perturbations caused by genetic and/or environmental risk factors for AD, compensatory responses to these perturbations, cellular injury, and induction of inflammatory responses which coincide with clinical manifestations of AD. All of these processes may occur simultaneously within an individual to a greater or lesser degree. In one model of AD, greater brain reserve (number of neurons and/or the density of their interconnections in youth, learned cognitive strategies, and amount of functional brain tissue that exists) has been proposed to buffer the clinical expression of AD *(57,268)*. Factors (genetic and/or environmental) that can keep the brain reserve above a minimum threshhold would appear to be protective against dementia.

Aberrant Biological Processes in the Alzheimer Brain

Aberrant biological processes associated with brain degeneration in all forms of AD include loss of up to half the brain mass, deposition of amyloid in "senile" plaques and blood vessels (meningeal and cerebral), and formation of neurofibrillary tangles (NFT) in certain neurons. A key molecular step underlying amyloid formation is the polymerization of the small Aβ peptide into amyloid fibrils. A key step underlying the development of the NFT is the accumulation of hyperphosphorylated tau molecules in neurons which bundle into paired helical filaments. Although Aβ and modified tau play a central role in Alzheimer pathology, it is becoming increasingly clear that AD results from a complex series of steps—"a pathogenic pathway"—that goes beyond the formation of amyloid and NFT. A loss of synaptic density in the AD brain has been observed consistently, although this feature is not usually assessed histopathologically because of methodological complexity *(206)*. Synaptic disconnection and neurodegenerative sprouting in AD correlate with overexpression of particular classes of neuronal thread proteins *(70–72)*.

Two independent lines of investigation have indicated that inflammation plays an important role in AD. First, there is evidence for a novel inflammatory response in the AD brain. Second, there is considerable epidemiological evidence (supported by some small clinical trials) that nonsteroidal antiinflammatory agents protect against AD *(3,37,38,247,249,275)*. The inflammatory process in the AD brain has been called the innate immune response to distinguish it from the classical peripheral cellular and humoral immune responses which require considerable time to become activated and to develop memory *(274)*. Evidence for a novel inflammatory response in the AD brain is reviewed in ref. *275*.

Possible Order of Events in the Alzheimer Pathogenic Pathway

A clue about early steps in the pathogenic pathway has been provided by studies of brains of people with Down syndrome. (The cells of people with Down syndrome carry an extra chromosome 21, which most often is the result of meiotic nondisjunction.) Almost all persons with Down syndrome develop brain pathology resembling that in AD and frequently dementia resembling AD by age 40–50 *(166,228)*. Trisomy 21 is known to be associated with excessive production of Aβ (which is derived from APP encoded on chromosome 21) and with an inflammatory reaction in the brain accompanied by the high expression of interleukin-1 (IL-1) and astroglial activation. These features also are characteristic of the Alzheimer brain *(121,122)*.

Genetic and biochemical studies of the Alzheimer and Down syndrome brain, the APP, α_1-antichymotrypsin (ACT) and ApoE genes and proteins, and of factors initiating the polymerization of Aβ peptide into amyloid filaments, have suggested that one of the earliest steps in this pathway is the diffuse accumulation of amorphous deposits of Aβ—the most widespread pathological change in AD. Diffuse (amorphous) amyloid deposits are thought to induce an inflammatory reaction involving microglial cells. The latter produce IL-1 which induces surrounding astrocytes to synthesize ACT and APP in response to IL-1 at the translational level *(323)*. There is evidence from in vitro experiments that ACT (and ApoE as well), in turn, promote the polymerization of soluble Aβ into the insoluble mature amyloid filaments which are found as deposits in blood vessel walls and in the more mature plaques, which contain a "core" *(17,60,224,225)*. ApoE also may regulate the phosphorylation of tau *(406)*, a process that is crucial for formation of the paired tau helical filaments. There is evidence that ApoE associates with the Aβ peptide to form novel monofibrils *(332)*, and that fibril formation is accelerated in vitro by ApoE. The ApoE4 isoform associates more efficiently than ApoE 3 *(414)*. CSF inhibits fibril formation *(413)*. Because amyloid plaques form before NFT which are comprised largely of phosphorylated, polymerized tau *(7)*, changes in particular species of Aβ or of APP in CSF might be among the earliest biomarkers of AD. However, because the overproduction of Aβ and phosphorylation of tau are characteristic of responses to injury, hypoxia, and senescence as well as of AD, changes in these markers may not be specific for AD *(39,79,103,242,319)*. A further complication in using APP and derivatives as a marker for AD, is the fact that changes in these markers may reflect metabolic perturbations resulting from genetic predisposing risk factors for AD rather than AD itself. Such metabolic perturbations do not constitute AD.

Mattson *(242)* has outlined how the APP and its Aβ derivatives might be involved in health and in AD. In neurons, APP is axonally transported and accumulates in presynaptic terminals and growth cones. A secreted form of APP (sAPP-α) is released from neurons in response to electrical activity; this is believed to be neuroprotective. A signaling pathway involving cyclic GMP is activated by sAPP-α and modulates the activity of potassium channels, *N*-methyl-D-aspartate receptors and the transcription factor NFκ-B. APP also may modulate cell adhesion and regulation of nonneuronal cells. Possibly as a response to injury, alternative enzymatic processing of APP liberates Aβ which has the tendency to form amyloid fibrils. Fibril formation leads to impairment of membrane transport systems including ATPases linked to ion movement, and glutamate and glucose transporters. Genetic and/or environmental factors that increase the production of Aβ and/or decrease the levels of neuroprotective sAPP-α are thought to promote neuronal degeneration in AD. In culture, Aβ has been found to be neurotrophic to undifferentiated hippocampal neurons at low concentrations and neurotoxic to mature neurons at high concentration. Amino acids 25 to 35 of Aβ mediate both of these effects and furthermore this region is homologous to the tachykinin neuropeptide family. In fact, both effects of Aβ have been mimicked by tachykinin antagonists and reversed by specific tachykinin agonists *(420)*. It has been suggested that effects of Aβ might be similar in vivo.

Oxidative Stress and Antioxidant Responses

There is substantial evidence that oxidative damage in the brain increases in normal aging, that it is greater in persons with AD, and greatest in the brain regions that are most vulnerable in AD, but the source of the oxidative stress resulting in these changes has been elusive *(50,231,364)*. Regions of the brain that degenerate in AD (e.g., cerebral cortices) have been found to have a significant increase of aluminum and iron compared with age-matched controls *(421)*. (See also ref. *251.*) Surprisingly, redox-active iron has been found to be reversibly associated with the plaques and tangles of the AD brain *(364)*. This iron may be a source of oxidative stress if there are not adequate levels of iron-binding proteins or antioxidants in the vicinity, since ferrous iron will catalyze the production of damaging hydroxyl or peroxyhydroxyl radicals in the presence of reactive oxygen species. High levels of RNA and protein for the inducible enzyme heme oxygenase-1 also are associated with AD plaques and tangles *(363,364)*. Because heme oxygenase-1 converts heme into antioxidant tetrapyrroles and free iron, heme may be a major source of the redox-active iron in plaques and tangles. Since there is evidence that plaques form at the site of microvascular aberrations *(40,131,162,172)*, leakage of blood from vasculoendothelial cells that are damaged by genetic and/or other risk factors for AD may be the source of the free heme. Accordingly, it is speculated that one function of plaques and tangles in the AD brain may be to reversibly immobilize free iron that is liberated from heme by heme oxygenase-1 until it can be sequestered and detoxified by ferritin and/or other iron-binding proteins. The iron-binding protein IRP2 which plays an important role in iron metabolism and in regulation of the levels of free iron, also colocalizes with AD plaques and tangles *(365)*.

Chronic oxidative stress should be accompanied by compensatory antioxidant processes. Although heme oxygenase-1 is a marker of oxidative stress, increased expression of heme oxygenase-1 in AD brain plays a key role in antioxidant defense because this enzyme catalyzes the production of antioxidant tetrapyrroles from heme. The enzyme Cu,Zn superoxide dismutase, which converts superoxide radicals into hydrogen peroxide, also plays a key role in antioxidant defense; its level increases in response to oxidative stress. Elevated levels of this enzyme have been reported in red cells of some AD patients and their first-degree relatives; these elevations may reflect increased peripheral antioxidant activity in AD *(343)*. Elevated levels of ferritin (which sequesters and stores iron) in CSF *(195)*, of P97 or melanotransferrin (which binds iron and zinc) in serum of AD patients *(186)*, or of changes in the plasma ratio of cysteine to sulfate *(134)*, similarly may be part of a spectrum of antioxidant defence that is upregulated in AD.

The Acute Phase Response and Alzheimer Disease

What is the Acute Phase Response?

The acute phase response (APR) is an orchestrated physiological response of the body to tissue injury, infection, or inflammation. A prominent feature of the APR is the induction of acute phase proteins, which are involved in the restoration of homeostasis. Cytokines [including interleukin-1 (IL-1), IL-6 and tumor necrosis factor-alpha (TNF-α)] are important mediators of the APR. Different signaling pathways are activated by different cytokine-receptor interactions. Eventually, cytokine-inducible transcription factors interact with their response elements in the promoter region of acute phase genes and their transcription is induced (or inhibited). The APR also involves activation of the hypothalamic–pituitary–adrenal (HPA) axis. Examples of serum proteins whose levels increase in a systemic APR are α_1-ACT, amyloids A and P, and ferritin (the major iron storage protein). Serum amyloid A is an acute phase protein that modulates proteoglycan synthesis in cultured murine macrophages *(86a)*. Serum amyloid P component controls chromatin degradation and prevents antinuclear autoimmunity *(22a)*. Examples of proteins whose levels decrease in an APR are transferrin (the major iron binding protein) and transferrin receptor (the major iron transporting protein) *(191,192)*.

Central Nervous System Acute Phase Response

The fact that various interleukins, α_1-ACT, and amyloids A and P are produced in the AD brain strongly suggests that the Alzheimer pathogenic pathway includes an APR in the CNS (or is one), since these substances are known to be an integral part of the APR in the periphery. Astrocytes, microglia, and the choroid plexus participate in the APR of the CNS. Measures of CSF cytokines and other factors involved in the CNS APR might be used as biomarkers of AD, although they would be expected to be relatively nonspecific indicators.

Peripheral Acute Phase Response

The fact that changes in serum levels of substances which are characteristic of a peripheral APR, including increases in inflammatory cytokines, α_1-ACT, amyloids A and P, and decreases in transferrin receptor, have been noted in some studies of AD patients suggests that a peripheral APR also is mounted in AD *(10,87,100,173)*. The peripheral APR in AD may not be typical, however. For example, AD is associated with activation of the HPA axis, which also is characteristic of a peripheral APR, but there is evidence that regulation of the HPA axis is aberrant in AD. For example, administration of cortisol reduces hippocampal glucose metabolism in the normal elderly but not in AD *(75)*. Peripheral markers of the APR may be induced in AD by excessive cytokine production in the CNS (particularly of IL-1), and possibly also by cytokine production by other tissues such as the thyroid *(119)* when AD is caused by genetic factors.

Interaction Between the Acute Phase Response and the Neuroendocrine Systems

There is mounting evidence that during the APR, the nervous, endocrine, immune, and inflammatory systems are bidirectionally interconnected and coordinated *(409,412)*. These bidirectional interactions are the key for linking together the myriad of changes that have been described in CSF and peripheral blood of AD patients and for understanding how changes in the AD brain can be reflected in the periphery, and how genetic and enviromental stressors might interact with the neuroendocrine and immune systems to predispose to AD. Furthermore, because of this bidirectional regulation, it is conceivable that specific neurodegenerative and other neurological diseases each will be associated with specific neuroendocrine and immune changes in blood.

The nervous, endocrine–immune, and inflammatory systems all express and respond to a large number of regulatory molecules in common. IL-1 and IL-6 are the most thoroughly characterized cytokines that function as regulators of neuroendocrine–immune communication; however, TNF-α, IL-2, interferon-gamma and other cytokines probably also play a role *(155,290)*. In addition to stimulation of the APR and the HPA axis, major actions of IL-1 and IL-6 in the neuroendocrine–immune network include stimulation of the sympathetic nervous system, the febrile response, modulation of sleep, mood and the immune and inflammatory responses; inhibition of growth and the hypothalamic-pituitary–gonadal (HPG) and hypothalamic–pituitary–thyroid (HPT) axes, and suppression of appetite and libido. Elevated serum IL-1 is thought to be characteristic of severe injury or stress, whereas elevated IL-6 is considered to be a marker of mild to moderate injury. There now is evidence that psychological stressors (which affect the CNS) and physical stressors (which affect the immune and inflammatory systems) also can perturb neuroendocrine–immune interactions; it is speculated that such stressors also may modulate the course of development of AD. The reader is referred to comprehensive review articles in which details of neuroendocrine–immune system interactions are provided *(48,90,409,412)*. A diagram showing how the neuroendocrine and immune systems may communicate in the APR is given in Fig. 2.

Dementia, Aging, and the Stress Control System

Elevated plasma levels of cortisol have been found in moderate to severe AD *(65,75,132,234,283,313)*. Orell and O'Dwyer *(283)* have explained that this may be initiated by excessive cytokine production by injured brain cells which trigger release of corticotropin releasing factor (CRF) from the hypothalamus. CRF stimulates corticotropin release from the pituitary which in turn stimulates glucocorticoid release from the adrenal glands. The activity of this loop is, in part, regulated by the binding of glucocorticosteroid to corticosteroid receptors in the hippocampus. In animals, aging is acompanied by an impairment in the ability of the hippocampus to inhibit corticotropin release, and is accompanied by a sustained high concentration of steroid production. In persons with AD, there is a delay in the decline of corticotropin concentration after challenge with dexamethasone. It is thought that the excessive and/or prolonged cortisol secretion in AD may result in the persistent downregulation of corticosteroid receptors in the hippocampus, which lead to further increases in corticosteroid concentration. Raised corticosteroids also may indirectly be toxic to neurons and lead to their destruction by leading to raised levels of excitatory amino acids (asparatate and glutamate) and to disruption of calcium homeostasis (excessive calcium is toxic to neurons). Very recent evidence suggests that corticocoids also decrease cytochrome c oxidase activity by a process that does not involve Ca^{2+} fluxes *(355)*. It is possible that AD might be an extreme variant of the normal aging process, and that continued injury of brain cells (due to a combination of genetic and/or environmental factors and long-standing metabolic perturbations) continues to drive the excessive production of cortisol which, in turn, further damages the hippocampus. (For further details see ref. *283*.)

Enhanced levels of cortisol have been found in major depression as well as in AD. However, after low-dose adrenocorticotropin stimulation, increased cortisol release was found to be characteristic of major depression but not AD. By contrast, an enhanced release of androgens after low-dose adrenocorticotropin stimulation has been found in patients with mild to moderate AD, but not in persons with depression *(313)*.

Decreased Blood Flow to the Brain

Recently, attention has been turning to the possibility that AD is primarily vascular in nature and results, at least in part, from reduced blood flow to the brain *(315)*. The reason for this is that clinical recovery of intellectual function in AD has been demonstrated after transposition of omentum from the peritoneal cavity to the affected brain *(116)*. This surgical procedure resulted in the apparent disappearance of amyloid plaque and enhanced vascularization of the affected brain region. Increased perfusion was seen of the ipsilateral and contralateral hemispheres adjacent to the transposed omentum. Reduced blood flow to the brain would result in a deficiency of oxygen, essential nutrients, and thyroxine, which regulates the metabolic rate of cells and which is essential for normal intellectual function. Thyroxine is thought to be transported from the blood stream to the CSF via transthyretin, which has been synthesized by the choroid plexus. Accordingly, it has been proposed that one of the physiological consequences of reduced blood flow to the brain would be a selective deficiency of thyroxine in the CNS. The observations that levels of transthyretin in the choroid plexus are much higher than normal in the AD brain support this hypothesis *(315)*. Brain imaging studies are now investigating the hypothesis that blood flow to the brain is reduced in AD. The literature suggests that this may be the case in late-onset AD but not in early-onset AD. Furthermore, there have been reports of orthostatic hypotension and low blood pressure in persons with AD *(125,289,354,404)*. It may be relevant that different regions of Aβ are reported to have different effects on vasoconstriction, although findings in this area are controversial *(54,187,386)*.

de la Torre *(73)* and Crawford *(54)* have summarized evidence that many risk factors for AD have a relationship or potential relationship with reduced cerebral blood flow.

Current Approaches for the Earlier Detection of Alzheimer's Disease

Overview

Many genetic and biological abnormalities are associated with AD. The challenge is to choose the markers which alone or in combination best predict the development of AD, or which best indicate the presence of AD at the earliest possible stage. The authors' conception of pathogenesis of AD is given in Figure 1. Figure 2 depicts the bidirectional interactions thought to occur between the neuroendocrine and immune systems during the acute phase response. Tables 2–10 summarize peripheral biological markers that have been reported to be associated with AD since 1993. Sensitivities and specificities have been provided in the present chapter only for markers that have been well-researched and confirmed. Studies carried out before 1993 are summarized in Ref. *294*. The reader also is referred to other reviews of peripheral markers of Alzheimer disease that have appeared recently *(15,18,25,26,76, 102,106,109,118,120,123a,139,149,185,190,202,221,241,244,321,398)*.

In this section we describe some peripheral biomarkers presently under investigation, and discuss their potential for the earlier detection of AD and their relation to the Alzheimer pathogenic pathway.

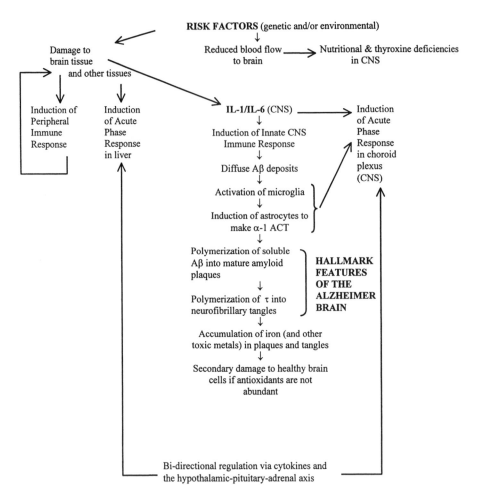

Fig. 1. Possible interactions between degenerating brain and peripheral tissues in Alzheimer disease. IL, interleukin; α-1 ACT, α-1 antichymotrypsin; τ, tau.

Genetic and Other Approaches in Combination

Introduction

The use of genetic and/or environmental risk factor information in combination with sensitive tests that monitor changes in the sensory systems and brain morphology and/or function is one approach that is being explored for direct and earlier AD diagnosis. In this section we explain how one genetic risk factor (the ApoE 4 allele) is being used in combination with other clinical information to increase the specificity of probable AD diagnosis. There now is evidence that persons with different ApoE genotypes react differently to certain Alzheimer drugs *(95,317)*. One problem

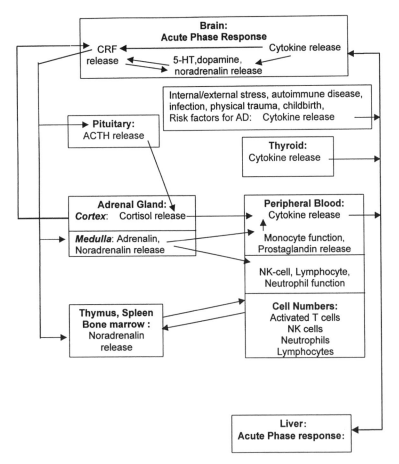

Fig. 2. Possible involvement of the neuroendocrine and immune systems in acute phase reaction in Alzheimer disease. CRF, corticotropin-releasing factor; 5-HT, seratonin; ACTH, adrenocorticotropin; NK, natured killer. (After ref. *48*.)

with using ApoE genotyping as a diagnostic adjunct is that the effects of the ApoE 4 allele are not the same in different ethnic groups *(181)*. Furthermore, there now is evidence for a nonrandom association between the ApoE and ACT loci in women which may have an important implication for the higher prevalence of AD in women *(175)*. Roses *(326)* has explained how more than one genetic risk factor (possibly in combination with environmental risk factors) and clinical tests might be used to classify participants in clinical trials into subgroups so that effects of drugs and treatments on persons with AD of different etiological origin can be examined. Tables 2 to 4 summarize published information about genetic and environmental risk factors for AD.

Table 4
Factors That Might Ameliorate Alzheimer Disease

Factors	Reference
Anti-oxidants (vitamin E, seligiline, estrogen)	*3*
Histamine H2-blocking drugs	*38*
Non-steroidal anti-inflammatory drugs (e.g., aspirin or ibuprofen)	*249*
and/or arthritis	*247, 248*
Education (risk of AD decreases 17% for each year of education)	*93*
Benzodiazepines	*96*
Increased blood flow to the brain	*315*

Nuclear Genetic Information

Genetic risk factors for AD may be nuclear (encoded on chromosomes in the nucleus) and/or mitochondrial. The nuclear genome is inherited from both parents whereas the mitochondral genome is inherited solely from the mother. In a small number of families (probably less than 50 worldwide), a variety of APP and PS-1 mutations have been found to be genetically linked to early onset familial AD *(55)*. Because their penetrance for AD is thought to be about 95%, these are being used as diagnostic aids in families in which they are present *(331)*. PS-2 mutations also have been found in association with familial AD; however, these are rare and variably penetrant *(351)*. As indicated in Table 2, there are a considerable number of other genetic variants and mutations which are "associated" with AD and/or modify the risk of acquiring AD.

The ApoE 4 allele appears to be a major genetic risk factor for AD in the general population. It is a risk factor for heart disease and for certain other neurological diseases. It also may affect survival. The frequency of ApoE 4 varies considerably from one population to another. A reading of the literature indicates that one E4 allele is carried by 16% to 30% of the population *(135)*. Two E4 alleles are carried by approximately 2% of the population. The ApoE 4 allele increases the risk for AD in a dose-dependent manner; persons with two E4 alleles tend to have an earlier age of onset of AD than those with one E4 (e.g., see ref. *326*). In persons with no symptoms of AD, identification of the ApoE 4 allele on its own is not a useful predictor of AD. However, longitudinal studies involving clinical diagnosis and brain autopsy suggest that ApoE genotyping increases the accuracy of a clinical diagnosis of probable AD *(244,326,327,333)*. In one study, all patients with probable AD who had at least one ApoE 4 allele were found at autopsy to have AD pathology *(333)*. In an ongoing longitudinal study which is monitoring changes in two cognitive domains that appear to be affected earliest in AD (memory and executive function ability) in persons with questionable AD, a preliminary analysis of the data has indicated that knowledge of the ApoE 4 status adds significant predictive power that an individual will ultimately develop clinical symptoms of probable AD *(4)*. High-exposure boxers with one or more ApoE 4 alleles appear to be at greater risk for developing more severe chronic brain injury than persons with other ApoE genotypes *(170)*, although head injury has not always been found to be a risk factor for AD *(275)*. The inclusion of ApoE genotype data did not improve the preclinical prediction of AD by single photon emission tomography (SPECT) *(168)*.

Other evidence that ApoE genotyping might have potential for very early predictive testing for AD comes from positron emission tomography (PET) scanning studies. PET scanning has detected "abnormalities" in brain glucose utilization in ApoE 4 positive individuals two decades before classical signs of dementia usually manifest. It is believed that these differences reflect a preclinical stage of AD rather than genetic differences in brain glucose utilization *(361,362)*. Longitudinal studies must now be done to determine the predictive power of such PET tests in conjunction with ApoE genotyping for AD. Since different ligands might be developed for use with PET, the potential of this technology for preclinical diagnosis in conjunction with ApoE genotyping in a variety of degenerative brain disorders seems enormous.

Mitochondrial DNA Mutations

The activity of the enzyme complex cytochrome c oxidase (CO) has been found to be decreased in brain and in peripheral tissues in late onset AD *(44,67)* but why is not known. Initially, it was thought that this phenomenon was the effect of CO1 and CO2 missense mutations in the mitochondrial genome, but this is no longer believed to be the case *(66,401)*. Nevertheless, there have been reports of mitochondrial DNA deletions and mutations in Alzheimer brain tissue *(51,147,380,400)*. A reduction in another mitochondrial marker—α-ketoglutarate dehydrogenase activity—has been found in fibroblasts from persons with familial AD *(334)*, but why is not known.

A recent hypothesis by de Grey *(69)* raises the possibility that mutations associated with low rates of oxidative phosphorylation might accumulate in affected brain tissue (and in other tissues as well) in AD. Free radicals are produced normally during oxidative phosphorylation; their rate of production varies with the rate of oxidative phosphorylation. If the free radicals are not neutralized, they can sequester electrons from DNA, protein, and lipids. Damage to DNA may result in some mutations associated with a low rate of oxidative phosphorylation. It is believed that when lipid damage in mitochondrial membranes reaches a certain level, the damaged mitochondria are engulfed and destroyed by lysosomes. It follows that the most slowly respiring mitochondria which inflict less damage to themselves, including those generated by somatic mutation, will preferentially survive, replicate, and accumulate over time. This aging process could be exacerbated by oxidative stresses external to the mitochondria that are thought to drive the pathogenesis of AD. Cells transformed by mitochondria from individuals with sporadic AD have been found to have altered Ca^{2+} homeostasis and increased reactive oxygen species production *(348)*. It is suggested that such mitochondria have excessive membrane damage caused by increased oxidative stress in the mitochondria donors.

Cerebrospinal Fluid Tests for Alzheimer Disease

Introduction

Three different biomarkers in CSF have been particularly well researched: neuronal thread protein, tau, and derivatives of APP (Table 5). Although these markers are distinguishing between persons with probable AD and healthy normal individuals, it remains to be determined if they have are sensitive and specific enough to aid with the earlier detection of AD.

Neuronal Thread Protein Test

NYMOX has developed a quantitative test for measuring levels of a specific type of neuronal thread protein (AD7c-NTP) in small samples of CSF *(70–72)*. This protein is overexpressed in brain neurons in AD. The promotional material of NYMOX indicates that in 80–90% of autopsy-verified cases of AD, the level of this protein exceeds a designated cut-off level, while less than 5% of control values exceed this level. This test is being advertised as the "first test proven to help physicians be certain in the diagnosis of Alzheimer's disease . . . now you can rule it out." Because interpathologist agreement for the diagnosis of AD by brain autopsy is about 85%, it has been suggested that the CSF test might be used as a "gold standard" against which other antemortem tests for AD are compared instead of brain autopsy. The 1992 publication had some important limitations. Around 70% of clinical patients with probable AD were reported to have AD7c-NTP levels >3 ng/mL in contrast to less than 5% of normal control individuals; however, the mean age of the AD patients was 76 years whereas the mean age of the normal controls was 54.5. The most recent publication of de la Monte and coworkers *(72)* is better controlled. CSF obtained in postmortem cases suggests that 84% of autopsied, confirmed AD cases have levels above 3 ng/mL, in contrast to only 5% of autopsied normal individuals. Only 19 normal control individuals were studied, however. In terms of cutoffs for the "living" sample, 62% of possible or probable AD patients, 0% of normal controls, 2% of multiple sclerosis patients (nonneurodegenerative disease controls), and 16% of Parkinson disease patients (neurodegenerative disease controls) exceeded levels of

Table 5
Well-Researched Cerebrospinal Fluid Markers in Patients With Probable Alzheimer Disease

Test	Accuracy	Reference
Aβ 1–40	Not useful	353
Aβ 1–42(43)	Levels significantly decreased in probable AD; considerable overlap with healthy normals	
CSF τ	SP: 0.94* ST: 0.31*	
Aβ ratio (Aβ 1–40/Aβ 1–42(43))	SP: 0.82* ST: 0.51*	
CSF τ + Aβ ratio	SP: 0.82*‡ ST: 0.58*‡	
CSF τ + Aβ deviation score index†	SP: 0.86* ST: 0.67*	
CSF τ × Aβ ratio	SP: 0.88* ST: 0.69*	
Aβ 1–42 + CSF τ	SP: 0.81–0.91* ST: 0.85*	146a
Neuronal thread protein ADC7c-NTP	Levels in postmortem CSF of 84% of autopsy-verified AD patients and 5% of autopsied healthy normal individuals exceeded 3 ng/ml. Levels in "living" CSF of 62% of possible or probable AD patients, 0% of normal controls, 2% of multiple sclerosis patients, and 16% of Parkison disease patients exceeded 3 ng/ml Levels in "living" CSF of 89% of possible/probable AD patients and 11% of normal controls exceeded 2 ng/ml.	72

*The specificity (SP) and sensitivity (ST) is given for living patients with probable AD relative to a healthy control group.
† The deviation score index = (deviation score of tau level + deviation score of Aβ ratio)/2. The deviation score in individuals = 10 $(x-$ mean)/ standard deviation + 50.
‡ SP is 0.83 and ST is 0.71 in Kanai's study (ref. 177).
    Additional references for CSF Aβ derivatives as markers: *6, 203, 269, 277, 308, 376. Additional references for CSF tau as a marker: 12, 14, 15, 106, 158, 202, 219, 318, 381, 395*

217

3 ng/mL, while 89% of possible/probable AD patients and 11% of normal controls had levels >2 ng/mL. Here again, only 18 normal controls were studied.

In summary, the apparent potential of the AD7c-NTP test as a biomarker for probable AD is considered by some researchers to be impressive. Furthermore, the assay appears to be technically reliable. However, the current claim made by NYMOX in their advertising to the medical community that the test can be used to rule out AD is not supported since examples of AD7c-NTP negative, AD positive cases were described in the 1997 publication. The authors state that low levels of AD7c-NTP in CSF of such patients could reflect either very early disesase or severe end-stage disease. Another possibility for the false negatives not mentioned by the authors is instability of AD7c-NTP in CSF due to long-term storage in the freezer, since some of the samples date back to 1979. Furthermore, as indicated above, the test is not specific for AD. The 1997 study clarifies that the size of AD7c-NTP in CSF is 41 kD rather than 21 kD as originally inferred. Evidence is presented that the AD7c-NTP cDNA is a novel gene that encodes a membrane spanning protein. The presence of particular sequences in the promoter region of the AD7c-NTP gene suggests that it may be involved in cell growth and possibly modified by growth factors or insulin stimulation. Transfection of neuronal cells in vitro results in neuritic growth as well as decreased cell viability.

Tau

Quite a number of studies have evaluated measures of CSF tau as an antemortem marker for AD. In most of these, total tau was measured, although assays for phosphorylated tau alone, or an internal repeat sequence of tau called the "core" antigen, have been used. Tau assays show promise in distinguishing persons with probable AD from healthy normal individuals. The reported sensitivity of CSF tau for AD detection (relative to healthy normal individuals) is 60–95% (see Table 5). High CSF levels of tau are not specific for AD and also have been found in non-AD dementias, other neurological control subjects, most patients with vascular dementia, and in large, acute stroke *(14,15,158,360)*. A strong ApoE 4 effect has been noted on CSF tau levels in some studies indicating that in the interpretation of CSF tau analysis, ApoE genotype should be taken into account *(14,381)*.

Published tau studies are characterized by unusually large interlaboratory differences in CSF concentrations. Potential sources of variability include the use of different types of tau preparations as standards, possible problems in reproducibility that plague many enzyme-linked immunoabsorbent assays, and different inclusion/exclusion criteria for the study participants. Other complicating factors appear to include a complex dependence of CSF tau levels on subject age, AD type and stage; there is evidence that tau is maximally elevated in early AD *(318)*. Finally, compared to brain tau, CSF tau has been shown to be proteolytically degraded; not clear is whether this process is physiological or an artifact of degradation in vitro *(184)*. It should be pointed out that correlative CSF-neuropathological studies of phosphorylated tau will be difficult, since agonal state and postmortem interval profoundly affect the phosphorylation state of tau in brain. A recent study has documented huge postmortem effects on tau levels in postmortem CSF, rendering tau studies on such samples questionable *(266)*. Despite the preceding caveats, the potential of CSF tau assays in earlier AD testing should be further investigated. Structural studies of tau suggest that there should be six different phosphorylated forms of tau in brain which may be differentially expressed and represented in CSF as AD develops. As indicated in Table 3 and below, measures of CSF tau in combination with measure of Aβ and/or other CSF substances appear to have better specificity for probable AD than any biomarker on its own.

Amyloid Precursor Protein and A Beta Peptides

Enzyme-linked immunoabsorbent (ELISA) and enzyme-linked sandwich-immunoabsorbent assays (ELSIA) have been established which distinguish between the major form of Aβ ending at amino acid 40 (Aβ 1–40) and the more amyloidogenic form ending at amino acid 42 or 43 [Aβ 1–42(43)] *(163,256)*. Measurements of total Aβ in CSF by these methods are thought not to be useful for the earlier detection of AD. However, measurements of specific Aβ derivatives presently are under investigation. A number of groups have reported that use of the ratio of Aβ 1–40 to Aβ 1–42(3) or measures of Aβ 1–42 in combination with tau results in a higher sensitivity and specificity of diagnosing probable AD than either test on their own (Table 5). Because AD cases with mild-to-moderate dementia have increased CSF Aβ 1–42 relative to controls *(146a,202,335)*, this latter approach may not be useful for the early detection of AD.

One of the metabolic pathways of APP involves the generation of soluble APP by α-secretase through amide bond cleavage at position 15/17 of Aβ, generating α-secretase derived soluble APP (SAPP-α). Preliminary studies suggest that SAPP-α may be a relevant marker for cognition in both AD and in healthy aging *(202,335)*, although probably not diagnostic or predictive of AD.

van Leeuwen et al. *(394)* recently described variant APP and ubiquitin-B proteins in the cerebral cortex of AD and DS patients which had (+1) frameshift mutations in their carboxyl terminus. These (+1) proteins were not found in young controls. Whether measurements of levels of such proteins in CSF or plasma might be useful in the earlier detection of AD should be investigated.

Factors complicating the measurements of APP derivatives in CSF include extreme instability to multiple freeze-thaw cycles, and low levels in CSF. There is evidence that soluble Aβ in normal human plasma and CSF is complexed to high density lipoprotein *(194)*. The data of Matsubara and coworkers *(236)* indicate that soluble Aβ complexes stoichiometrially to apolipoprotein J. These observations might explain the instability of APP derivatives in plasma and CSF to freeze-thawing. Plasma should be harvested from blood at room temperature in order to keep lipid-Aβ complexes solubilized. Furthermore, frozen samples of plasma or CSF should be warmed to room temperature and care taken to solubilize the lipid before analyses are undertaken. See Olson *(281)* for a review of lipoprotein metabolism.

Pitschke and colleagues *(308)* recently reported that fluorescence correlation spectroscopy can detect single amyloid aggregates in CSF. Aggregates were found in samples from 15 patients with AD and from one with cerebral amyloid angiopathy, but not in 19 normal individuals. Not known is how early in AD such aggregates appear, or if the test can distinguish between AD and related disorders.

Other CSF Tests

As indicated in Table 6, a wide spectrum of aberrations other than neuronal thread protein, tau and Aβ have been noted in CSF in AD. Several additional CSF biomarkers that appear worthy of further exploration include: CSF autoantibodies to microglia and other brain constituents, increased pyruvate and cleavage of high molecular weight kininogen. Blennow and Vanmechelen *(26)* have proposed that a battery of different CSF markers should be used in combination to increase the specificity of CSF testing for AD.

Blood Tests

Introduction

Blood based tests for AD would be preferable to CSF-based tests for the sake of patient comfort. Serum or plasma based tests would be more convenient than red cell, platelet or white-cell based tests because serum/plasma can be easily prepared and readily stored. A list of abnormalities that are not immunological in nature and that have been identified in blood of AD patients is given in Table 7.

Serum P97 (Melanotransferrin)

A promising peripheral blood marker for AD involves measuring serum levels of a novel iron and zinc-binding protein called P97 or melanotransferrin *(186)*. The levels of P97 in serum refrigerated for 24 hours were reported to be elevated in all AD patients compared to levels in frozen serum from healthy control individuals. (P97 levels also were elevated in AD CSF.) In a longitudinal study, serum levels of P97 increased with AD progression over a 2- to 3-year period and correlated significantly with scores of cognitive function, suggesting that it might be an early marker for AD or used as an endpoint in clinical intervention protocols. As yet, there have been no published follow-up reports by the authors of this first report or by others of P97 as an early marker of AD.

One possible concern with this published study is that the serum samples from the AD patients and normal individuals were not prepared under the same conditions. Samples from the patients were analyzed without freezing; samples from the normal individuals had been frozen. Moreover, the authors did not provide details about how the serum samples were prepared from the blood samples. In particular, they did not indicate whether the clotted blood samples were refrigerated before recovering the serum, a factor which is known to leach material from blood cells. In any case/control study it is imperative that data on cases and controls be obtained in exactly the same way. Furthermore, sufficient technical detail should be provided so that the study can be replicated. There is no published information about interassay, inter-person, or intraperson variability in the P97 test, or if P97 values also are elevated in neurological and non-neurological controls. Comments about the sensitivity and specificity of P97 for the earlier detection of AD thus are premature, although in the published study the sensitivity was 1.0!

How serum P97 is related to the AD pathogenic pathway is not clear. P97 is believed to have one iron-binding site and one zinc-binding site *(108)* and is thought to be involved in a pathway for iron uptake into cells that is independent of the transferrin receptor *(186)*. P97 occurs both in circulating and cell-bound forms. In the AD brain, P97 is highly localized to capillary endothelium (along with the transferrin receptor) and it also is present in a subset of reactive microglia associated with senile plaques. Aside from these facts, and the observation that iron levels are increased in degenerating areas of the AD brain *(304)*, there is no direct rationale for measuring P97 levels in serum.

It is speculated that P97 may play an important role in maintaining iron and zinc homeostasis in the acute phase response and in chronic inflammatory states including AD. There would be an advantage to keeping the circulating levels of these elements low in these conditions, but nevertheless bioavailable. High levels of free iron and zinc which have been documented in the AD brain *(50)* could catalyze the production of hydroxyl radicals from reactive oxygen species which are increased in inflammatory processes and lead to unscheduled "bystander" oxidation.

Table 6
Other Cerebrospinal Fluid Abnormalities in Alzheimer Disease

Abnormality	Reference
Autopsy brain localization of immune antigens	
IL-6, α_2-macroglobulin, C-reactive protein CD4, CD8, LA,	214, 358,
IL-1, IL2-R, TNF, HLA-DR, complement proteins, S100, serum	415
amyloid A and P	
Cerebrospinal fluid volumes	
Increased in EOAD and LOAD; greater increase in EOAD	374
Acute phase reaction/neuroendocrine-immune markers	
Ferritin: increased compared to Parkinson's patients and controls	195
α_1-ACT: closely associated with late onset AD	130
α_1-ACT: elevated in early and late onset AD but not vascular	215, 216
dementia; levels correlate negatively with stage of severity of AD	
IL-1β: increased in sporadic AD and in de novo Parkinson's patients	28
IL-6: significantly decreased in early onset AD; increased in sporadic	417
AD and in de novo Parkinson's patients; increased in AD, AIDS	28
dementia complex, multiple sclerosis, systemic lupus erythymatosis,	124
CNS trauma, viral and bacterial meningitis	
IL-6: no change in first degree relatives and patients with AD	129
Antibodies to:	
*Microglia	252
*Variety of substances (should be further studied with reference	382
to subgrouping and prognosis)	
Amino acids	
D-Amino acids: increased in AD	101
Methionine and alanine: significantly increased	263
CSF/serum ratios for alanine and glycine: significantly increased	
Significant negative correlations between MMSE score and	
alanine, urea, arginine and alpha-amino butyric acid	
Amino acids: high glycine, low GABA in pooled AD CSF	226
(done by microcapillary electrophoresis)	
Other substates	
*Pyruvate: remarkably increased in DAT	287
*Indicators of mitochondrial function—lactate: significantly increased	314
succinate, fumarate and glutamine: significantly decreased	
Neurotransmitters and their metabolites	
Nitrate levels: decreased in AD, Parkinson's and multiple systems	196
atrophy patients	
Neuropeptide changes in dementia are controversial	391
Somatostatin-like immunoreactivity: significant negative correlation	260
with severity of dementia	
Norepinephrine: decreased substantially;	89
Epinephrine, dopamine: decreased moderately	89

Table 6 *(continued)*

Abnormality	Reference
Serotonin: decreased	89
Norepinephrine:increased in earlier AD and continues to increase as AD progresses	88
Correlations between P300 components and various neurotransmitters	264
3-methoxy-4-hydroxy-phenylglycol (MHPG): higher in DAT and inversely correlated with cognitive function, but not significantly	349
Lipids	
ApoE: no difference	209
ApoE: increased	219, 257, 329
Ventricular fluid lipoprotein composition altered in autopsy samples	265
Longitudinal values of ApoE: decreased in AD patients with an ApoE4 allele; stayed the same in AD patients without an ApoE4 allele	307
Proteins	
APP derivatives	⎫
Tau	⎬ See text and Table 4
Neuronal thread protein	⎭
Acid phosphatase: 40% of AD samples but 0% of controls were positive	282
Ubiquitin: increased	158
Cathepsin D: increased levels of inactive enzyme in AD versus Huntington patients and other degenerative diseases	338
Chromogranin A: no difference or lower levels in AD patients, mean age 60 years	279, 27
Synaptotagmin: decreased	61
Transthyretin: lower in late onset AD	342
*Massive cleavage of high molecular weight kininogen (suggests activation of the contact system due to interaction of β-amyloid with factor XII with kallikrein generation)	22
Alanyl-amino peptidase: decreased	159
Mannan-binding lectin: decreased	204
Vitamins	
Vitamin E: reduced	167
Markers of oxidative stress	
Hydroxynonenol in ventricular fluid: increased in AD	223
Superoxide dismutase activity: decreased in total dementia, DAT, and non-DAT dementia groups	68

α_1-ACT, α_1-antichymotrypsin; DAT, dementia of the Alzheimer type; EOAD, early onset Alzheimer disease; GABA, γ-amino butyric acid; IL, interleukin; LOAD, late onset Alzheimer disease; TNF, tumor necrosis factor. Abnormalities denoted with an asterisk are striking and merit further investigation.

Table 7
Nonimmunological Serum/Plasma Abnormalities in Alzheimer's Disease

Abnormality	Reference
Amino acids and metabolites	
Taurine and glutamate: increased	*19*
*Cysteine to sulfate ratios: increased in patients with motor neuron disease, Parkinson's disease, and AD	*134*
*Glutamate and metabolites: altered levels distinguish patients with AD from normals and others with dementia	*262*
Basal plasma 3-methoxy-4-hydroxyphenylglycol (MHPG): inverse relation with cognitive function in AD	*207*
Fasting plasma ornithine and arginine: increased	*311*
Total serum homocysteine: increased in SDAT; independent of nutritional status	*169, 246*
Abnormal amino acid metabolism in early stage probable AD (decreased plasma tryptophan and methionine; increased plasma tyrosine/large neutral amino acid ratio; increased plasma taurine/methionine serine ratio)	*97*
Enzymes/Proteins	
APP in plasma: decreased in most sporadic AD	*233*
Sialyl transferase: decreased	*227*
Urokinase-type plasminogen activity in euglobulin fraction: increased in severe AD	*8*
Hemostasis abnormalities in vascular dementia and AD (e.g., high von Willebrand factor, activated factor VIII)	*229*
Glutamyl aminopeptidase activity: decreased in sporadic AD	*193*
Neuroendocrine markers	
Plasma cortisol: increased in moderate and severe AD	*64, 234, 2, 132*
*Abnormalities in adrenal androgens, but not of glucocorticoids in early AD	*272*
Blunted adrenocorticotropin and increased adrenal steroid response to human CRH	*273*
Dehydroepiandrosterone (DHEA) and DHEA-sulfate/DHEA ratio decreased in patients with AD and cerebrovascular dementia	*419*
Total 7 α-hydroxydehydroepiandrosterone: increased	*16*
Fat metabolism	
Serum apolipoprotein AI and AII: low in AD	*199*
Plasma ApoE: increased in AD	*375*
High density lipid (HDL) phospholipid and HDL cholesterol have decreased concentrations of arachadonic acid	*52*
Vitamin status	
Vitamin B_{12}: frequently low in dementia	*41, 259, 383*
Vitamin B_{12} and folate: low in AD;	*46*
Total homocysteine: increased in AD	*46*

Table 7 *(continued)*

Abnormality	Reference
Markers of oxidative status	
Glutathione peroxidase activity and selenium: increased	*43*
Mn-SOD level: significantly decreased	*388*
Total radical-trapping antioxidant activity of plasma: significantly decreased in AD	*74*
Mineral metabolism	
Plasma levels of: aluminum, mercury, cadmium, selenium: increased; iron and manganese: decreased	*20*
Serum aluminum levels: increased in probable AD relative to other senile dementias and age-matched controls	*422*
Aluminum absorption: increased from normal dietary intake	*320*
*p97(melanotransferrin): increased in AD	*186;* see text
*Ceruloplasmin oxidative activity: strikingly decreased	*367*

ApoE, apolipoprotein E; APP, amyloid precursor protein; CRH, corticotropin releasing hormone; Mn-SOD, manganese-containing superoxide dismutase (mitochondrial); PD, Parkinson's disease.

*These abnormalities are striking and merit further investigation.

Other Serum and Plasma Markers

Attention is drawn to several other plasma/serum tests with possible biomarker potential. In one study, early morning plasma cysteine to sulfate ratios were reported to be 4- to 5-fold elevated in patients with motor neuron disease, Parkinson's disease, and AD *(85,134)*. Although this phenomenon has been interpreted to be a "defect" in endogenous sulfur metabolism, it may be indicative of upregulated antioxidant defenses in these conditions, since cysteine is a reducing agent and sulfate is an oxidizing agent. In another study, plasma concentrations of glutamate dehydrogenase, aspartate, glutamate, and α-ketoglutarate were found to be significantly elevated in institutionalized persons with previously diagnosed AD compared to people with non-AD dementia. Discriminant analysis based on these four significantly different compounds was suggested as the basis for a plasma screening test for AD *(262)*. Recently, serum levels of ceruloplasmin oxidative activity were found to be strikingly low in AD *(367)*.

Red Cell Markers

A number of different approaches have revealed that red blood cells are modified in AD patients (Table 8). For example, Prasher *(310)* has suggested that increases in the volume of red cells might be used as an indicator of AD in Down syndrome. Kay and Goodman *(182)* have described various phe-

Table 8
Reported Abnormalities in Different Cells and Tissues Other Than White Blood Cells in Alzheimer Disease

Cell or Tissue Type	Reference
Blood	
Advanced glycation end-products: trends to lower values	*387*
Increased blood mercury levels: correlate with levels of Aβ in CSF	*140*
Platelets	
Enzymes	
Altered antimycin A-insensitive NADH-cytochrome c reductase	*424*
Monoamine oxidase B activity: increased in LOAD; correlates with emotional deterioration	*286*
Increased specific activity of monoamine oxidase in demented patients; positive correlation with dementia severity in Parkinsonian and demented patients	*32*
Increased phenolsulfotransferase activity; correlation between enzyme activity and disease severity	*29*
Function	
Smooth endoplasmic reticulum structure (proliferation) and function (calcium homeostasis) is abnormal	*127*
Hyperacidification and aberrant granule secretion in response to thrombin in males with severe AD	*62*
Decreased serotonin uptake with altered kinetics (decreased K_m and V_{max})	*157*
Decreased serotonin	*345*
Decreased binding of platelet activating factor in AD and MID patients	*137*
Increased membrane fluidity	*425*
Decreased B_{max} for benzodiazepine binding	*31*
Platelet activation differences: in moderate and advanced AD	*63, 64*
Increased unstimulated activation	*345*
Amyloid related-phenomena	
Abnormal pattern of platelet APP isoforms in AD: ratio between intensity of the 130 kDa and 106-110 kDa isoforms is significantly lower in AD than in controls and non-AD dementia patients; significant correlation of isoform ratio with severity of disease	*78*
Altered amyloid protein processing	*325*
Red Blood Cells	
Oxidative processes	
Cu/Zn SOD and catalase: increased in DAT	*305*
Cu/Zn SOD: increased in some AD patients and first degree relatives; complex dependence on age	*343*
Hydroxyl radicals: increased in DAT and VAD	*154*
Cu/Zn SOD activity and specific activity: significantly decreased in DAT and VAD	
Cu/Zn SOD activity: increased	*74*
MnSOD mRNA levels: increased	
Antioxidant status: decreased	

Table 8 *(continued)*

Cell or Tissue Type	Reference
Cu/Zn SOD activity significantly decreased	*367*
Enzymes	
Butyrylcholinesterase activity: reduced in sporadic AD	*156*
Increased transketolase activity coefficient; increased affinity of transketolase for thiamine pyrophosphate	*86*
Decreased methionine adenosyl transferase activity	*117*
Structural changes	
Decreased membrane fluidity or no change	*127*
Structural changes in anion transporter protein band-3	*35, 182*
Increased electrophoretic mobility	*403*
Disruption of phospholipid asymmetry and increased turnover	*403*
Increase in mean cell volume	*310*
Altered membrane properties (see text)	*330*
Skin fibroblasts	
Enzymes	
40 kDa form of interferon-inducible (2′,5) oligoadenylate synthetase and its mRNA: absent	*188*
Cu/Zn protein and mRNA levels: increased in EOAD; decreased in LOAD	*390*
Deficient α-ketoglutarate dehydrogenase complex activity, but normal glutamate metabolism	*49*
Calcium and potassium-related abnormalities	
Calcium uptake by mitochondria: decreased; mitochondrial sensitivity to free radicals increased	*198*
Altered internal Ca^{2+} mobilization	*160*
At least one calcium compartment is abnormal	*114*
Potassium channel abnormalities	*91, 92*
Potassium channel abnormalities not a useful screening test	*240*
Calcium homeostasis and autofluorescence: abnormal	*47*
Altered signal transduction	
Memory-associated GTP-binding protein Cp20: decreased	*189*
Changes in transduction systems and APP metabolism	*118*
High molecular weight Gs α isoform of G protein subunit: decreased in a subset of FAD patients	*347*
Reduced levels of protein kinase Cα	*21*
Other	
Glucose and glutamine oxidation: altered	*368*
Fluorescent light-induced chromatid breaks: increased in AD and in first-degree relatives	*288*
Urine	
Truncated nerve growth factor receptor: increased in mildly-demented AD patients	*220*
Trypsin inhibitors: increased	*370*
Neuronal thread protein: increased	*111a*
Skin	
Impaired skin vessel reactivity to acetylcholine	*5*

DAT, dementia of the Alzheimer type; GTP, guanosine triphosphate; Cu/Zn SOD, copper/zinc containing red cell superoxide dismutase; MnSOD, manganese-containing superoxide dismutase of mitochondria; VAD, vascular dementia.

nomena associated with anion transport band 3 in red cells of AD patients that parallel those observed in the AD brain. Furthermore, serum autoantibodies to band 3 peptides are increased in AD patients. Sabolovic and colleagues *(330)* have reported that red cells from AD patients can be effectively distinguished from those of age- and gender-matched nondemented patients on the basis of a combination of several different physicochemical properties using logistic analysis. Parameters used in the logistic analysis included measures of annexin V-binding, glycerol resistance, and cell rigidity as demonstrated by their filterability. This approach allowed the assignment of 95% of the AD patients to the correct group. The high annexin binding suggests that AD cells have a disruption of the phospholipid asymmetry; the high glycerol resistance and low rigidity are characteristic of young red blood cells, suggesting that their turnover is enhanced in AD. Whether such tests will have potential for the earlier detection of AD is not known. Red cell-based tests would not be as convenient as serum or plasma-based tests for direct AD diagnosis.

Platelet Membrane Fluidity and Other Platelet Tests

Numerous AD-associated phenomena have been described in platelets (Table 8). An increase in the fluidity of platelet membranes in persons with early-onset and late-onset AD using fluorescence spectroscopy has been most extensively studied, and furthermore has been evaluated in a longitudinal study *(427)*. To study platelet membrane fluidity, purified platelets obtained from fasting blood samples are collected in the morning in a plastic syringe containing EDTA as an anticoagulant and a protease inhibitor are labeled with the lipid probe 1,6-diphenyl-1,3,5-hexatriene (DPH), and the steady-state anisotropy of the DPH labeled membranes is determined at 37°C. An increase in platelet membrane fluidity is reflected by a decrease in the steady-state anisotropy of the labeled membranes. In 1987, 71% of patients were reported to have lower anisotropy values than 8% of the controls. The alteration in platelet fluidity parallels clinical severity as measured by the Mini-Mental State Exam (MMSE) Score, but there appears to be no effect of depresssion, mania, or multiinfarct dementia on this. In a prospective longitudinal study of initially asymptomatic first-degree relatives of probands with AD, subject age, a family history of AD, and increased platelet membrane fluidity made significant and independent contributions to the risk of developing AD. The 95% confidence intervals were large, however, indicating that the test is not really useful as a predictor *(425)*. An apparent gender effect was not statistically significant in this study. The effect of ApoE genotype has not yet been investigated. There is no published information about the interassay, intraperson, or interperson variation of this assay. This platelet phenomenon has been independently confirmed by several research groups worldwide. Only one study has failed to find an association between platelet membrane fluidity and AD *(197)*. An inspection of the methodology used in the latter study suggests that a reason for failure might have been due to omission of protease inhibitor from the EDTA solution used to collect the blood.

The cause of increased platelet membrane fluidity in AD and other of the platelet phenomena listed in Table 8 is not known.

Immune and Inflammatory Markers

There is considerable evidence for altered immune and inflammatory functions in many AD patients. This field has been reviewed by Singh *(356–358)* and Singh and Guthikonda *(359)*. It has been proposed that a cell-mediated autoimmune response against brain antigens may explain immune abnormalities in at least a subset of AD patients. This model involves activation of CD8+ cells (activated cytotoxic T lymphocytes). Antibrain antibodies may contribute to neurodegeneration through a cell-specific autoimmune assault. A summary of immune parameters that have been investigated in AD is given in Table 9. Shalit and associates *(346)* have suggested that T-lymphocyte subpopulations and markers correlate with the severity of AD. Very striking are observations that soluble and spontaneously aggregating Aβ activate peripheral T cells and antigen-producing cells, respectively, in normal individuals but not in AD patients, suggesting that Aβ is recognized as a "self" antigen in patients with AD! Neuroautoimmune phenomena associated with AD should be further investigated. As well as being relevant to the immunopathogenesis of AD, they also might be utilized in AD diagnostics or in therapy for AD. Recently, immunization with amyloid-beta has been found to attenuate AD-like pathology in the PDAPP transgenic mouse which overexpresses mutant human APP (in which the amino acid at position 717 is phenylalanine instead of the normal valine) *(349a)*. Whether PDAPP mice really are analogous to humans with AD, in whom amyloid disposition might occur in response to injury, is debatable, however. That levels of CSF or serum cytokines, and cytokine secretion by monocytes, are altered in AD might be predicted from our understanding of neuroimmune regulation, and the fact that inflammatory cytokine production is characteristic of the AD brain. As in other biomarker studies, effects of AD subtype, stage, and duration of disease must be taken into account in future studies of neuroimmune involvement in AD. Examples of irreproducibility of observations in the literature indicate that attention must be paid to quality control. Whether any of the reported AD-associated immune and inflammatory markers reflect nutritional deficiency, which affects about one-third of the elderly, is not known.

Table 9
Immune and White Blood Cell Abnormalities in Blood in Alzheimer Disease

Abnormality	Reference
Immunogenetics	
Increased frequency of HLA-BW15 + cytomegalovirus	*316*
Increased frequency of certain HLA haplotypes and G_m allotypes	
Association of HLA-linked C4*B2 allele	
Association of HLA-A2 variant	See Table 2
Association of HLA DR 1,2,3 variants (protective against AD)	
Association of HLA DR 4,5,6 variants	
Abnormalities of blood lymphocytes/lymphoblastoid cells	
APP-related phenomena	
Abnormal and deficient processing of APP in FAD lymphoblastoid cells	*237–239*
Ratio of lymphocyte APP751:APP770 mRNA lower	*80*
*Soluble Aβ induces IL-2 receptor and proliferation of peripheral T cells of young and old healthy individuals but not AD cases	*389*
*Spontaneously aggregating Aβ (25–31) does not activate antigen-producing cells	*358*
APP content of lymphocytes is increased	*285*
Ca^{2+}-related phenomena	
Basal and activated intracellular Ca^{2+} levels significantly higher in mononuclear cells in AD patients compared to elderly controls or patients with unipolar depression	*1a*
Amplifying effect of Aβ Ca^{2+} signalling in lymphocytes is reduced	*81*
Inhibition of the PHA-induced Ca^{2+} response by tetraethylammonium is reduced	*81*
Altered Ca^{2+} homeostasis in lymphoblasts from patients with late-onset AD	*150*
Diminished Ca^{2+} uptake in mitogen-activated lymphocytes	*358*
Receptor changes	
Increased IgM on T cells	*183*
Decreased T cell interferon-gamma binding	*30*
Decreased lymphocyte benzodiazepine binding	*31*
Increased T cell TNF-α p60 and p80 receptors	*33*
Increased T cell IL-6 receptor binding in late onset AD	*34*
Function	
Decreased mitotic index of lymphocytes in presence of glutamine in AD and DS	*293*
T lymphocyte subpopulations and activation markers correlate with AD severity	*346*
Suppressed lymphocyte proliferation to T-cell mitogens	*358*
Increased level of activated T cells (IL-2R+ and HLA-DR+)	*358*
Increased ratio of CD8+ T cells (suppressor/cytotoxic) to CD4+ (helper/inducer) cells	*358*

Table 9 *(continued)*

Abnormality	Reference
Increased Con A-induced T suppressor (Ts) cell function	358
Enzymes and proteins	
Decreased acetylcholinesterase and butyrylcholinesterase activity in lymphocytes	156
Decreased actin in lymphocytes	241
Increased proteolytic activity in lymphocytes	180
Decreased β-adrenoceptor-stimulated adenylyl cyclase activity	107
Increased expression of S100 protein (on CD8+ cells)	358
Other	
Heat shock protein 70 mRNA levels in mononuclear blood cells decreased in DAT	399
Increased oxidative damage in lymphocytes	255
Decreased lymphocyte counts	358
MnSOD mRNA level in lymphocytes is significantly increased	74
Greater amplitude of intracellular pH changes under acid-loading conditions in lymphoblasts from patients with AD	151
Cytokine production by monocytes	
Decreased IL-3 and TNF-α in mild AD	145
Increased production of IL-2 and INF-γ in moderately severe AD and vascular dementia	145
Increased production of IL-6 in PHA-stimulated cells in mild and moderately severe AD vs vascular dementia and normals	146
Increased production of IL-1, IL-2, and IL-6	358
Serum immune activation antigens	
Increased sCD8 and sCAM	357
Decreased TNFα (EOAD, LOAD)	10
Increased TNF receptor	208
Increased IL-1β (EOAD)	10
Increased IL-2 receptor	208
Increased IL-6 in severe, late-onset sporadic AD	173
Increased levels of IL-6 but normal levels of INF-α, INF-γ and IL-12	358
No changes in IL-6	13
Decreased IL-6 soluble receptor	
Increased histamine (EOAD, LOAD)	10
Increased levels of S100-α and S100-β proteins	358
Serum Ig	
Normal IgG and IgA but decreased IgM	358
IgG3 isotype significantly increased	358
IgA increased	208

(continued)

Table 9 (continued)

Abnormality	Reference
Autoantibodies in serum/plasma	
To:	
Histones	253
Neurofilament heavy chain	369
GFAP, S100	254
Nuclear antigen, gastric parietal cells, CNS antigen, gangliosides, laminin, keratin	337
Thyroglobulin and thyroid microsomes in FAD	94, 110
Choroid plexus	341
Aβ	416
Erythrocyte anion transporter protein, band 3	182
Many other substances	222, 294, 358
Acute phase reactants in serum/plasma	
α_1-AT increased	410
α_1-ACT increased in probable AD; increases with age in controls but not in AD patients	138
α_1-ACT increased in EOAD and LOAD	217, 235
α_1-ACT increased in a subset of nondemented first degree relatives of AD patients	9
α_1-ACT levels in AD remain elevated, but return to normal in non-AD inflammatory conditions	218
Amyloid P decreased	276
*p97(melanotransferrin): greatly increased	186; see text
*Ceruloplasmin oxidative activity: greatly decreased	367

AT, anti-trypsin; ACT, antichymotrypsin; EOAD, early-onset Alzheimer disease; HLA, human leukocyte antigens; LOAD, late-onset Alzheimer disease.
*These abnormalities are striking and worthy of further exploration.

Markers of Cultured Fibroblasts and Skin

Cutaneous biopsy has been of great value in the diagnosis of certain neurodegenerative diseases—especially neurometabolic and inborn errors of metabolism (153). This approach is currently not favored in AD diagnostics because it is thought that skin and fibroblast-related AD abnormalities are metabolic perturbations caused by genetic predisposing factors for AD rather than AD effects. Although this concern may apply to fibroblasts, it is possible that circulating cytokines, APP derivatives, and other substances that reflect brain changes in AD may induce AD-specific changes in vascularized epithelium. Abnormalities that have been found in cultured skin fibroblasts in people with AD are listed in Table 8. A problem with some of these studies is that the cell lines that have been examined are not generally representative of AD, and in some reports members of one large pedigree with early onset familial AD have been overrepresented (e.g., see *91,92,113*).

There is evidence that processes involved in cell division may be abnormal in persons with AD. This hypothesis is supported by the demonstration that presenilins 1 and 2 physically localize to the nuclear membrane, interphase kinetochores, and centrosomes *(213)*. It has been proposed that defective presenilin function associated with PS-1 and PS-2 mutations could cause chromosome missegration in dividing microglia and astrocytes in the brain, resulting in excessive spontaneous cell death (apoptosis) or excessive chromosomal aneuploidy (including trisomy 21 mosaicism) which could trigger inflammation and initiate characteristic AD lesion formation as in Down syndrome *(213)*. Primary fibroblasts from persons with familial AD carrying presenilin 1 or 2 mutations have been reported to have significant aneuploidy including trisomy 21 mosacism compared to chromosomes from normal individuals (see ref. *213*), although these studies have not yet been independently confirmed. The possibility should be considered that the chromosome 21 gain observed in AD in the general population and the chromosome 21 loss observed in older people with Down syndrome *(303)* are adaptive phenomena which are protective in nature rather than destructive.

Urinary Markers

Researchers have begun to explore the possibility that urine analysis can be used in testing for AD (Table 8). Increased levels of truncated nerve growth factor receptor previously were described in the urine of mildly demented patients with Alzheimer disease, a marker also present in the urine of patients with diabetic neuropathy *(220)*. Urinary acid-stable proteinase inhibitors (kallikrein and trypsin inhibitors) also have been examined and their levels compared in the urine of healthy and Alzheimer subjects *(370)*. The levels of antikallikrein activity were similar in both groups. By contrast, urinary levels of trypsin inhibitors were significantly increased in both males and females with AD. These data raise the possibility that an imbalance in acid-stable proteolytic enzyme inhibitors may be involved in the pathogenesis of AD and that levels of these inhibitors in urine might be further explored as markers of the disease. Normal urine has been shown to contain low levels of soluble Aβ (1–40), but it presently is not known if urinary levels of this or other derivatives of Aβ in urine are potentially useful as markers of AD *(112)*. There now is a published report that neuronal thread protein antigen AD7c-NTP is elevated in the urine of AD patients, and that the specificity and sensitivity of a bioassay for urinary AD7c-NTP is comparable to that of CSF AD7c-NTP in AD diagnosis *(111a)*.

The Pupil Assay

There is a deficiency of the neurotransmitter acetylcholine in the brain of persons with AD and also in older persons with Down syndrome (who are at greatly increased risk of developing AD-like brain changes and also clinical dementia resembling AD). Based on additional observations that the neuronal controls of the heart and iris of persons with DS are hypersensitive to a class of drug that inhibited acetylcholine-mediated neurotransmission as evidenced by an abnormally increased heart rate and a hypersensitive pupillary response to atropine (or its synthetic analog, tropicamide), Scinto and associates *(339),* hypothesized that persons with AD might respond similarly. As testing the heart response is potentially dangerous, the decision was made to focus on the pupillary response. As anticipated, the pupillary response to a very low concentration of tropicamide instilled in the eye indeed was found to be hypersensitive in persons with AD. Furthermore, one "false positive" case developed dementia within a year of admission into the study suggesting that the pupil assay might be reflecting early signs of AD. Because of the obvious potential importance of a non-invasive eye test for AD which could be administered in an outpatient setting, a flurry of activity to confirm and extend these preliminary findings has resulted. Although some groups have obtained evidence for a hypersensitive pupillary response in persons with AD, others have not (e.g., see Ref. *123).* Nevertheless, on balance, the positive findings in conjunction with one report that a hypersensitive response is associated with an ApoE 4 genotype, suggests that the phenomenon indeed is real, but that unidentified factors are contributing to the variability, the test may be very sensitive, and that it works only when it is done "right."

On the basis of published experiences and information, factors resulting in "irreproducibility" in the pupil assay probably include: accuracy of reporting groups in diagnosing possible or probable AD, choice of control individuals (in some studies controls have been prescreened for early signs of AD and questionable cases excluded from the study), subject age, whether the pupil test is done in a lighted or dark room, when the test is begun after instillation of the eye drops, effects of ApoE genotype, eye color, and the type and stage of the AD. Whether stress associated with the testing or time of day the test is done affects the results is not known. It would be advisable to conduct tests at the same time of day and also to monitor the patients' heart rate and blood pressure for signs of anxiety. How the acetylcholine antagonist solution is prepared also may be crucial for success of the test. Inherent chemical instability or loss of solute by adherence to the surface of the storage container (especially in dilute solutions) can lead to a progressive decrease of reagent concentration. The need for a standardized test reagent may be particularly great in this case. A large-scale longitudinal study presently being conducted by the

Harvard group should resolve the current controversies about the usefulness and reliability of the pupil assay as an early marker for AD, and whether it is an indicator that is independent of an ApoE 4 effect. The pupil assay and recent literature on the assay are reviewed in greater detail in Chapter 10.

Brain Imaging Tests

The potential of in vivo functional brain imaging to quantify and localize functional defects associated with AD has recently been summarized by Robles *(321)* (Table 10). Rapoport *(312)* has reported that discriminant analysis of PET resting metabolic patterns can identify patients at risk for AD with mild memory deficits as having probable AD. It was suggested that activation studies using PET studies might augment the power of this discriminant analysis. Importantly, PET scanning has detected abnormalities in brain glucose utilization in ApoE 4-positive individuals two decades before classical signs of dementia usually manifest, but it is not clear if these differences reflect

Table 10
Neuropsychological and Brain Imaging Markers of Probable Alzheimer Disease

Markers	Uses	Accuracy	Reference
Neuropsychologic Delayed recall profiles	Dx PREDT	SP: 0.91-0.98 ST: 0.96-1	*179, 321*
MRI Hippocampal atrophy	Dx	ST: 0.82-1	*321*
SPECT Bilateral posterior temporoparietal hypoperfusion	Dx	SP: 0.87-0.96 ST: 0.42-0.88	*321*
MRI + SPECT	Dx	SP: 0.92 ST: 0.95	*321*
PET Bilateral posterior temporoparietal hypometabolism	Dx	SP: 0.85-0.88 ST: 0.38-0.92	*321*
Discriminant analysis of resting metabolic patterns	PREDT		*312*
1H-MRI-Spectroscopy $\downarrow$ NAA + $\uparrow$ ml	Dx	?	*321*

Dx, diagnostic; ml, myoinositol; NAA, *n*-acetylaspartic acid + other acetyl-containing molecules; PREDT, predictive; SP, specificity; ST, sensitivity (for living patients with probable AD relative to a healthy control group).
After ref. *321.* See also refs. *378,428,429,* and Chapter 7.

a preclinical stage of AD or genetic differences in brain glucose utilization *(361,362)*. Longitudinal studies must now be done to determine the predictive power of such PET tests. Since different ligands are under development for use with PET, the potential of PET for preclinical diagnosis in a variety of degenerative brain diseases seems inherently enormous. Other approaches that might increase the sensitivity and specificity of PET for early AD detection include pharmacological challenges of short-acting cholinergic agents and sensory activation during functional scanning. SPECT also may have potential for the preclinical diagnosis of AD *(24,168,259)*. The role of functional imaging in early diagnosis is reviewed in Chapter 7.

Dementia Test Batteries

Although labor-intensive, dementia test batteries are promising for the earlier diagnosis of AD (see Chapter 8). Furthermore, the prescreening for AD almost certainly will continue to involve some type of neuropsychological or neurobehavioral test. Certain neuropsychological profiles on their own have been shown to predict regional neuropathology 5 years later *(179,371)*. To facilitate the early diagnosis of AD with a dementia test battery, persons might be evaluated at least once in early adulthood (say by age 25 years) to establish a record of baseline cognitive functioning. A comparison of existing baseline data with current test data would indicate the nature and magnitude of deterioration in various areas of functioning. Tests administered in the baseline assessment might include those functions that are known to decline with dementia, that is, memory, executive functions, visual spatial skills, motor function, and skills of daily living. Such approaches are currently being used to evaluate the development of AD-like dementia in persons with Down syndrome.

Tests in Combination for the Earlier Detection of Alzheimer's Disease

At this time, it appears that there is unlikely to be a single biomarker that can be used to directly distinguish persons with AD from those with non-AD among a group of persons with possible AD or before any clinical symptoms appear. It is suggested that different types of readily available information be used for diagnosis. When different tests are applied independently, the misclassification rate inevitably increases. A procedure is needed to combine multiple pieces of information into a single index that can be used to estimate the probability that a person with questionable symptoms of AD is developing definite AD. The powerful technique of logistic discrimination is ideal for separating populations on the basis of overlapping, quantitative characteristics.

In order to determine logistic coefficients for combining multiple pieces of information in the best possible way, two different types of longitudinal studies should be carried out. Implicit in this approach are that guidelines be used for diagnosing definite AD at autopsy and for classifying "possible" AD, that the patients with possible AD in both studies are comparable, and that the same biomarker information be obtained for all participants. It is important to clarify that a diagnosis of "possible" AD is not restricted to the classification scheme of McKhann and coworkers *(250)*. The term "possible" AD could refer to a diagnosis of either possible AD or probable AD using these guidelines, or to some other classification scheme. In practice, it would be sensible to begin an evaluation of biomarkers using the McKhann et al. diagnosis of probable AD. If this approach were successful, then an evaluation might be conducted, for example, using threshhold values in a neuropsychological/neurobehavioral screening test to classify people as having "possible" AD. Of importance is that some suitable protocol for diagnosis of people with questionable symptoms of AD be implemented and be used consistently throughout the investigation. The classification scheme that is used to diagnose the study participants will depend upon available knowledge of the sensitivity and specificity of the biomarkers under evaluation for diagnosing AD.

For study 1, a group of patients diagnosed as having possible AD according to a protocol should be identified, for example, in an Alzheimer clinic. This group will consist of persons who are developing AD and others with conditions that can mask as AD. These individuals should be followed through to autopsy, which will distinguish those with definite AD from the others. Logistic regression, using biological data taken at the time of entry into the study, should be applied to all of the deceased. This will identify the biomarkers that best predict definite AD, and generate a set of coefficients that will enable calculation of the probability of definite AD, given the risk factors, among a population with possible AD.

For study 2, a group of healthy individuals ranging in age from 70 to 80 years who reside in housing for elders (for example) would be selected and followed for (say) 4 years until a reasonable proportion developed possible AD. Logistic regression should be applied to the biological data taken at year 1 from all patients. This will generate a second set of coefficients that will enable calculation of the probability of developing possible AD given that a person is in the high-risk population.

To determine whether a person with symptoms of possible AD has definite AD, the battery of tests would be applied. The test data would be transformed into two separate probability indices using the two sets of logistic coefficients described above. The probability that the person with symptoms of possible

AD has definite AD, given his/her set of biomarker data, would be obtained by multiplying the probability index obtained using the first set of coefficients by the probability index obtained using the second set of coefficients.

Such an approach would make the most of available data, and avoid the use of arbitrary cut-off values to classify persons as definitely affected with AD or not. In such studies, one or a combination of biomarkers, age, gender, presence of the ApoE 4 allele, family history of AD, results from neurocognitive tests or other suitable tests might be evaluated. For the diagnosis of possible AD, it might be convenient to use threshhold values in a neuropsychological/neurobehavioral screening test. The reader is referred to ref. *296* for further information about deriving logistic coefficients and calculating probabilities from biological data.

Summary and Discussion

Although considerable progress is being made in biomarker research in the Alzheimer field, particularly with regard to CSF and serum/plasma markers, a review of the literature has revealed many examples of irreproducible results. Since lack of reproducibility reflects the use of differing protocols and/or methodology, factors known to contribute to variability in the biomarker field have been reviewed to aid with quality control in the Alzheimer field. These include specification of inclusion/exclusion criteria for study participants, identification of biological, environmental, and technical factors, which can produce variability in test results, controlling for the effects of these variables through proper experimental design and quality control procedures, and application of appropriate statistical procedures to achieve the best possible interpretation of test data.

The issue of whether to lump cases into one group or split them into subgroups is controversial but critical to many biomedical case/control studies. Although AD has been treated as a single entity for many years, there is undeniable evidence for genetic and biological heterogeneity in this disorder. At the clinical level there are familial and sporadic forms of AD with differing ages of onset. AD researchers must be aware not only of possible complicating effects of AD subtypes, but also of genetic and/or environmental risk factors, subject age and gender, ethnic background, and disease severity, duration and stage on biomarker expression, so that data can be utilized in the most effective way. Regardless of the research design that ultimately is chosen, it is crucial that characteristics of the study participants be specified in sufficient detail so that the study can be independently replicated, and that the sample size is sufficiently large for "effects" to be properly evaluated.

Biomarker tests for early AD diagnosis must not only be adequately sensitive and specific, but be tolerable for the patient and cost-effective. The quest for a single, sensitive biomarker that reflects the presence of AD should be continued. However, because the histopathological diagnosis of AD requires the synthesis of more than one type of information, it is unlikely that only one biomarker will be adequate for the antemortem diagnosis of AD. As discussed, it should be possible to combine different types of information into a predictive index for dementia that reflects dementia severity and/or that detects dementia earlier than any single parameter alone. Readily obtainable data such as age, gender, family history information, and Mini-Mental State Exam scores, should not be overlooked. Biomarker researchers are urged to collaborate with statisticians or epidemiologists to ensure the most appropriate experimental design and to make the most of the experimental data. To facilitate the achieving of common goals, the sharing of protocols, methodological details, specialized reagents and different types of standards (including positive and negative pools of biological samples), and the establishment of banks of biological samples taken longitudinally from well-characterized subjects who go on to autopsy, are encouraged. Because of postmortem effects on biomarkers, the use of CSF and blood samples from deceased individuals may not yield reliable results.

Not clear at present is to what extent many so-called biomarkers of AD are independent of effects of the ApoE 4 allele, which is a prevalent and significant risk factor for AD, but is not a reliable predictor of AD on its own. It has been recommended that ApoE genotyping be included as part of the screening battery in any biomarker study so that this matter may be clarified.

At the present time, no single biomarker has yet been found in blood, CSF or other tissues which has been proven to be predictive of definite AD at the possible AD stage. Currently, biomarkers in tissues other than brain can be used only as diagnostic aids at the probable AD stage. However, there is evidence that neuropsychological profiles on their own and certain types of brain imaging are predictive of probable AD at the possible AD stage. It therefore is likely that both of these latter approaches for directly measuring function will continue to be adapted for the earlier and earlier direct testing for AD.

The demonstration that ApoE genotyping in combination with other tests can improve the predictive power in AD diagnosis raises the possibility that other genetic risk factors for AD might similarly be exploited *(181,326)*. The development of new technologies for rapidly identifying genetic variants and mutations such as "microchip" assays *(45,84,152)*, capillary electrophoresis *(261)*, and other novel approaches, in addition to promising AD therapeutics, are expected to drive this approach. Whether society will allow such genetic information to be utilized remains to be determined. The disclosure of genetic test results can be associated with complex and unexpected psychological, legal, social, and medical insurance issues (see Chapter 12). As with other serious genetic disorders, genetic testing in AD must continue to be carried out according to the highest of ethical standards and include genetic counseling and other backup support.

Acknowledgments

Grants to M.E.P. from the Queen Elizabeth Hospital Research Institute (Toronto, Canada), the Ontario Mental Health Foundation, the Alzheimer Society of Canada, the U.S. Alzheimer's Society, Health Canada, the University of Toronto Work Study and Life Sciences (Physiology) Programs, the Scottish Charitable Rite Foundation of Canada, and the Federal Government Summer Student Career Development Awards Program, to D.F.A. from the Natural Sciences and Engineering Research Council, and to H.P. from NIH and NIA supported the authors' investigative studies of risk factors in Alzheimer's disease. We thank the editors of this book for providing peer-reviews of this chapter and for their helpful comments, and Simon Wong for assistance with preparation of the figures and tables.

References

1. Adler MJ, Coronel C, Shelton E, Seegmiller JE, Dewji NN. Increased gene expression of Alzheimer disease beta-amyloid precursor protein in senescent cultured fibroblasts. *Proc. Natl. Acad. Sci.* U.S.A. 1991;88:16–20.

1a. Adunsky A, Diver-Haber A, Becker D, Hershkowitz M. Basal and activated intracellular calcium concentrations in mononuclear cells of Alzheimer's disease and unipolar depression. *J. Gerontol. A Biol. Med. Sci.* 1995;50:B201–B204.

2. Ahlskog JE, Uitti RJ, Tyce GM, O'Brien JF, Petersen RC, Kokmen E. Plasma catechols and monoamine oxidase metabolites in untreated Parkinson's and Alzheimer's diseases. *J. Neurol. Sci.* 1996;136:62–168.

3. Aisen PS. Inflammation and Alzheimer disease. *Mol. Chemical. Neuropathol.* 1996;28:83–88.

4. Albert MS. Cognitive and neurobiologic markers of early Alzheimer disease. *Proc. Natl. Acad. Sci.* U.S.A. 1996;93:13,547–13,551.

5. Algotsson A, Nordberg A, Almkvist O, Winblad B. Skin vessel reactivity is impaired in Alzheimer's disease. *Neurobiol. Aging* 1995;16:577–582.

6. Almkvist O, Basun H, Wagner SL, Rowe BA, Wahlund LO, Lannfelt L. Cerebrospinal fluid levels of alpha-secretase-cleaved soluble amyloid precursor protein mirror cognition in a Swedish family with Alzheimer disease and a gene mutation: cerebrospinal fluid levels of alpha-secretase soluble amyloid precursor protein mirror cognition in a Swedish family with Alzheimer disease and a gene mutation. *Arch. Neurol.* 1997;54:641–644.

7. Alonso AD, Grundke-Iqbal I, Barra HS, Iqbal K. Abnormal phosphorylation of tau and the mechanism of Alzheimer neurofibrillary degeneration: sequestration of

microtubule-associated proteins 1 and 2 and the disassembly of microtubules by the abnormal tau. *Proc. Natl. Acad. Sci. U.S.A.* 1997;94:298–303.

8. Alonso DF, Farias EF, Famulari AL, Dominguez RO, Kohan S, de Lustig ES. Excessive urokinase-type plasminogen activator activity in the euglobulin fraction of patients with Alzheimer-type demenetia. *J. Neurol. Sci.* 1996;139:83–88.

9. Altstiel LD, Lawlor B, Mohs R, Schmeidler J, Dalton A, Mehta P, Davis K. Elevated alpha 1-antichymotrypsin serum levels in a subset of nondemented first-degree relatives of Alzheimer's disease patients. *Dementia* 1995;6:17–20.

10. Alvarez XA, Franco A, Fernandez-Novoa L, Cacabelos R. Blood levels of histamine, IL-1 beta, and TNF-alpha in patients with mild to moderate Alzheimer disease. *Mol. Chem. Neuropathol.* 1996;29:237–252.

11. Alzheimer Disease Collaborative Group. The structure of the presenilin 1 (S182) gene and identification of six novel mutations in early onset families. *Nature Genet.* 1995;11:219–222.

12. Andreasen N, Vanmechelen E, Van de Voorde A, Davidsson P, Hesse C, Tarvonen S, Raiha I, Sourander L, Winblad B, Blennow K. Cerebrospinal fluid tau protein as a biochemical marker for Alzheimer's disease: a community based follow up study. *J. Neurol. Neurosurg. Psychiatry* 1998;64:298–305.

13. Angelis P, Scharf S, Mander A, Vajda F, Christopihidis N. Serum interleukin-6 and interleukin-6 soluble receptor in Alzheimer's disease. *Neurosci. Lett.* 1998; 244:106–108.

14. Arai H, Terajima M, Miura M, Higuchi S, Muramatsu T, Matsushita S, Machida N, Nakagawa T, Lee VM, Trojanowski JQ, Sasaki H. Effect of genetic risk factors and disease progression on the cerebrospinal fluid tau levels in Alzheimer's disease. *J. Am. Geriatr. Soc.* 1997;45:1228–1231.

15. Arai H, Clark CM, Ewbank DC, Takase S, Higuchi S, Miura M, Seki H, Higuchi M, Matsui T, Lee VM, Trojanowski JQ, Sasaki H. Cerebrospinal fluid tau protein as a potential diagnostic marker in Alzheimer's disease. *Neurobiol. Aging* 1998; 19:125–126.

16. Attal-Khemis S, Dalmeyda V, Michot JL, Roudier M, Morfin R. Increased total 7 alpha-hydroxydehydroepiandrosterone in serum of patients with Alzheimer's disease. *J. Gerontol. A. Biol. Sci. Med. Sci.* 1998;53:B125–B132.

17. Bales KR, Verina T, Dodel RD, Du Y, Altsteil L, Bender M, Hyslop P, Johnstone EM, Little SP, Cummins DJ, Piccardo P, Ghetti B, Paul SM. Lack of apolipoprotein E dramatically reduces amyloid beta-peptide deposition. *Nature Genet.* 1997; 17:263–264.

18. Bancher C, Jellinger K, Wichart I. Biological markers for the diagnosis of Alzheimer's disease. *J. Neural Transm. Suppl.* 1998;53:185–197.

19. Basun H, Forssell LG, Almkvist O, Cowburn RF, Eklof R, Winblad B, Wetterberg L. Amino acid concentrations in cerebrospinal fluid and plasma in Alzheimer's disease and healthy control subjects. *J. Neural Transm. Park. Dis. Dement. Sect.* 1990;2:295–304.

20. Basun H, Forssell LG, Wetterberg L, Winblad B. Metals and trace elements in plasma and cerebrospinal fluid in normal aging and Alzheimer's disease. *J. Neural Transm. Park. Dis. Dement. Sect.* 1991;3:231–258.

21. Benussi L, Govoni S, Gasparini L, Binetti G, Trabucchi M, Bianchetti A, Racchi

M. Specific role for protein kinase C alpha in the constitutive and regulated secretion of amyloid precursor protein in human skin fibroblasts. *Neurosci. Lett.* 1998;240:97–101.

22. Bergamaschini L, Parnetti L, Pareyson D, Canziani S, Cugno M, Agostoni A. Activation of the contact system in cerebrospinal fluid of patients with Alzheimer's disease. *Alzheimer Dis. Assoc. Disord.* 1998;12:102–108.

22a. Bickerstaff MC. Serum amyloid P component controls cromatin degradation and prevents antinuclear autoimmunity. *Nat. Med.* 1999;5:694–697.

23. Blacker D, Wilcox MA, Laird NM, Rodes L, Horvath SM, Go RC, Perry R, Watson B Jr, Bassett SS, McInnis MG, Albert MS, Hyman BT, Tanzi RE. Alpha-2 macroglobulin is genetically associated with Alzheimer disease. *Nature Genet.* 1998;19:357–360.

24. Blanco A, Alberra R, Marques Lopez-Dominguez JM, Gil Neciga E, Carrizosa E. Usefulness of SPECT in the study of Alzheimer's disease. *Neurologia* 1998; 13:63–68.

25. Blass JP, Gibson GE, Sheu KF. Peripheral markers of Alzheimer's disease. *Aging (Milano)* 1997;9(4 Suppl):55–56.

26. Blennow K, Vanmechelen E. Combination of the different biological markers for increasing specificity of in vivo Alzheimer's testing. *J. Neural Transm. Suppl.* 1998;53:223–235.

27. Blennow K, Davidsson P, Wallin A, Ekman R. Chromogranin A in cerebrospinal fluid: a biochemical marker for synaptic degeneration in Alzheimer's disease? *Dementia* 1995;6:306–311.

28. Blum-Degen D, Muller T, Kuhn W, Gerlach M, Przuntek H, Riederer P. Interleukin-1 beta and interleukin-6 are elevated in the cerebrospinal fluid of Alzheimer's and de novo Parkinson's patients. *Neurosci. Lett.* 1995;202:17–20.

29. Bongioanni P, Donato M, Castagna M, Gemignani F. Platelet phenolsulphotransferase activity, monoamine oxidase activity and peripheral-type benzodiazepine binding in demented patients. *J. Neural Transm.* 1996;103:491–501.

30. Bongioanni P, Boccardi B, Borgna M, Castagna M, Mondino C. T-cell interferon gamma binding in patients with dementia of the Alzheimer type. *Arch. Neurol.* 1997;54:457–462.

31. Bongioanni P, Castagna M, Mondino C, Boccardi B, Borgna M. Platelet and lymphocyte benzodiazepine binding in patients with Alzheimer's disease. *Exp. Neurol.* 1997;146:560–566.

32. Bongioanni P, Gemignani F, Boccardi B, Borgna M, Rossi B. Platelet monoamine oxidase molecular activity in demented patients. *Ital. J. Neurol. Sci.* 1997;18:151–156.

33. Bongioanni P, Romano MR, Sposito R, Castagna M, Boccardi B, Borgna M. T-cell tumour necrosis factor-alpha receptor binding in demented patients. *J. Neurol.* 1997;244:418–425.

34. Bongioanni P, Boccardi B, Borgna M, Rossi B. T-lymphocyte interleukin 6 receptor binding in patients with dementia of Alzheimer type. *Arch. Neurol.* 1998; 55:1305–1308.

35. Bosman GJ, Bartholomeus IG, de Man AJ, van Kalmthout PJ, de Grip WJ. Erythrocyte membrane characteristics indicate abnormal cellular aging in patients with Alzheimer disease. *Neurobiol. Aging* 1991;12:13–18.

36. Bowler JV, Munoz DG, Merskey H, Hachinski V. Fallacies in the pathological confirmation of the diagnosis of Alzheimer's disease. *J. Neurol. Neurosurg. Psychiatry* 1998;64:18–24.

37. Breitner JC. Inflammatory processes and antiinflammatory drugs in Alzheimer's disease: a current appraisal. *Neurobiol. Aging* 1996;17:789–794.

38. Breitner JC, Welsh KA, Helms MJ, Gaskell PC, Gau BA, Roses AD, Pericak-Vance MA, Saunders AM. Delayed onset of Alzheimer's disease with nonsteroidal anti-inflammatory and histamine H2 blocking drugs. *Neurobiol. Aging* 1995;16:523–530.

39. Brugg B, Dubreuil YL, Huber G, Wollman EE, Delhaye-Bouchard N, Mariani J. Inflammatory processes induce beta-amyloid precursor protein changes in mouse brain. *Proc. Natl. Acad. Sci. U.S.A.* 1995;92:3032–3035.

40. Buee L, Hof PR, Bouras C, Delacourte A, Perl DP, Morrison JH, Fillit HM. Pathological alterations of the cerebral microvasculature in Alzheimer's disease and related dementing disorders. *Acta Neuropathol. (Berl.)* 1994;87:469–480.

41. Carmel R, Gott PS, Waters CH, Cairo K, Green R, Bondareff W, DeGiorgio CM, Cummings JL, Jacobsen DW, Buckwalter G, et al. The frequently low cobalamin levels in dementia usually signify treatable metabolic, neurologic and electro-physiologic abnormalities. *Eur. J. Haematol.* 1995;54:245–253.

42. Carr DB, Goate A, Phil D, Morris JC. Current concepts in the pathogenesis of Alzheimer's disease. *Am. J. Med.* 1997;103:3S–10S.

43. Ceballos-Picot I, Merad-Boudia M, Nicole A, Thevenin M, Hellier G, Legrain S, Berr C. Peripheral antioxidant enzyme activities and selenium in elderly subjects and in dementia of Alzheimer's type—place of the extracellular glutathione per-oxidase. *Free Radic. Biol. Med.* 1996;20:579–587.

44. Chandrasekaran K, Giordano T, Brady DR, Stoll J, Martin LJ, Rapoport SI. Impairment in mitochondrial cytochrome oxidase gene expression in Alzheimer disease. Brain Research. *Mol. Brain Res.* 1994;24:336–340.

45. Cheng J, Waters LC, Fortina P, Hvichia G, Jacobson SC, Ramsey JM, Kricka LJ, Wilding P. Degenerate oligonucleotide primed-polymerase chain reaction and capillary electrophoretic analysis of human DNA on microchip-based devices. *Anal. Biochem.* 1998;257:101–106.

46. Clark R, Smith AD, Jobst KA, Refsum H, Sutton L, Ueland PM. Vitamin B12, and serum total homocysteine levels in confirmed Alzheimer disease. *Arch. Neurol.* 1997;55:1449–1455.

47. Connolly GP. Fibroblast models of neurological disorders: fluorescence measure-ment studies. *Trends Pharmacol. Sci.* 1998;19:171–177.

48. Connor TJ, Leonard BE. Minireview. Depression, stress and immunological acti-vation: the role of cytokines in depressive disorders. *Life Sci.* 1998;62:583–606.

49. Cooper AL, Sheu KF, Blass JP. Normal glutamate metabolism in Alzheimer's dis-ease fibroblasts deficient in alpha-ketoglutarate dehydrogenase complex activity. *Dev. Neurosci.* 1996;18:499–504.

50. Cornett CR, Markesbery WR, Ehmann WD. Imbalances of trace elements related to oxidative damage in Alzheimer's disease brain. *Neurotoxicology* 1998;19:339–345.

51. Corral-Debrinski M, Horton T, Lott MT, Shoffner JM, McKee AC, Beal MF, Graham BH, Wallace DC. Marked changes in mitochondrial DNA deletion levels in Alzheimer brains. *Genomics* 1994;23:471–476.

52. Corrigan FM, Mowat B, Skinner ER, Van Rhijn AG, Cousland G. High density lipoprotein fatty acids in dementia. *Prostagland. Leukot. Essent. Fatty. Acids.* 1998;58:125–127.

53. Crawford JG. Alzheimer's disease risk factors as related to cerebral blood flow: additional evidence. *Med. Hypothe.* 1998;50:25–36.

54. Crawford F, Suo Z, Fang C, Mullan M. Characteristics of the in vitro vasoactivity of beta-amyloid peptides. *Exp. Neurol.* 1998;150:159–168.

55. Cruts M, van Duijn CM, Backhovens H, Van den Broeck M, Wehnert A, Serneels S, Sherrington R, Hutton M, Hardy J, St. George-Hyslop PH, Hofman A, Van Broeckhoven C. Estimation of the genetic contribution of presenilin-1 and -2 mutations in a population-based study of presenile Alzheimer disease. *Hum. Mol. Genet.* 1998;7:43–51.

56. Csaszar A, Kalman J, Szalai C, Janka Z, Romics L. Association of the apolipoprotein A-IV codon 360 mutation in patients with Alzheimer's disease. *Neurosci. Lett.* 1997;230:151–154.

57. Cummings JL, Vinters HV, Cole GM, Khachaturian ZS. Alzheimer's disease: etiologies, pathophysiology, cognitive reserve, and treatment opportunities. *Neurology* 1998;51:S2–S17.

58. Curran M, Middleton D, Edwardson J, Perry R, McKeith I, Morris C, Neill D. HLA-DR antigens associated with major genetic risk for late-onset Alzheimer's disease. *NeuroReport* 1997;8:1467–1469.

59. Dalton AJ, Selzer GB, Adlin MS, Wisniewski HM. Association between Alzheimer disease and Down syndrome: clinical observations. In Berg JM, Karlinsky H, Holland AJ, editors. *Alzheimer Disease, Down Syndrome and Their Relationship.* Oxford: Oxford University Press, 1993;53–59.

60. Das S, Potter H. (1995). Expression of the Alzheimer amyloid-promoting factor antichymotrypsin is induced in human astrocytes by IL-1. *Neuron* 1995;14:447–456.

61. Davidsson P, Jahn R, Bergquist J, Ekman R, Blennow K. Synaptotagmin, a synaptic vesicle protein, is present in human cerebrospinal fluid: a new biochemical marker for synaptic pathology in Alzheimer disease? *Mol. Chem. Neuropathol.* 1996;27:195–210.

62. Davies TA, Fine RE, Johnson RJ, Levesque CA, Rathburn WH, Seetoo KF, Smith SJ, Strohmeier G, Volicer L, Delva L, et al. Non-age related differences in thrombin responses by platelets from male patients with advanced Alzheimer's disease. *Biochem. Biophys. Res. Commun.* 1993;194:537–543.

63. Davies TA, Long HJ, Sgro K, Rathbun WH, McMenamin ME, Seetoo K, Tibbles H, Billingslea AM, Fine RE, Fishman JB, Levesque CA, Smith SJ, Wells JM, Simons ER. Activated Alzheimer disease platelets retain more beta amyloid precursor protein. *Neurobiol. Aging* 1997;18:147–153.

64. Davies TA, Long HJ, Tibbles HE, Sgro KR, Wells JM, Rathbun WH, Seetoo KF, McMenamin ME, Smith SJ, Feldman RG, Levesque CA, Fine RE, Simons ER. Moderate and advanced Alzheimer's patients exhibit platelet activation differences. *Neurobiol. Aging* 1997;18:155–162.

65. Davis BM, Mohs RC, Greenwald BS, Mathe AA, Johns CA, Horvath TB, Davis KL. Clinical studies of the cholinergic deficit in Alzheimer's disease. I. Neurochemical and neuroendocrine studies. *J. Am. Geriatr. Soc.* 1985;33:741–748.

66. Davis JN 2nd, Parker WD Jr. Evidence that two reports of mtDNA cytochrome C oxidase "mutations" in Alzheimer's disease are based on mDNA pseudogenes of recent evolutionary origin. *Biochem. Biophys. Res. Commun.* 1998;244:877–883.

67. Davis RE, Miller S, Herrnstadt C, Ghosh SS, Fahy E, Shinobu LA, Galasko D, Thal LJ, Beal MF, Howell N, Parker WD Jr. Mutations in mitochondrial cytochrome c oxidase genes segregate with late-onset Alzheimer disease. *Proc. Natl. Acad. Sci. U.S.A.* 1997;94:4526–4531.

68. de Deyn PP, Hiramatsu M, Borggreve F, Goeman J, D'Hooge R, Saerens J, Mori A. Superoxide dismutase activity in cerebrospinal fluid of patients with dementia and some other neurological disorders. *Alzheimer Dis. Assoc. Disord.* 1998; 12:26–32.

69. de Grey AD. A proposed refinement of the mitochondrial free radical theory of aging. *Bioessays* 1997;19:161–166.

70. de la Monte SM, Wands JR. Neuronal thread protein over-expression in brains with Alzheimer's disease lesions. *J. Neurol. Sci.* 1992;113:152–164.

71. de la Monte SM, Carlson RI, Brown NV, Wands JR. Profiles of neuronal thread protein expression in Alzheimer's disease. *J. Neuropathol. Exp. Neurol.* 1996;55: 1038–1050.

72. de la Monte SM, Ghanbari K, Frey WH, Beheshti I, Averback P, Hauser SL, Ghanbari HA, Wands JR. Characterization of the AD7c-NTP cDNA expression in Alzheimer's disease and measurement of a 41 kD protein in cerebrospinal fluid. *J. Clin. Invest.* 1997;100:3093–3104.

73. de la Torre JC. (1997). Hemodynamic consequences of deformed microvessels in the brain in Alzheimer's disease. *Ann. N.Y. Acad. Sci.* 1997;8:75–91.

74. de Leo ME, Borrello S, Passantino M, Palazzotti B, Mordente A, Daniele A, Filippini V, Galeotti J, Masullo C. Oxidative stress and overexpression of manganese superoxide dismutase in patients with Alzheimer's disease. *Neurosci. Lett.* 1998;250:173–176.

75. de Leon MJ, McRae T, Rusinek H, Convit A, De Santi S, Tarshish C, Golomb J, Volkow N, Daisley K, Orentreich N, McEwen B. Cortisol reduces hippocampal glucose metabolism in normal elderly, but not in Alzheimer's disease. *J. Clin. Endocrinol. Metab.* 1997;82:3251–3259.

76. de Lustig ES, Kohan S, Famulari AL, Dominguez RO, Serra JA. Peripheral markers and diagnostic criteria in Alzheimer's disease: critical evaluations. *Rev. Neurosci.* 1994;5:213–225.

77. de Rijk R, Michelson D, Karp B, Petrides J, Galliven E, Deuster P, Paciotti G, Gold PW, Sternberg EM. Exercise and circadian rhythm-induced variations in plasma cortisol differentially regulate interleukin-1 beta (IL-1 beta), IL-6, and tumor necrosis factor-alpha (TNF alpha) production in humans: high sensitivity of TNF alpha and resistance of IL-6. *J. Clin. Endocrinol. Metabol.* 1997;82:2182–2191.

78. Di Luca M, Pastorino L, Bianchetti A, Perez J, Vignolo LA, Lenzi GL, Trabucchi M, Cattabeni F, Padovani A. Differential level of platelet amyloid beta precursor protein isoforms: an early marker for Alzheimer disease. *Arch. Neurol.* 1998; 55:1195–1200.

79. Du Yan S, Zhu H, Fu J, Yan SF, Roher A, Tourtellotte WW, Rajavashisth R, Chen X, Godman GC, Stern D, Schmidt AM. Amyloid-beta peptide-receptor for ad-

vanced glycation endproduct interaction elicits neuronal expression of macrophage-colony stimulating factor: a proinflammatory pathway in Alzheimer disease. *Proc. Natl. Acad. Sci. U.S.A.* 1997;94:5296–5301.

80. Ebstein RP, Nemanov L, Lubarski G, Dano M, Trevis T, Korczyn AD. Changes in expression of lymphocyte amyloid precursor protein mRNA isoforms in normal aging and Alzheimer's disease. *Brain Res. Mol. Brain Res.* 1996;35:260–268.

81. Eckert A, Fiorstl H, Zerfass R, Hartmann H, Muller WE. Lymphocytes and neutrophils as peripheral models to study the effect of beta-amyloid on cellular calcium signalling in Alzheimer's disease. *Life Sci.* 1996;59:499–510.

82. Edland SD, Silverman JM, Peskind ER, Tsuang D, Wijsman E, Morris JC. Increased risk of dementia in others of Alzheimer's disease cases: evidence for maternal inheritance. *Neurology* 1996;47:254–256.

83. Egensperger R, Kosel S, Schnopp NM, Mehraein P, Graeber MB. (1997). Association of the mitochondrial tRNA(A4336G) mutation with Alzheimer's and Parkinson's diseases. *Neuropathol. Appl. Neurobiol.* 1996;23:315–321.

84. Eggers M, Ehrlich D. A review of microfabricated devices for gene-based diagnostics. *Hematol. Pathol.* 1995;9:1–15.

85. Eisen A, Calne D. Amyotrophic lateral sclerosis, Parkinson's disease and Alzheimer's disease: phylogenetic disorders of the human neocortex sharing many characteristics. *Can. J. Neurol. Sci.* 1992;19:117–123.

86. Eisinger J, Arroyo P, Braquet M, Arroyo H, Ayavou T. Erythrocyte transketolases and Alzheimer disease. *Rev. Med. Interne.* 1994;15:387–389.

86a. Botto M, Hutchinson WL, Herbert J, et al. Serum amyloid A, an acute-phase protein, modulates proteoglycan synthesis in cultured murine peritoneal macrophages. *Biochem. Biophys. Res. Comm.* 1999;261:298–301.

87. Elovaara I, Maury CP, Palo J. Serum amyloid A protein, albumin and prealbumin in Alzheimer's disease and in demented patients with Down's syndrome. *Acta Neurol. Scand.* 1986;74:245–250.

88. Elrod R, Peskind ER, DiGiacomo L, Brodkin KI, Veith RC, Raskind MA. Effects of Alzheimer's disease severity on cerebrospinal fluid norepinephrine concentration. *Am. J. Psychiatry* 1997;154:25–30.

89. Engelborghs S, De Deyn PP. The neurochemistry of Alzheimer's disease. *Acta Neurol. Belg.* 1997;97:67–84.

90. Engler R. Acute phase protein in inflammation. *C.R. Seances Soc. Biol. Fil.* 1995;189:563–78.

91. Etcheberrigaray E, Gibson GE, Alkon DL. Molecular mechanisms of memory and the pathophysiology of Alzheimer's disease. *Ann. N.Y. Acad. Sci.* 1994;747:245–255.

92. Etcheberrigaray R, Payne JL, Alkon DL. Soluble beta-amyloid induces Alzheimer's disease features in human fibroblasts and in neuronal tissues. *Life Sci.* 1996;59:491–498.

93. Evans DA, Hebert LE, Beckett LA, Scherr PA, Albert MS, Chown MJ, Pilgrim DM, Taylor JO. Education and other measures of socioeconomic status and risk of incident Alzheimer disease in a defined population of older persons. *Arch. Neurol.* 1997;54:1399–1405.

94. Ewins DL, Rossor MN, Butler J, Roques PK, Mulla MJ, McGregor AM. Association between autoimmune thyroid disease and familial Alzheimer's disease. *Clin. Endocrinol.* 1991;35:93–96.

95. Farlow MR, Lahiri DK, Poirier J, Davignon J, Schneider L, Hui SL. Treatment outcome of tacrine therapy depends on apolipoprotein genotype and gender of the subjects with Alzheimer's disease. *Neurology* 1998;50:669–677.

96. Fastbom J, Forsell Y, Winblad B. Benzodiazepines may have protective effects against Alzheimer disease. *Alzheimer Dis. Assoc. Disord.* 1998;12:14–17.

97. Fekkes D, van der Cammen RJ, van Loon CP, Verschoor C, van Harskamp F, de Koning I, Schudel WJ, Pepplinkhuizen L. Abnormal amino acid metabolism in patients with early stage Alzheimer dementia. *J. Neural Transm.* 1998;105:287–294.

98. Feychting M, Pedersen NL, Svedberg P, Floderus B, Gatz M. Dementia and occupational exposure to magnetic fields. *Scand. J. Work Environ. Health* 1998; 24:46–53.

99. Finch CE, Marchalonis JJ. Evolutionary perspectives on amyloid and inflammatory features of Alzheimer disease. *Neurobiol. Aging* 1996;17:809–815.

100. Fischer P, Gotz ME, Danielczyk W, Gsell W, Riederer P. Blood transferrin and ferritin in Alzheimer's disease. *Life Sci.* 1997;60:2273–2278.

101. Fisher GH, Petrucelli L, Gardner C, Emory C, Frey WH 2nd, Amaducci L, Sorbi S, Sorrentino G, Borghi M, D'Aniello A. Free D-amino acids in human cerebrospinal fluid of Alzheimer disease, multiple sclerosis, and healthy control subjects. *Mol. Chem. Neuropathol.* 1994;23:1115–1124.

102. Foster NL. The development of biological markers for the diagnosis of Alzheimer's disease. *Neurobiol. Aging* 1998;19:127–129.

103. Fowler CJ, Cowburn RF, Joseph JA. Alzheimer, ageing and amyloid: an absurd allegory? *Gerontology* 1997;43:132–142.

104. Frecker MF, Pryse-Phillips WE, Strong HR. Immunological associations in familial and non-familial Alzheimer patients and their families. *Can. J. Neurol. Sci.* 1994;21:112–119.

105. French BM, Dawson MR, Dobbs AR. Classification and staging of dementia of the Alzheimer type: a comparison between neural networks and linear discriminant analysis. *Arch. Neurol.* 1997;54:1001–1009.

106. Galasko D. Cerebrospinal fluid levels of A beta 42 and tau: potential markers of Alzheimer's disease. *J. Neural Transm. Suppl.* 1998;53:209–221.

107. Garlind A, Johnston JA, Algotsson A, Winblad B, Cowburn RF. Decreased beta-adrenoceptor-stimulated adenylyl cyclase activity in lymphocytes from Alzheimer's disease patients. *Neurosci. Lett.* 1997;226:37–40.

108. Garratt RC, Jhoti H. A molecular model for the tumour-associated antigen, p97, suggests a Zn-binding function. *FEBS Lett.* 1992;305:55–61.

109. Gasparini L, Racchi M, Binetti G, Trabucchi M, Solerte SB, Alkon D, Etcheberrigaray R, Gibson G, Blass J, Paoletti R, Govani S. Peripheral markers in testing pathophysiological hypotheses and diagnosing Alzheimer's disease. *FASEB J.* 1998;12:17–34.

110. Genovesi G, Paolini P, Marcellini L, Vernillo E, Salvati G, Polidori G, Ricciardi D, de Nuccio I, Re M. Relationship between autoimmune thyroid disease and Alzheimer's disease. Panminerva Med 1996;38:61–63.

111. Gentleman SM, Greenberg BD, Savage MJ, Noori M, Newman SJ, Roberts GW, Griffin WS, Graham DI. A beta 42 is the predominant form of amyloid beta-protein in the brains of short-term survivors of head injury. *NeuroReport* 1997;8:1519–1522.

111a. Ghanbari H, Ghanbari K, Beheshti I, Munzar M, Vasauskas A, Averback P. Biochemical assay for AD7c-NTP in urine as an Alzheimer's disease marker. *J. Clin. Lab. Anal.* 1998;12:285–288.

112. Ghiso J, Calero M, Matsubara E, Governale S, Chuba J, Beavis R, Wisniewski T, Frangione B. Alzheimer's soluble amyloid beta is a normal component of human urine. *FEBS Lett.* 1997;408:105–108.

113. Gibson G, Martins R, Blass J, Gandy S. Altered oxidation and signal transduction systems in fibroblasts from Alzheimer patients. *Life Sci.* 1996;59:477–489.

114. Gibson GE, Zhang H, Toral-Barza L, Szolosi S, Tofel-Grehl B. Calcium stores in cultured fibroblasts and their changes with Alzheimer's disease. *Biochim. Biophys. Acta* 1996;1316:71–77.

115. Goate A, Chartier-Harlin MC, Mullan M, Brown J, Crawford F, Fidani L, Giuffra L, Haynes A, Irving N, James L, et al. Segregation of a missense mutation in the amyloid precursor protein gene with familial Alzheimer's disease. *Nature* 1991; 349:704–706.

116. Goldsmith HS. Omental transposition for Alzheimer's disease. *Neurol. Res.* 1996; 18:103–108.

117. Gomes Trolin C, Regland B, Oreland L. Decreased methionine adenosyltransferase activity in erythrocytes of patients with dementia disorders. *Eur. Neuropsychopharmacol.* 1995;5:107–114.

118. Govoni S, Gasparini L, Racchi M, Trabucchi M. Peripheral cells as an investigational tool for Alzheimer's disease. *Life Sci.* 1996;59:461–468.

119. Graebert KS, Lemansky P, Kehle T, Herzog V. Localization and regulated release of Alzheimer amyloid precursor-like protein in thyrocytes. *Lab. Invest.* 1995;72: 513–523.

120. Green RC, Clarke VC, Thompson NJ, Woodard JL, Letz R. Early detection of Alzheimer disease: methods, markers, and misgivings. *Alzheimer Dis. Assoc. Disord.* 1997;11(Suppl 5):S1–S5.

121. Griffin W, Stanley LC, Ling C, White L, MacLeod V, Perrot LJ, White CL 3rd, Araoz C. Brain interleukin 1 and S-100 immunoreactivity are elevated in Down syndrome and Alzheimer disease. *Proc. Natl. Acad. Sci. U.S.A.* 1989;86:7611–7615.

122. Griffin WS, Sheng JG, Royston MC, Gentleman SM, McKenzie JE, Graham DI, Roberts GW, Mrak RE. Glial-neuronal interactions in Alzheimer's disease: the potential role of a 'cytokine cycle' in disease progression. *Brain Pathol.* 1998;8:65–72.

123. Growdon JH, Graefe K, Tennis M, Hayden D, Schoenfeld D, Wray SH. Pupil dilation to tropicamide is not specific for Alzheimer disease. *Arch. Neurol.* 1997;54:841–844.

123a. Growdon JH. Biomarkers of Alzheimer disease. *Arch. Neurol.* 1999;56:281–283.

124. Gruol DL, Nelson TE. Physiological and pathological roles of interleukin-6 in the central nervous system. *Mol. Neurobiol.* 1997;15:307–339.

125. Guo Z, Viitanen M, Fratiglioni L, Winblad B. Blood pressure and dementia in the elderly: epidemiologic perspectives. *Biomed. Pharmacother.* 1997;51:68–73.

126. Gutacker M, Valsangiacomo C, Balmelli T, Bernasconi MV, Bouras C, Piffaretti JC. Arguments against the involvement of Borrelia burgdorferi sensulato in Alzheimer's disease. *Res. Microbiol.* 1997;149:31–37.

127. Hajimohammadreza I, Brammer MJ, Eagger S, Burns A, Levy R. Platelet and

erythrocyte membrane changes in Alzheimer's disease. *Biochim. Biophys. Acta* 1990;1025:208–214.

128. Hampel H, Kotter HU, Moller HJ. Blood-cerebrospinal fluid barrier dysfunction for high molecular weight proteins in Alzheimer disease and major depression: indication for disease subsets. *Alzheimer Dis. Assoc. Disord.* 1997;11:78–87.

129. Hampel H, Schoen D, Schwarz MJ, Kotter HU, Schneider C, Sunderland T, Dukoff R, Levy J, Padberg F, Stubner S, Buch K, Muller N, Moller HJ. Interleukin-6 is not altered in cerebrospinal fluid of first-degree relatives and patients with Alzheimer disease. *Neurosci. Lett.* 1997;228:143–146.

130. Harigaya Y, Shoji M, Nakamura T, Matsubara E, Hosoda K, Hirai S. Alpha 1-antichymotrypsin level in cerebrospinal fluid is closely associated with late onset Alzheimer's disease. *Intern. Med.* 1995;34:481–484.

131. Hart MN, Merz P, Bennett-Gray J, Menezes AH, Goeken JA, Schelper RL, Wisniewski HM. Beta-amyloid protein of Alzheimer's disease is found in cerebral and spinal cord vascular malformations. *Am. J. Pathol.* 1988;132:167–172.

132. Hartmann A, Veldhuis JD, Deuschle M, Standhardt H, Heuser I. (1997) Twenty-four hour cortisol release profiles in patients with Alzheimer's and Parkinson's disease compared to normal controls: ultradian secretory pulsatility and diurnal variation. *Neurobiol. Aging* 18:285–289.

133. Hayflick L. Aging under glass. *Mutat. Res.* 1991;256:69–80.

134. Heafield MT, Fearn S, Steventon GB, Waring RH, Williams AC, Sturman SG. Plasma cysteine and sulphate levels in patients with motor neurone, Parkinson's and Alzheimer's disease. *Neurosci. Lett.* 1990;110:216–220.

135. Helisalmi S, Linnaranta K, Lehtovirta M, Mannermaa A, Heinonen O, Ryynanen M, Riekkinen P Sr, Soininen H. Apolipoprotein E polymorphism in patients with different neurodegenerative disorders. *Neurosci. Lett.* 1996;205:61–64.

136. Henderson AS, Jorm AF, Korten AE, Creasey H, McCusker E, Broe GA, Longley W, Anthony JC. Environmental risk factors for Alzheimer's disease: their relationship to age of onset and to familial or sporadic types. *Psychol. Med.* 1992;22:429–436.

137. Hershkowitz M, Adunsky A. Binding of platelet-activating factor to platelets of Alzheimer's disease and multiinfarct dementia patients. *Neurobiol. Aging* 1996;17:865–868.

138. Hinds TR, Kukull WA, Van Belle G, Schellenberg GD, Villacres EL, Larson EB. Relationship between serum alpha 1-antichymotrypsin and Alzheimer's disease. *Neurobiol. Aging* 1994;15:21–27.

139. Hock C. Biological markers of Alzheimer's disease. *Neurobiol. Aging* 1998;19:149–151.

140. Hock C, Drasch G, Golombowski S, Muller-Spahn F, Willershausen-Zonnchen B, Schwarz P, Hock U, Growdon JH, Nitsch RM. Increased blood mercury levels in patients with Alzheimer's disease. *J. Neural. Transm.* 1998;105:59–68.

141. Holland AJ. Down syndrome and the links to Alzheimer's disease. *Neurol. Neurosurg. Psychiatry* 1995;59:111–114.

142. Hooijer C, Jonker C, Posthuma J, Visser SL. Reliability, validity and follow-up of the EEG in senile dementia: sequelae of sequential measurement. *Electroencephalogr. Clin. Neurophysiol.* 1990;76:400–412.

143. Hoshi M, Takashima A, Murayama M, Yasutake K, Yoshida N, Ishiguro K, Hoshino T, Imahori K. Non-toxic amyloid beta peptide 1-42 suppresses acetylcholine synthesis: possible role in cholinergic dysfunction in Alzheimer's disease. *J. Biol. Chem.* 1997;272:2038–2041.

144. Houlden H, Crook R, Backhovens H, Prihar G, Baker M, Hutton M, Rossor M, Martin JJ, Van Broeckhoven C, Hardy J. ApoE genotype is a risk factor in nonpresenilin early-onset Alzheimer's disease families. *Am. J. Med. Genet.* 1998;81: 117–121.

145. Huberman M, Shalit R, Roth-Deri I, Gutman B, Brodie C, Kott E, Sredni B. Correlation of cytokine secretion by mononuclear cells of Alzheimer patients and their disease stage. *J. Neuroimmunol.* 1994;52:147–152.

146. Huberman M, Sredni B, Stern L, Kott E, Shalit F. IL-2 and IL-6 secretion in dementia: correlation with type and severity of disease. *J. Neurol. Sci.* 1995;130: 161–164.

146a. Hulstaert F, Blennow K, Ivanoiu A, et al. Improved discrimination of AD patients using beta-amyloid (1-42) and tau levels in CSF. *Neurology* 1999;52:1555–1562.

147. Hutchin T, Cortopassi G. A mitochondrial DNA clone is associated with increased risk for Alzheimer disease. *Proc. Natl. Acad. Sci. U.S.A.* 1995;92:6892–6895.

148. Hutton M, Lendon CL, Rizzu P, Baker M, Froelich S, Houlden H, Pickering-Brown S, Chakraverty S, et al. Association of missense and 4′ splice-site mutations in tau with the inherited dementia FTDP-17. *Nature* 1998;393:702–705.

149. Hyman BT. Biomarkers in Alzheimer's disease. *Neurobiol. Aging* 1998; 19:159–160.

150. Ibarreta D, Parrilla R, Ayuso MS. Altered Ca 2+ homeostasis in lymphoblasts from patients with late-onset Alzheimer disease. *Alzheimer Dis. Assoc. Disord.* 1997;11:220–227.

151. Ibarreta D, Urcelay E, Parrilla R, Ayuso MS. Distinct pH homeostatic features in lymphoblasts from Alzheimer's disease patients. *Ann. Neurol.* 1998;44:216–222.

152. Ibrahim MS, Lofts RS, Jarhling PB, Henchal EA, Weedn VS, Northrup MA, Belgrader P. Real-time microchip PCR for detecting single-base differences in viral and human DNA. *Anal. Chem.* 1998;70:2013–2017.

153. Idoate Gastearena MA, Vega Basquez F. Diagnosis of neurometabolic and neurodegenerative diseases by cutaneous biopsy. *Rev. Neurol.* 1997;25:S269–S280.

154. Ihara Y, Hayabara T, Sasaki K, Fujisawa Y, Kawada R, Yamamoto T, Nakashima Y, Yoshimune S, Kawai M, Kibata M, Kuroda S. Free radicals and superoxide dismutase in blood of patients with Alzheimer's disease and vascular dementia. *J. Neurol. Sci.* 1997;153:76–81.

155. Imura H, Fukata J-I, Mori T. Cytokines and endocrine function: an interaction between the immune and neuroendocrine systems. *Clin. Endocrinol.* 1991;35:107–115.

156. Inestrosa NC, Alarcon R, Arriagada J, Donoso A, Alvarez J, Campos EO. Blood markers in Alzheimer disease: subnormal acetylcholinesterase and butyrylcholinesterase in lymphocytes and erythrocytes. *J. Neurol. Sci.* 1994;122:1–5.

157. Inestrosa NC, Alarcon R, Arriagada J, Donoso A, Alvarez J. Platelet of Alzheimer patients: increased counts and subnormal uptake and accumulation of [14]5-hydroxytryptamine. *Neurosci. Lett.* 1993;163:8–10.

158. Iqbal K, Grundke-Iqbal I. Elevated levels of tau and ubiquitin in brain and cerebrospinal fluid in Alzheimer's disease. *Int. Psychogeriatr.* 1997;9:289–296.

159. Iribar MC, Montes J, Gonzalez Maldonado R, Peinado JM. Alanyl-aminopeptidase activity decrease in cerebrospinal fluid of Alzheimer patients. *Dement. Geriatr. Cogn. Disord.* 1998;9:44–49.

160. Ito E, Oka K, Etcheberrigaray R, Nelson TJ, McPhie DL, Tofel-Grehl B, Gibson GE, Alkon D. Internal Ca2+ mobilization is altered in fibroblasts from patients with Alzheimer disease. *Proc. Natl. Acad. Sci. U.S.A.* 1994;91:534–538.

161. Itzhaki RF, Lin WR, Shang D, Wilcock GK, Faragher B, Jamieson GA. Herpes simplex virus type 1 in brain and risk of Alzheimer's disease. *Lancet* 1997;349: 241–244.

162. Iwamoto N, Nishiyama E, Ohwada J, Arai H. Distribution of amyloid deposits in the cerebral white matter of the Alzheimer's disease brain: relationship to blood vessels. *Acta Neuropathol. (Berl.)* 1997;93:334–340.

163. Iwatsubo T. Amyloid beta protein in plasma as a diagnostic marker for Alzheimer's disease. *Neurobiol. Aging* 1998;19:161–163.

164. Jellinger KA, Bancher C. Proposals for re-evaluation of current autopsy criteria for the diagnosis of Alzheimer's disease. *Neurobiol. Aging* 1997;18:S55–S65.

165. Jendroska K, Poewe W, Daniel SE, Pluess J, Iwerssen-Schmidt H, Paulsen J, Barthel S, Schelosky L, Cervos-Navarro J, DeArmond SJ. Ischemic stress induces deposition of amyloid beta immunoreactivity in human brain. *Acta Neuropathol. (Berl.)* 1995;90:461–466.

166. Jervis GA. Early senile dementia in mongoloid idiocy. *Am. J. Psychiatry* 1948; 105:102–106.

167. Jimenez-Jimenez FJ, de Bustos F, Molina JA, Benito-Leon J, Tallon-Barranco A, Gasalla T, Orti-Pareja M, Guillamon F, Rubio JC, Arenas J, Enriquez-de-Salamanca R. Cerebrosopinal fluid levels of alpha-tocopherol (vitamin E) in Alzheimer's disease. *J. Neural Transm.* 1997;104:703–710.

168. Johnson KA, Jones K, Holman BL, Becker JA, Spiers PA, Satlin A, Albert MS. Preclinical prediction of Alzheimer's disease using SPECT. *Neurology* 1998; 50:1563–1571.

169. Joosten E, Lesaffre E, Riezler R, Ghekiere V, Dereymacker L, Pelemans W, Dejaeger E. Is metabolic evidence for vitamin B-12 and folate deficiency more frequent in elderly patients with Alzheimer's disease? *J. Gerontol. A Biol. Sci. Med. Sci.* 1997;52:M76–79.

170. Jordan BD, Relkin NR, Ravdin LD, Jacobs AR, Bennett A, Gandy S. Apolipoprotein E epsilon 4 associated with chronic traumatic brain injury in boxing. *JAMA* 1997;278:136–140.

171. Jorm AF. Alzheimer's disease: risk and protection. *Med. J. Aust.* 1997;167: 443–446.

172. Kalaria RN. Cerebrovascular degeneration is related to amyloid-beta protein deposition in Alzheimer's disease. *Ann. N.Y. Acad. Sci.* 1997;826:263–271.

173. Kalman J, Juhasz A, Laird G, Dickens P, Jardanhazy T, Rimanoczy A, Boncz I, Parry-Jones WL, Janka A. Serum interleukin-6 levels correlate with the severity of dementia in Down syndrome and in Alzheimer's disease. *Acta Neurol. Scand.* 1997;96:236–240.

174. Kamboh MI, Sanghera DK, Ferrell RE, De Kosky ST. APOE4-associated Alzheimer's disease risk is modified by alpha 1-antichymotrypsin polymorphism. *Nature Genet.* 1995;10:486–488.

175. Kamboh MI, Sanghera DK, Aston CE, Bunker CH, Hamman RF, Ferrell RE, DeKosky ST. Gender-specific nonrandom association between the alpha 1-antichymotrypsin and apolipoprotein E polymorphisms in the general population and its implication for the risk of Alzheimer's disease. *Genet. Epidemiol.* 1997;14:169–180.

176. Kamboh MI, Ferrell RE, DeKosky ST. Genetic association studies between Alzheimer's disease and two polymorphisms in the low density lipoprotein receptor-related protein gene. *Neurosci. Lett.* 1998;244:65–68.

177. Kanai M, Matsubara E, Isoe K, Urakami K, Nakashima K, Arai H, Sasaki H, Abe K, Iwatsubo T, Kosaka T, Watanabe M, Tomidokoro Y, Shizuka M, Mizushima K, Nakamura T, Igeta Y, Ikeda Y, Amari M, Kawarabayashi T, Ishiguro K, Harigaya Y, Wakabayashi K, Okamoto K, Hirai S, Shoji M. Longitudinal study of cerebrospinal fluid levels of tau, A beta1-40, and A beta 1-42(43) in Alzheimer's disease: a study in Japan. *Ann. Neurol.* 1998;44:17–26.

178. Kang DE, Saitoh T, Chen X, Xia Y, Masliah E, Hansen LA, Thomas RG, Thal LJ, Katzman R. Genetic association of the low-density lipoprotein receptor-related protein gene (LRP), an apolipoprotein E receptor, with late-onset Alzheimer's disease. *Neurology* 1997;49:56–61.

179. Kanne SM, Balota DA, Storandt M, McKeel DW Jr, Morris JC. Relating anatomy to function in Alzheimer's disease: neuropsychological profiles predict regional neuropathology 5 years later. *Neurology* 1998;50:979–985.

180. Karlsson JO, Blennow K, Janson I, Blomgren K, Karlsson I, Regland B, Wallin A, Gottfries CG. Increased proteolytic activity in lymphocytes from patients with early onset Alzheimer's disease. *Neurobiol. Aging* 1995;16:901–906.

181. Katzman R, Kang D, Thomas R. Interaction of apolipoprotein E epsilon 4 with other genetic and non-genetic risk factors in late onset Alzheimer disease: problems facing the investigator. *Neurochem. Res.* 1998;23:369–376.

182. Kay MM, Goodman J. Brain and erythrocyte anion transporter protein, band 3, as a marker for Alzheimer's disease: structural changes detected by electron microscopy, phosphorylation, and antibodies. *Gerontology* 1997;43:44–66.

183. Kell SH, Allman TM, Harrell LE, Liu T, Solvason N. Association between Alzheimer's disease and bound autochthonous IgM on T cells. *J. Am. Geriatr. Soc.* 1996;44:1362–1365.

184. Kenessey A, Nacharaju PM, Ko LW, Yen SH. Degradation of tau by lysosomal enzyme cathepsin D: implication for Alzheimer neurofibrillary degeneration. *J. Neurochem.* 1997;69:2026–2038.

185. Kennard M. Diagnostic markers for Alzheimer's disease. *Neurobiol. Aging* 1998;19:131–132.

186. Kennard ML, Feldman H, Yamada T, Jefferies WA. Serum levels of the iron binding protein p97 are elevated in Alzheimer's disease. *Nature Med.* 1996;2:1230.

187. Khalil Z, Chen H, Helme RD. Mechanisms underlying the vascular activity of beta-amyloid protein fragment (beta A (4) 25-35) at the level of skin microvasculature. *Brain Res.* 1996;736:206–216.

188. Khanna KK, An SS, Wu JM, Landolfo S, Hovanessian AG. Absence of the 40-kDa form of (2′-5′) oligoadenylate synthetase and its corresponding mRNA from skin fibroblasts derived from Alzheimer disease patients. *Proc. Natl. Acad. Sci. U.S.A.* 1991;88:5852–5856.

189. Kim CS, Han YF, Etcheberrigaray R, Nelson TJ, Olds JL, Yoshioka T, Alkon DL. Alzheimer and beta-amyloid treated fibroblasts demonstrate a decrease in a memory-associated GTP-binding protein, Cp20. *Proc. Natl. Acad. Sci. U.S.A.* 1995;92:3060–3064.

190. Klunk WE. Biological markers of Alzheimer's disease. *Neurobiol. Aging* 1998; 19:145–147.

191. Koj A. Initiation of acute phase response and synthesis of cytokines. *Biochim. Biophys. Acta* 1996;1317:84–94.

192. Koj A. Termination of acute phase response: role of some cytokines and anti-inflammatory drugs. *Gen. Pharmacol.* 1998;31:9–18.

193. Kuda T, Shoji M, Arai H, Kawashima S, Saido TC. Reduction of plasma glutamyl aminopeptidase activity in sporadic Alzheimer's disease. *Biochem. Biophys. Res. Commun.* 1997;231:526–530.

194. Kudinova NV, Kudinov AR, Berezov TT. Beta amyloid in blood and cerebrospinal fluid is associated with high density lipoproteins. *Vopr. Med. Khim.* 1996;42: 253–262.

195. Kuiper MA, Mulder C, van Kamp GJ, Scheltens P, Wolters EC. Cerebrospinal fluid ferritin levels of patients with Parkinson's disease, Alzheimer's disease, and multiple system atrophy. *J. Neural Transm. Park. Dis. Dement. Sect.* 1994;7: 109–114.

196. Kuiper MA, Visser JJ, Bergmans PL, Scheltens P, Wolters. Decreased cerebrospinal fluid nitrate levels in Parkinson's disease, Alzheimer's disease and multiple system atrophy patients. *J. Neurol. Sci.* 1994;121:46–49.

197. Kukull WA, Hinds TR, Schellenberg GD, van Belle G, Larson EB. Increased platelet membrane fluidity as a diagnostic marker for Alzheimer's disease: a test in population-based cases and controls. *Neurology* 1992;42:607–614.

198. Kumar U, Dunlop DM, Richardson JS. Mitochondria from Alzheimer's fibroblasts show decreased uptake of calcium and increased sensitivity to free radicals. *Life Sci.* 1994;54:1855–1860.

199. Kuriyama M, Takahashi K, Yamano T, Hokezu Y, Togo S, Osame M, Igakura T. Low levels of serum apolipoprotein AI and AII in senile dementia. *Jpn. J. Psychiatry Neurol.* 1994;48:589–593.

200. Kuusisto J, Koivisto K, Mykkanen L, Helkala EL, Vanhanen M, Hanninen T, Kervinen K, Kesaniemi YA, Riekkinen PJ, Laakso M. Association between features of the insulin resistance syndrome an Alzheimer's disease independently of apolipoprotein E4 phenotype: cross sectional population based study. *BMJ* 1997;315:1045–1049.

201. Lambert JC, Pasquier F, Cottel D, Frigard B, Amouyel P, Chartier-Harlin MC. A new polymorphism in the APOE promoter associated with risk of developing Alzheimer's disease. *Hum. Mol. Genet.* 1998;7:533–540.

202. Lannfelt L. Biochemical diagnostic markers to detect early Alzheimer's disease. *Neurobiol. Aging* 1998;19:165–67.

203. Lannfelt L, Basun H, Wahlund LO, Rowe BA, Wagner SL. Decreased alpha-secretase-cleaved amyloid precursor protein as a diagnostic marker for Alzheimer's disease. *Nature Med.* 1995;1:829–832.

204. Lanzrein AS, Jobst KA, Thiel S, Jensenius JC, Sim RB, Perry VH, Sim E. Mannan-binding lectin in human serum, cerebrospinal fluid and brain tissue and its role in Alzheimer's disease. *NeuroReport* 1998;9:1491–1495.

205. Lanzrein AS, Johnston CM, Perry VH, Jobst KA, King EM, Smith ADL. Longitudinal study of inflammatory factors in serum, cerebrospinal fluid, and brain tissue in Alzheimer disease:interleukin-1 beta, interleukin-6, interleukin-1 receptor antagonist, tumor necrosis factor-alpha, the soluble tumor necrosis factor receptor I and II and alpha 1-antichymotrypsin. *Alzheimer Dis. Assoc. Disord.* 1998;12:215–217.

206. Lassmann H, Fischer P, Jellinger K. Synaptic pathology of Alzheimer's disease. *Ann. N. Y. Acad. Sci.* 1993;695:59–64.

207. Lawlor BA, Bierer LM, Ryan TM, Schmeidler J, Knott PJ, Williams LL, Mohs RC, Davis KL. Plasma 3-methoxy-4-hydroxyphenylglycol (MPHG) and clinical symptoms in Alzheimer's disease. *Biol. Psychiatry* 1995;38:185–188.

208. Leblhuber F, Walli J, Tilz GP, Wachter H, Fuchs D. Systemic changes of the immune system in patients with Alzheimer's dementia. *Dtsch. Med. Wochenschr.* 1998;123:787–791.

209. Lefranc D, Vermersch P, Dallongeville J, Daems-Monpeurt C, Petit H, Delacourte A. Relevance of the quantification of apolipoprotein E in the cerebrospinal fluid in Alzheimer's disease. Neurosci Lett 1996;212:91–94.

210. Lehmann DJ, Johnston C, Smith AD. Synergy between the genes for butyrylcholinesterase K variant and apolipoprotein E4 in late-onset confirmed Alzheimer's disease. *Hum. Mol. Genet.* 1997;6:1933–1936.

211. Levy-Lahad E, Wasco W, Poorkaj P, Romano DM, Oshima J, Pettingell WH, Yu CE, Jondro PD, Schmidt SD, Wang K, et al. Candidate gene for chromosome 1 familial Alzheimer's disease locus. *Science* 1995;269:973–977.

212. Li J, Ma J, Potter H. Identification and expression analysis of a potential familial Alzheimer disease gene on chromosome 1 related to AD3. *Proc. Natl. Acad. Sci. U.S.A.* 1995;92:12180–184.

213. Li J, Xu M, Zhou H, Ma J, Potter H. Alzheimer presenilins in the nuclear membrane, interphase kinetochores, and centrosomes suggest a role in chromosome segregation. *Cell* 1997;90:917–927.

214. Liang JS, Sloane JA, Wells JM, Abraham CR, Fine RE, Sipe JD. Evidence for local production of acute phase response apolipoprotein serum amyloid A in Alzheimer's disease brain. *Neurosci. Lett.* 1997;225:73–76.

215. Licastro F, Morini MC, Polazzi E, Davis LJ. Increased serum alpha 1-antichymotrypsin in patients with probable Alzheimer's disease: an acute phase reactant without the peripheral acute phase response. *J. Neuroimmunol.* 1995;57:71–75.

216. Licastro F, Parnetti L, Morini MC, Davis LJ, Cucinotta D, Gaita A, Senin U. Acute phase reactant alpha 1-antichymotrypsin is increased in cerebrospinal fluid and serum of patients with probable Alzheimer disease. *Alzheimer Dis. Assoc. Disord.* 1995;9:112–118.

217. Licastro F, Sirri V, Trere D, Davis LJ. Monomeric and polymeric forms of alpha-1 antichymotrypsin in sera from patients with probable late onset Alzheimer's disease. *Dement. Geriatr. Cogn. Disord.* 1997;8:337–342.

218. Lieberman J, Schleissner L, Tachiki KH, Kling AS. Serum alpha 1-antichymotrypsin level as a marker for Alzheimer-type dementia. *Neurobiol. Aging* 1995;16:747–753.

219. Lindh M, Blomberg M, Jensen M, Basun H, Lannfelt L, Engvall B, Scharnagel H, Marz W, Wahlund LO, Cowburn RF. Cerebrospinal fluid apolipoprotein E (apoE) levels in Alzheimer's disease patients are increased at follow up and show a correlation with levels of tau protein. *Neurosci. Lett.* 1997;229:85–88.

220. Lindner MD, Gordon DD, Miller JM, Tariot PN, McDaniel KD, Hamill RS, DiStefano PS, Loy R. Increased levels of truncated nerve growth factor receptor in urine of mildly demented patients with Alzheimer's disease. *Arch. Neurol.* 1993;50:1054–1060.

221. Litvan I. Methodological and research issues in the evaluation of biological diagnostic markers for Alzheimer's disease. *Neurobiol. Aging* 1998;19:121–123.

222. Lopez OL, Rabin BS, Huff FJ, Rezek D, Reinmuth OM. Serum autoantibodies in patients with Alzheimer's disease and vascular dementia and in nondemented control subjects. *Stroke* 1992;23:1078–1083.

223. Lovell MA, ehmann WD, Mattson MP, Markesbery WR. Elevated 4-hydroxynonenal in ventricular fluid in Alzheimer disease. *Neurobiol. Aging* 1997;18:457–461.

224. Ma J, Yee A, Brewer HB Jr, Das S, Potter H. Amyloid-associated proteins alpha 1-antichymotrypsin and apolipoprotein E promote assembly of Alzheimer beta-protein into filaments. *Nature* 1994;372:92–94.

225. Ma J, Brewer HB Jr, Potter H. Alzheimer A beta neurotoxicity: promotion by antichymotrypsin, ApoE4; inhibition by A beta-related peptides. *Neurobiol. Aging* 1996;17:773–780.

226. MacTaylor CE, Ewing AG. Profiling of amino acids in human cerebrospinal fluid that requires no sample clean-up: a comparison of Alzheimer's patients with normal controls. *Beckman Times* Issue 4, Summer, 1997.

227. Maguire TM, Gillian AM, O'Mahony D, Coughlan CM, Dennihan A, Breen KC. A decrease in serum sialyltransferase levels in Alzheimer's disease. *Neurobiol. Aging* 1994;15:99–102.

228. Mann DM, Iwatsubo T. Diffuse plaques in the cerebellum and corpus striatum in Down's syndrome contain amyloid beta protein (A beta) only in the form of A beta 42 (43). *Neurodegeneration* 1996;5:115–120.

229. Mari D, Parnetti L, Coppola R, Bottasso B, Reboldi GP, Senin U, Mannucci PM. Hemostasis abnormalities in patients with vascular dementia and Alzheimer's disease. *Thromb. Haemost.* 1996;75:216–218.

230. Mark RJ, Pang Z, Geddes JW, Uchida K, Mattson MP. Amyloid beta-peptide impairs glucose transport in hippocampal and cortical neurons: involvement of membrane lipid peroxidation. *J. Neurosci.* 1997;17:1046–1054.

231. Markesbery WR. Oxidative stress hypothesis in Alzheimer's disease. *Free Radic. Biol. Med.* 1997;23:134–147.

232. Markesbery WR. Neuropathological criteria for the diagnosis of Alzheimer's disease. *Neurobiol. Aging* 1997;18:S13–S19.

233. Martins RN, Muir J, Brooks WS, Creasey H, Montgomery P, Sellers P, Broe GA. Plasma amyloid precursor protein is decreased in Alzheimer's disease. *NeuroReport* 1993;4:757–759.

234. Masugi F, Ogihara T, Sakaguchi K, Otsuka A, Tsuchiya Y, Morimoto S, Kumahara Y, Saeki S, Nishide M. High plasma level of cortisol in patients with senile dementia of the Alzheimer's type. *Methods Find. Exp. Clin. Pharmacol.* 1989; 11:707–710.

235. Matsubara E, Hirai S, Amari M, Shoji M, Yamaguchi H, Okamoto K, Ishiguro K, Harigaya Y, Wakabayashi K. Alpha 1-antichymotrypsin as a possible biochemical marker for Alzheimer-type dementia. *Ann. Neurol.* 1990;28:561–567.

236. Matsubara E, Frangione B, Ghiso J. Characterization of apolipoprotein J-Alzheimer's A beta interaction. *J. Biol. Chem.* 1995;270:7563–7567.

237. Matsumoto A. Altered processing characteristics of beta-amyloid-containing peptides in cytosol and in media of familial Alzheimer's disease cells. *Biochim. Biophys. Acta* 1994;1225:304–310.

238. Matsumoto A, Fujiwara Y. Abnormal and deficient processing of beta-amyloid precursor protein in familial Alzheimer's disease lymphoblastoid cells. *Biochem. Biophys. Res. Commun.* 1991;175:361–365.

239. Matsumoto A, Matsumoto R. Familial Alzheimer's disease cells abnormally accumulate beta-amyloid-harbouring peptides preferentially in cytosol but not in extracellular fluid. *Eur. J. Biochem.* 1994;225:1055–1062.

240. Matsuyama SS, Yamaguchi DT, Vergara Y, Jarvik LF. Tetraethylammonium-induced calcium concentration changes in skin fibroblasts from patients with Alzheimer disease. *Dementia* 1995;6:241–244.

241. Mattila KM, Frey H. Two-dimensional analysis of qualitative and quantitative changes in blood cell proteins in Alzheimer's disease: search for extraneuronal markers. *Appl. Theor. Electrophor.* 1995;4:189–196.

242. Mattson MP. Cellular actions of beta-amyloid precursor protein and its soluble and fibrillogenic derivatives. *Physiol. Rev.* 1997;77:1081–1132.

243. Mattson MP, Barger SW, Furukawa K, Bruce AJ, Wyss-Coray T, Mark RJ, Mucke L. Cellular signaling roles of TGF beta, TNF alpha and beta APP in brain injury responses and Alzheimer's disease. *Brain. Res. Brain. Res. Rev.* 1997;23:47–61.

244. Mayeux R. Evaluation and use of diagnostic tests in Alzheimer's disease. *Neurobiol. Aging* 1998;19:139–143.

245. Mayeux R, Saunders AM, Shea S, Mirra S, Evans D, Roses AD, Hyman BT, Crain B, Tang MX, Phelps CH. Utility of the apolipoprotein E genotype in the diagnosis of Alzheimer's disease: Alzheimer's Disease Centers Consortium on Apolipoprotein E and Alzheimer's Disease. *N. Engl. J. Med.* 1998;338:506–511.

246. McCaddon A, Davies G, Hudson P, Tandy S, Cattell H. Total serum homocysteine in senile dementia of the Alzheimer type. *Int. J. Geriatr. Psychiatry* 1998; 13:235–239.

247. McGeer PL, McGeer EG. Anti-inflammatory drugs in the fight against Alzheimer's disease. *Ann. N.Y. Acad. Sci.* 1996;777:213–20.

248. McGeer EG, McGeer PL. The role of the immune system in neurodegenerative disorders. *Mov. Disord.* 1997;12:855–858.

249. McGeer PL, Schulzer M, McGeer EG. Arthritis and anti-inflammatory agents as possible protective factors for Alzheimer's disease: a review of 17 epidemiologic studies. *Neurology* 1996;47:425–432.

250. McKhann G, Drachman D, Folstein M, Katzman R, Price D, Stadlan EM. Clinical diagnosis of Alzheimer's disease: Report of the NINCDS-ADRDA Work Group under the auspices of Department of Health and Human Services Task Force on Alzheimer's disease. *Neurology* 1984;34:939–944.

251. McLachlan DR, Bergeron C, Smith JE, Boomer D, Rifat SL. Risk for neuropathologically confirmed Alzheimer's disease and residual aluminum in municipal drinking water employing weighted residential histories. *Neurology* 1996;46:401–405.

252. McRae A, Ling EA, Wigander A, Dahlstrom A. Microglial cerebrospinal fluid antibodies. Significance for Alzheimer disease. *Mol. Chem. Neuropathol.* 1996;28: 89–95.

253. Mecocci P, Ekman R, Parnetti L, Senin U. Antihistone and anti-dsDNA autoantibodies in Alzheimer's disease and vascular dementia. *Biol. Psychiatry* 1993;34: 380–385.

254. Mecocci P, Parnetti L, Romao G, Scarelli A, Chionne F, Cecchetti R, Polidori MC, Palumbo B, Cherubini A, Senin U. Serum GFAP and anti-S100 autoantibodies in brain aging, Alzheimer's disease and vascular dementia. *J. Neuroimmunol.* 1995; 57:165–170.

255. Mecocci P, Cherubini A, Senin U. Increased oxidative damage in lymphocytes of Alzheimer's disease patients. *J. Am. Geriatr. Soc.* 1997;45:1536–1537.

256. Mehta PD, Dalton AJ, Mehta SP, Kim KS, Sersen EA, Wisniewski HM. Increased plasma amyloid beta protein 1-42 levels in Down syndrome. *Neurosci. Lett.* 1998;241:13–16.

257. A, Blain H, Visvikis S, Herbeth B, Jeandel C, Siest G. Cerebrospinal fluid apolipoprotein E level is increased in late-onset Alzheimer's disease. *J. Neurol. Sci.* 1997;145:33–39.

258. Miklossy J, Kasas S, Janzer RC, Ardizzoni F, Van der Loos H. Further ultrastructural evidence that spirochaetes may play a role in the etiology of Alzheimer's disease. *NeuroReport* 1994;5:1201–1204.

259. Mikosch P, Gallowitsch HJ, Gomez I, Kresnik E, Plob H, Lind P. Diagnosis of SDAT by HMPAO SPECT and vitamin B12 serum concentration. *Nuklearmedizin* 1995;34:104–109.

260. Minthon L, Edvinsson L, Gustafson L. Correlation between clinical characteristics and cerebrospinal fluid neuropeptide Y levels in dementia of the Alzheimer type and frontotemporal dementia. *Alzheimer Dis. Assoc. Disord.* 1996;10:197–203.

261. Mitchelson KR, Cheng J, Kricka LJ. The use of capillary electrophoresis for point-mutation screening. *Trends Biotechnol.* 1997;15:448–458.

262. Miulli DE, Norwell DY, Schwartz FN. Plasma concentrations of glutamate and its metabolites in patients with Alzheimer's disease. *J. Am. Osteopath. Assoc.* 1993; 93:670–676.

263. Mochizuki Y, Oishi M, Hara M, Takasu T. Amino acid concentration in dementia of the Alzheimer type and multi-infarct dementia. *Ann. Clin. Lab. Sci.* 1996;26: 275–278.

264. Mochizuki YL, Oishi M, Takasu T. Correlations between P300 components and neurotransmitters in the cerebrospinal fluid. *Clin. Electroencephalogr.* 1998; 29:7–9.

265. Montine TJ, Montine KS, Swift LL. Central nervous system lipoproteins in Alzheimer's disease. *Am. J. Pathol.* 1997;151:1571–1575.

266. Morihara T, Kudo T, Ikura Y, Kashiwagi Y, Miyamae Y, Nakamura Y, Tanaka Y, Shinozaki K, Nishikawa T, Takeda M. Increased tau protein level in postmortem cerebrospinal fluid. *Psychiatry Clin. Neurosci.* 1998;52:107–110.

267. Morris JC. Clinical dementia rating: a reliable and valid diagnostic and staging measure for dementia of the Alzheimer type. *Int. Psychogeriatr.* 1997;9(Suppl 1): 173–176.

268. Mortimer JA. Brain reserve and the clinical expression of Alzheimer's disease. *Geriatrics* 1997;52:S50–S53.

269. Motter R, Vigo-Pelfrey C, Kholodenko D, Barbour R, Johnson-Wood K, Galasko D, Chang L, Miller B, Clark C, Green R, et al. Reduction of beta-amyloid peptide 42 in the cerebrospinal fluid of patients with Alzheimer's disease. *Ann. Neurol.* 1995;38:643–648.

270. Mullan M, Houlden H, Windelspecht M, fidani L, Lombardi C, Diaz P, Rossor M, Crook R, Hardy J, Duff K, et al. A locus for familial early-onset Alzheimer's disease on the long arm of chromosome 14, proximal to the alpha 1-antichymotrypsin gene. *Nature Genet.* 1992;2:340–342.

271. Namekata K, Imagawa M, Terashi A, Phta S, Oyama F, Ihara Y. Association of transferrin C2 allele with late-onset Alzheimer's disease. *Hum. Genet.* 1997; 101:126–129.

272. Nasman B, Olsson T, Seckl JR, Eriksson S, Viitanen M, Bucht G, Carlstrom K. Abnormalities in adrenal androgens, but not of glucocorticoids, in early Alzheimer's disease. *Psychoneuroendocrinology* 1995;20:83–94.

273. Nasman B, Olsson T, Fagerlund M, Eriksson S, Viitanen M, Carlstrom K. Blunted adrenocorticotropin and increased adrenal steroid response to human corticotropin-releasing hormone in Alzheimer's disease. *Biol. Psychiatry* 1996; 39:311–318.

274. Nerl C, Mayeux R, O'Neill GJ. HLA-linked complement markers in Alzheimer's and Parkinson's disease: C4 variant (C4B2). A possible marker for senile dementia of the Alzheimer type. *Neurology* 1984;34:310–314.

275. Nilsson L, Rogers J, Potter H. The essential role of inflammation and induced gene expresion in the pathogenic pathway of Alzheimer's disease. *Front. Biosci.* 1998;3:436–446.

276. Nishiyama E, Iwamoto N, Kimura M, Arai H. Serum amyloid P component level in Alzheimer's disease. *Dementia* 1996;7:256–259.

277. Nitsch RM, Rebeck GW, Deng M, Richardson UI, Tennis M, Schenk DB, Vigo-Pelfrey C, Lieberburg IK, Wurtman RJ, Hyman BT, et al. Cerebrospinal fluid levels of amyloid beta-protein in Alzheimer's disease: inverse correlation with severity of dementia and effect of apolipoprotein E genotype. *Ann. Neurol.* 1995; 37:512–18.

278. Notkola IL, Sulkava R, Pekkanen J, Erkinjuntti T, Ehnholm C, Kivinen P, Tuomilehto J, Nissinen A. Serum total cholesterol, apolipoprotein E epsilon 4 allele, and Alzheimer's disease. *Neuroepidemiology* 1998;17:14–20.

279. O'Connor DT, Kailasam MT, Thal LJ. Cerebrospinal fluid chromogranin A is unchanged in Alzheimer dementia. *Neurobiol. Aging* 1993;14:267–269

280. Ogura H, Fujii R, Hamano M, Kuzuya M, Nakajima H, Ohata R, Mori T. Detection of HeLa cell contamination—presence of human papillomavirus 18 DNA as He La marker in JTC-3, OG and OE cell lines. *Jpn. J. Med. Sci. Biol.* 1997;50:161–167.

281. Olson RE. Discovery of the lipoproteins, their role in fat transport and their significance as risk factors. *J. Nutr.* 1998;128:439S–443S.

282. Omar R, Pappola M, Argani I, Davis K. Acid phosphatase activity in senile plaques and cerebrospinal fluid of patients with Alzheimer's disease. *Arch. Pathol. Lab. Med.* 1993;117:166–169.

283. Orrell MW, O'Dwyer A-M. Dementia, aging, and the stress control system. *Lancet* 1995;345:666–667.

284. Ott A, Stolk RP, Hofman A, van Harskamp F, Grobbee DE, Breteler MM. Association of diabetes mellitus and dementia: the Rotterdam Study. *Diabetologia* 1996;39:1392–1397.

285. Pallister C, Jung SS, Shaw I, Nalbantoglu J, Gauthier S, Cashman NR. Lymphocyte content of amyloid precursor protein is increased in Down's syndrome and aging. *Neurobiol. Aging* 1997;18:97–103.

286. Parnetti L, Reboldi GP, Santucci C, Santucci A, Gaiti A, Brunetti M, Cecchetti R, Senin U. Platelet MAO-B activity as a marker of behavioural characteristics in dementia disorders. *Aging* 1994;6:201–207.

287. Parnetti L, Gaiti A, Polidori MC, Brunetti M, Palumbo B, Chionne F, Cadini D, Cecchetti R, Senin UI. Increased cerebrospinal fluid pyruvate levels in Alzheimer's disease. *Neurosci. Lett.* 1995;199:231–233.

288. Parshad RP, Sanford KK, Price FM, Melnick LK, Nee LE, Schaprio MB, Tarone RE, Robbins JH. Fluorescent light-induced chromatid breaks distinguish Alzheimer disease cells from normal cells in tissue culture. *Proc. Natl. Acad. Sci. U.S.A.* 1996;93:5146–5150.

289. Passant U, Warkentin S, Gustafson L. Orthostatic hypotension and low blood pressure in organic dementia: a study of prevalence and related clinical characteristics. *Int. J. Geriatr. Psychiaty* 1997;12:395–403.

290. Path G, Bornstein SR, Ehrhart-Bornstein M, Scherbaum WA. Interleukin-6 and the interleukin-6 receptor in the human adrenal gland: expression and effects on steroidogenesis. *J. Clin. Endocrinol. Metab.* 1997;82:2343–2349.

291. Payami H, Schellenberg GD, Zareparsi S, Kaye J, Sexton GJ, Head MA, Matsuyama SS, Jarvik LF, Miller B, McManus DQ, Bird TD, Katzman R, Heston L, Norman D, Small GW. Evidence for association of HLA-A2 allele with onset age of Alzheimer's disease. *Neurology* 1997;49:512–518.

292. Payami H, Grimslid H, Oken B, Camicioli R, Sexton G, Dame A, Howieson D, Kaye J. A prospective study of cognitive health in the elderly (Oregon Brain Aging Study): effects of family history and apolipoprotein E genotype. *Am. J. Hum. Genet.* 1997;60:948–956.

293. Peeters MA, Salabelle A, Attal N, Rethore MO, Mircher C, Laplane D, Lejeune J. Excessive glutamine sensitivity in Alzheimer's disease and Down syndrome lymphocytes. *J. Neurol. Sci.* 1995;133:31–41.

294. Percy ME. Peripheral biological markers as confirmatory or predictive tests for Alzheimer disease in the general population and in Down syndrome. In Berg JM,

Karlinsky H, Holland AJ, editors. *Alzheimer Disease, Down Syndrome and Their Relationship.* Oxford: Oxford University Press, 1993;199–223.

295. Percy ME, Andrews DF. Risk estimation in X-linked recessive genetic diseases: theory and practice. *Can. J. Public. Health.* 1986;77(Suppl 1):174–183.

296. Percy ME, Andrews DF, Thompson MW. Duchenne muscular dystrophy carrier detection using logistic discrimination: serum creatine kinase and hemopexin in combination. *Am. J. Med. Genet.* 1981;8:397–409.

297. Percy ME, Andrews DF, Thompson MW. Serum creatine kinase in the detection of Duchene muscular dystrophy carriers: effects of season and multiple testing. *Muscle Nerve* 1982;5:58–64.

298. Percy ME, Pichora GA, Chang LS, Manchester KE, Andrews DF. Serum myoglobin in Duchenne muscular dystrophy carrier detection: a comparison with creatine kinase and hemopexin using logistic discrimination. *Am. J. Med. Genet.* 1984;18:279–287.

299. Percy ME, Andrews DF, Brasher PM, Rusk AC. Making the most of multiple measurements in estimating carrier probability in Duchenne muscular dystrophy: the Bayesian incorporation of repeated measurements using logistic discrimination. *Am. J. Med. Genet.* 1987;26:851–861.

300. Percy ME, Rusk AC, Garvey MB, Freedman JJ, Teitel JM, Blake P, Carter C, Andrew M, Johnson M, Inwood M, et al. Carrier detection in hemophilia A: ABO blood group, multiple measurements, and application of logistic discrimination. *Am. J. Med. Genet.* 1988;31:871–879.

301. Percy ME, Dalton AJ, Markovic VD, McLachlan DR, Hummel JT, Rusk AC, Andrews DF. Red cell superoxide dismutase, glutathione peroxidase and catalase in Down syndrome patients with and without manifestations of Alzheimer disease. *Am. J. Med. Genet.* 1990;35:459–467.

302. Percy ME, Markovic VD, Crapper McLachlan DR, Berg JM, Hummel JT, Laing ME, Dearie TG, Andrews DF. Family with 22-derived marker chromosome and late-onset dementia of the Alzheimer type: I. Application of a new model for estimation of the risk of disease associated with the marker. *Am. J. Med. Genet.* 1991;39:307–313.

303. Percy ME, Markovic VD, Dalton AJ, McLachlan DR, Berg JM, Rusk AC, Somerville MJ, Chodakowski B, Andrews DF. Age-associated chromosome 21 loss in Down syndrome: possible relevance of mosaicism and Alzheimer disease. *Am. J. Med. Genet.* 1993;45:584–588.

304. Percy ME, Wong S, Bauer S, Liaghati-Nasseri N, Perry MD, Chauthaiwale VM, Dhar M, Joshi JG. Iron metabolism and human ferritin heavy chain cDNA from adult brain with an elongated untranslated region: new findings and insights. *Analyst* 1998;123:41–50.

305. Perrin R, Briancon S, Jeandel C, Artur Y, Minn A, Penin F, Siest G. Blood activity of Cu/Zn superoxide dismutase, glutathione peroxidase and catalase in Alzheimer's disease: a case-control study. *Gerontology* 1990;36:306–313.

306. Piccini C, Pecori D, Campani D, Falcini M, Piccininni M, Manfredi G, Amaducci L, Bracco L. Alzheimer's disease: patterns of cognitive impairment at different levels of disease severity. *J. Neurol. Sci.* 1998;156:59–64.

307. Pirtilla T, Koivisto K, Mehta PD, Reinikainen K, Kim KS, Kilkka O, Heinonen E, Soininen H, Riekkinen P Sr, Wisniewski HM. Longitudinal study of cerebrospinal

fluid amyloid proteins and apolipoprotein E in patients with probable AD. *Neurosci. Lett.* 1998;249:21–24.

308. Pitschke M, Prior R, Haupt M, Riesner D. Detection of single amyloid beta-protein aggregates in the cerebrospinal fluid of Alzheimer's patients by fluorescence correlation spectroscopy. 1998;*Nature Med* 4:832–834.

309. Poorkaj P, Bird TD, Wijsman E, Nemens E, Garruto RM, Anderson L, Andreadis A, Wiederholt WC, Raskind M, Schelleberg GD. Tau is a candidate gene for chromosome 17 frontotemporal dementia. *Ann. Neurol.* 1998;43:815–825.

310. Prasher VP. Increase in mean cell volume—a possible peripheral marker for Alzheimer's disease? *Int. J. Geriatr. Psychiatry* 1997;12:130–131.

311. Prior RL, Crim MC, Castaneda C, Lammi-Keefe C, Dawson-Hughes B, Rosen CJ, Spindler AA. Conditions altering plasma concentrations of urea cycle and other amino acids in elderly human subjects. *J. Am. Coll. Nutr.* 1996;15:237–247.

312. Rapoport SI. Discriminant analysis of brain imaging data identified subjects with early Alzheimer's disease. *Int. Psychogeriatr.* 1997;9(Suppl) 1:229–235.

313. Rasmuson S, Nasman B, Eriksson S, Carlstrom K, Olsson T. Adrenal responsivity in normal aging and mild to moderate Alzheimer's disease. *Biol. Psychiatry* 1998;43:401–407.

314. Redjems-Bennani N, Jeandel C, Lefebvre E, Blain H, Vidailhet M, Gueant JL. Abnormal substrate levels that depend upon mitochondrial function in cerebrospinal fluid from Alzheimer patients. *Gerontology* 1998;44:300–304.

315. Regelson W, Harkins SW. "Amyloid is not a tombstone" - a summation. The primary role for cerebrovascular and CSF dynamics as factors in Alzheimer's disease (AD): DMSF, fluorocarbon oxygen carriers, thyroid hormonal, and other suggested therapeutic measures. *Ann. N.Y. Acad. Sci.* 1997;826:348–374.

316. Renvoize EB, Hambling MH. Cytomegalovirus infection and Alzheimer's disease. *Age Ageing* 1984;13:205–209.

317. Riekkinen P Jr, Soininen H, Partanen J, Paakkonen A, Helisalmi S, Riekkinen R Sr. The ability of THA treatment to increase cortical alpha waves is related to apolipoprotein E genotype of Alzheimer disease patients. *Psychopharmacology (Berl.)* 1997;129:285–288.

318. Riemenschneider M, Buch K, Schmolke M, Kurz A, Guder WG. Diagnosis of Alzheimer's disease with cerebrospinal fluid tau protein and aspartate aminotransferase. *Lancet* 1997;350:784.

319. Roberts GW, Gentleman SM, Lynch A, Murray L, Landon M, Graham DI. Beta amyloid protein deposition in the brain after severe head injury: implications for the pathogenesis of Alzheimer's disease. *J. Neurol. Neurosurg. Psychiatry* 1994; 57:419–25.

320. Roberts NB, Clough A, Bellia JP, Kim JY. Increased absorption of aluminium from a normal dietary intake in dementia. *J. Inorg. Biochem.* 1998;69:171–176.

321. Robles A. Some remarks on biological markers of Alzheimer's disease. *Neurobiol. Aging* 1998;19:153–157.

322. Rogaev EI, Sherrington R, Rogaeva EA, Levesque G, Ikeda M, Liang Y, Chi H, Lin C, Holman K, Tsuda T, et al. Familial Alzheimer's disease in kindreds with missense mutations in a gene on chromosome 1 related to the Alzheimer's disease type 3 gene. *Nature* 1995;376:775–778.

323. Rogers JT, Leiter L, McPhee J, Cahill CM, Zhan SS, Potter H, Nilsson L. Amyloid precursor protein is regulated by interleukin 1 at the translational level by 5′un-translated sequences.1999;274:6421–6431.

324. Rosenberg RN, Richter RW, Risser RC, taubman K, Prado-Farmer I, Ebalo E, Posey J, Kingfisher D, Dean D, Weiner MF, Svetlik D, Adams P, Honig LS, Cullum CM, Schaefer FV, Schellenberg GD. Genetic factors for the development of Alzheimer disease in the Cherokee Indian. *Arch. Neurol.* 1996;53:997–1000.

325. Rosenberg RN, Baskin F, Fosmire JA, Risser R, Adams P, Svetlik D, Honig LS, Cullum CM, Weiner MF. Altered amyloid protein processing in platelets of patients with Alzheimer disease. *Arch. Neurol.* 1997;54:139–144.

326. Roses AD. Review: apolipoprotein E, a gene with complex biological interactions in the aging brain. *Neurobiol. Dis.* 1997;4:170–186.

327. Roses AD, Saunders AM. Apolipoprotein E genotying as a diagnostic adjunct for Alzheimer's disease. *Int. Psychogeriatr.* 1997;9:277–288.

328. Roses A, Saunders AM. ApoE, Alzheimer's disease, and recovery from brain stress. *Ann. N.Y. Acad. Sci.* 1997;826:200–212.

329. Rosler N, Wichart I, Jellinger KA. Intra vitam lumbar cerebrospinal fluid and serum and postmortem ventricular immunoreactive apolipoprotein E in patients with Alzheimer's disease. *J. Neurol. Neurosurg. Psychiatry* 1996;60:452–454.

330. Sabolovic D, Roudier M, Boynard M, Pautou C, Sestier C, Fertil B, Geldwerth D, Roger J, Pons JN, Amri A, Halbreich A. Membrane modifications of red blood cells in Alzheimer's disease. *J. Gerontol. A Biol. Sci. Med. Sci.* 1997;52:B217–B220.

331. St. George-Hyslop PH. Role of genetics in tests of genotype, status and disease progression in early-onset Alzheimer's disease. *Neurobiol. Aging* 1998;19: 133–137.

332. Sanan DA, Weisgraber KH, Russell SJ, Mahley RW, Huang D, Saunders A, Schmechel D, Wisniewski T, Frangione B, Roses AD, et al. Apolipoprotein E associates with beta amyloid peptide of Alzheimer's disease to form novel monofibrils: isoform apoE4 associates more efficiently than apoE3. *J. Clin. Invest.* 1994;94: 860–869.

333. Saunders AM, Hulette O, Welsh-Bohmer KA, Schmechel DR, Crain B, Burke JR, Alberts MJ, Stritmatter WJ, Breitner JC, Rosenberg C. Specificity, sensitivity and predictive value of apolipoprotein-E genotyping for sporadic Alzheimer's disease. *Lancet* 1996;348:90–93.

334. Scheu KF, Cooper AJ, Koike K, Koike M, Lindsay JG, Blass JP. Abnormality of the alpha-ketoglutarate dehydrogenase complex in fibroblasts from familial Alzheimer's disease. *Ann. Neurol.* 1994;35:312–318.

335. Scheuner D, Eckman C, Jensen M, Song X, Citron M, Suzuki N, Bird TD, Hardy J, Hutton M, Kukull W, Larson E, Levy-Lahad E, Viitanen M, Peskind E, Poorhaj P, Schellenberg G, Tanzi R, Wasco W, Lannfelt L, Selkoe D, Younkin S. Secreted amyloid beta-protein similar to that in the senile plaques of Alzheimer's disease is increased in vivo by the presenilin 1 and 2 and APP mutations linked to familial Alzheimer's disease. *Nature Med.* 1996;2:854–870.

336. Schofield PW, Logroscino G, Andrews HF, Albert S, Stern Y. An association between head circumference and Alzheimer's disease in a population-based study of aging and dementia. *Neurology* 1997;49:30–37.

337. Schott K, Wormstall H, Dietrich M, Klein R, Batra A. Autoantibody reactivity in serum of patients with Alzheimer's disease and other age-related dementias. *Psychiatry Res.* 59:251–254.

338. Schwagerl AL, Mohan PS, Cataldo AM, Vonsattel JP, Kowall NW, Nixon RA. Elevated levels of the endosomal-lysosomal proteinase cathepsin D in cerebrospinal fluid in Alzheimer disease. *J. Neurochem.* 1995;64:443–446.

339. Scinto LF, Daffner KR, Dressler d, Ransil BI, Rentz D, Weintraub S, Mesulam M, Potter H. A potential noninvasive neurobiological test for Alzheimer's disease. *Science* 1994;266:1051–1054.

340. Selkoe DJ. Cell biology of the amyloid beta-protein precursor and the mechanism of Alzheimer's disease. *Annu. Rev. Cell. Biol.* 1994;10:373–403.

341. Serot JM, Bene MC, Foliguet B, Faure GC. Altered choroid plexus basement membrane and epithelium in late-onset Alzheimer's disease: an ultrastructural study. *Ann. N.Y. Acad. Sci.* 1997;826:507–509.

342. Serot JM, Christmann D, Dubost T, Couturier M. Cerebrospinal fluid transthyretin: aging and late onset Alzheimer's disease. *J. Neurol. Neurosurg. Psychiatry* 1997;63:506–508.

343. Serra JA, Famulari AL, Kohan S, Marschoff ER, Dominguez RO, de Lustig ES. Copper-zinc superoxide dismutase activity in red blood cells in probable Alzheimer's patients and their first-degree relatives. *J. Neurol. Sci.* 1994;122:179–188.

344. Seshadri S, Wolf PA, Beiser A, Au R, McNulty K, White R, D'Agostino RB. Lifetime risk of dementia and Alzheimer's disease. The impact of mortality on risk estimates in the Framingham Study. *Neurology* 1997;49:1498–1504.

345. Sevush S, Jy W, Horstman LL, Mao WW, Kolodny L, Ahn YS. Platelet activation in Alzheimer disease. *Arch. Neurol.* 1998;55:530–536.

346. Shalit F, Sredni B, Brodie C, Kott E, Huberman M. T lymphocyte subpopulations and activation markers correlate with severity of Alzheimer's disease. *Clin. Immunol. Immunopathol.* 1995;75:246–250.

347. Shanahan C, Gibson GE, Cowburn RF, Johnston JA, Wiehager B, Lannfelt L, O'Neill C. G protein subunit levels in fibroblasts from familial Alzheimer's disease patients: lower levels of high molecular weight Gs alpha isoform in patients with decreased beta-adrenergic receptor stimulated cAMP formation. *Neurosci. Lett.* 1997;232:33–36.

348. Sheehan JP, Swerdlow RH, Miller SW, Davis RE, Parks JK, Parker WD, Tuttle JB. Calcium homeostasis and reactive oxygen species production in cells transformed by mitochondria from individuals with sporadic Alzheimer's disease. *J. Neurosci.* 1997;17:4612–4622.

349. Sheline YI, Miller K, Bardgett ME, Csernansky JG. Higher cerebrospinal fluid MHPG in subjects with dementia of the Alzheimer type: relationship with cognitive dysfunction. *Am. Geriatr. Psychiatr.* 1998;6:155–161.

349a. Schenk D, Barbour R, Dunn W, et al. *Nature* 1999;400:173–177.

350. Sherrington R, Rogaev EI, Liang Y, Rogaeva EA, Levesque G, Ikeda M, Chi H, Lin C, Li G, Holman K, et al. Cloning of a gene bearing missense mutations in early-onset familial Alzheimer's disease. *Nature* 1995;375:754–760.

351. Sherrington R, Froelich S, Sorbi S, Campion D, Chi H, Rogaeva EA, Levesque G, Rogaev EI, Lin C, Liang Y, Ikeda M, Mar L, Brice A, Agid Y, Percy ME, Clerget-

Darpoux F, Piacentini S, Marcon G, Nacmias B, Amaducci L, Frebourg T, Lannfelt L, Rommens JM, St. George Hyslop PH. Alzheimer's disease associated with mutations in presenilin 2 is rare and variably penetrant. *Hum. Mol. Genet.* 1996;5:985–988.

352. Shoffner JM, Brown MD, Torroni A, Lott MT, Cabell MF, Mirra SS, Beal MF, Yang CC, Gearing M, Salvo R, et al. Mitochondrial DNA variants observed in Alzheimer disease and Parkinson disease patients. *Genomics* 1993;17:171–184.

353. Shoji M, Matsubara E, Kanai M, Watanabe M, Nakamura T, Tomidokoro Y, Shizuka M Wakabayashi K, Igeda Y, Mizushima K, Amari M, Ishiguro K, Kawarabayashi T, Harigaya Y, Okamoto K, Hirat S. Combination assay of CSF tau, A beta 1-40 and A beta 1-42(43) as a biochemical marker of Alzheimer's disease. *J. Neurol. Sci.* 1998;158:134–40.

354. Siennicki-Lantz A, Lilja B, Rosen I, Elmstahl S. Cerebral blood flow in white matter is correlated with systolic blood pressure and EEG in senile dementia of the Alzheimer type. *Dement. Geriatr. Cogn. Disord.* 1998;9:29–38.

355. Simon N, Jolliet P, Morin C, Zini R, Urien S, Tillement JP. Glucocorticoids decrease cytochrome c oxidase activity of isolated rat kidney mitochondria. *FEBS Lett.* 1998;435:25–28.

356. Singh VK. Studies of neuroimmune markers in Alzheimer's disease. *Mol. Neurobiol.* 1994;9:73–81.

357. Singh VK. Immune-activation model in Alzheimer disease. *Mol. Chem. Neuropathol.* 1996;28:105–11.

358. Singh VK. Neuroautoimmunity: pathogenic implications for Alzheimer's disease. *Gerontology* 1997;43:79–94.

359. Singh VK, Guthikonda P. Circulating cytokines in Alzheimer's disease. *J. Psychiatr. Res.* 1997;31:657–660.

360. Slooter AJ, Tang MX, van Duijn CM, Stern Y, Ott A, Bell K, Breteler MM, Van Broeckhoven C, Tatemichi TK, Tycko B, Hofman A, Mayeux R. Apolipoprotein E epsilon 4 and the risk of dementia with stroke. A population-based investigation. *JAMA* 1997;277:818–821.

361. Small GW, Komo S, La Rue A, Saxena S, Phelps ME, Mazziotta JC, Saunders AM, Haines JL, Pericak-Vance MA, Roses AD. Early detection of Alzheimer's disease by combining apolipoprotein E and neuroimaging. *Ann. N.Y. Acad. Sci.* 1996;802:70–78.

362. Small BJ, Herlitz A, Fratiglioni L, Almkvist O, Backman L. Cognitive predictors of incident Alzheimer's disease: a prospective longitudinal study. *Neuropsychology* 1997;11:413–420.

363. Smith MA, Richey PL, Kutty RK, Wiggert B, Perry G. Ultrastructural localization of heme oxygenase-1 to the neurofibrillary pathology of Alzheimer disease. *Mol. Chem. Neuropathol.* 1995;24:227–230.

364. Smith MA, Harris PL, Sayre LM, Perry G. Iron accumulation in Alzheimer disease is a source of redox-generated free radicals. *Proc. Natl. Acad. Sci. U.S.A.* 1997;94:9866–9868.

365. Smith MA, Wehr K, Harris PLR, Siedlak SL, Connor JR, Perry G. Abnormal localization of iron regulatory protein in Alzheimer's disease. *Brain Res.* 1998; 788:232–236.

366. Smith RP, Broze GJ Jr. Characterization of platelet-releasable forms of beta-amyloid precursor proteins: the effect of thrombin. *Blood* 1992;80:2252–2260.
367. Snaedal J, Kristinsson J, Gunnarsdottir S, Olafsdottir, Baldvinsson M, Johannesson T. Copper, ceruloplasmin and superoxide dismutase in patients with Alzheimer's disease: a case control study. *Dement. Geriatr. Cogn. Disord.* 1998;9:239–242.
368. Sorbi S, Piacentini S, Latorraca S, Piersanti P, Amaducci L. Alterations in metabolic properties in fibroblasts in Alzheimer disease. *Alzheimer Dis. Assoc. Disord.* 1995;9:73–77.
369. Soussan L, Tchernakov K, Bachar-Lavi O, Yuvan T, Wertman E, Michaelsom DM. Antibodies to different isoforms of the heavy neurofilament protein (NF-H) in normal aging and Alzheimer's disease. *Mol. Neurobiol* 1994;9:83–91.
370. Sparro G, Bonaiuto S, Galdenzi G, Eleuteri AM, Angeletti M, Lupidi G, Tacconi R, Giannandrea E, Vesprini A, Fioretti E. Acid-stable serine proteinase inhibitors in the urine of Alzheimer disease subjects. *Dis. Markers* 1996;13:31–41.
371. Stern RG, Mohs RC, Davidson M, Schmeidler J, Silverman J, Kramer-Ginsberg E, Searcey T, Bierer L, Davis KL. A longitudinal study of Alzheimer's disease: measurement, rate, and predictors of cognitive deterioration. *Am. J. Psychiatry* 1994;151:390–396.
372. Stern Y, Tang MX, Denaro J, Mayeux R. Increased risk of mortality in Alzheimer's disease patients with more advanced educational and occupational attainment. *Ann. Neurol.* 1995;37:590–595.
373. Strittmatter WJ, Saunders AM, Schmechel D, Pericak-Vance M, Enghild J, Salvesen GS, Roses AD. Apolipoprotein E: high avidity binding to beta-amyloid and increased frequency of type 4 allele in late-onset familial Alzheimer disease. *Proc. Natl. Acad. Sci. U.S.A.* 1993;90:1977–1981,
374. Sullivan EV, Shear PK, Mathalon DH, Lim KO, Yesavage JA, Tinklenberg JR, Pfefferbaum A. Greater abnormalities of brain cerebrospinal fluid volumes in younger than in older patients with Alzheimer's disease. *Arch. Neurol.* 1993;50:359–373.
375. Taddei K, Clarnette R, Gandy SE, Martins RN. Increased plasma apolipoprotein E (apoE) levels in Alzheimer's disease. *Neurosci. Lett.* 1997;223:29–32.
376. Tamaoka A. Characterization of amyloid beta protein species in the plasma, cerebrospinal fluid and brains of patients with Alzheimer's disease. *Nippon Ronen Igakkai Zasshi* 1998;35:273–277.
377. Tanaka S, Chen X, Xia Y, Kang DE, Matoh N, Sundsmo M, Thomas RG, Katzman R, Thal LJ, Trojanowski JQ, Saitoh T, Ueda K, Masliah E. Association of CYP2D microsatellite polymorphism with Lewy body variant of Alzheimer's disease. *Neurology* 1998;50:1556–1562.
378. Tanaka S, Kawamata J, Shimohama S, Akaki H, Akiguchi I, Kimura J, Ueda K. Inferior temporal lobe atrophy and APOE genotypes in Alzheimer's disease: x-ray computed tomography, magnetic resonance imaging and Xe-133 SPECT studies. *Dement. Geriatar. Cogn. Disord.* 1998;9:90–98.
379. Tang MX, Maestr G, Tsai WY, Liu XH, Feng L, Chung WY, Chun M, Schofield P, Stern Y, Tycko B, Mayeux R. Effect of age, ethnicity, and head injury on the association between APOE genotypes and Alzheimer's disease. *Ann. N.Y. Acad. Sci.* 1996;802:6–15.

380. Tanno Y, Okuizumi K, Tsuji S. (1998). mtDNA polymorphisms in Japanese sporadic Alzheimer's disease. *Neurobiol. Aging* 1998;19(1 Suppl):S47–S51.
381. Tapiola T, Lehtovirta M, Ramberg J, Helisalmi S, Linnaranta K, Riekkinen P Sr, Soininen H. CSF tau is related to apolipoprotein E genotype in early Alzheimer's disease. *Neurology* 1998;50:169–174.
382. Terryberry JW, Thor G, Peter JB. Autoantibodies in neurodegenerative diseases: antigen-specific frequencies and intrathecal analysis. *Neurobiol. Aging* 1998;19: 205–216.
383. Teunisse S, Bollen AE, van Gool WA, Walstra GJ. Dementia and subnormal levels of vitamin B12: effects of replacement therapy on dementia. *J. Neurol.* 1996; 243:522–529.
384. The Canadian Study of Health and Aging: risk factors for Alzheimer's disease in Canada. *Neurology* 1994;44:2073–2080.
385. The Ronald and Nancy Reagan Research Institute of the Alzheimer's Association and the National Institute on Aging Working Group. Consensus report of the Working Group on: Molecular and Biochemical Markers of Alzheimer's Disease. *Neurobiol. Aging* 1998;19:109–116.
386. Thomas T, Thomas G, McLendon C, Sutton T, Mullan M. beta-Amyloid-mediated vasoactivity and vascular endothelial damage. *Nature* 1996;380:168–171.
387. Thome J, Munch G, Muller R, Schinzel R, Kornhuber J, Blum-Degen D, Sitzmann L, Rosler M, Heidland A, Riederer P. Advanced glycation endproducts-associated parameters in the peripheral blood of patients with Alzheimer's disease. *Life Sci.* 1996;59:679–685.
388. Thome J, Gsell W, Rosler M, Kornhuber J, Frolich L, Hashimoto E, Zielke B, Wisbeck GA, Riederer P. Oxidative-stress associated parameters (lactoferrin, superoxide dismutases) in serum of patients with Alzheimer's disease. *Life Sci.* 1997;60:13–9.
389. Trieb K, Ransmayr G, Sgone R, Lassmann H, Grubeck-Loebenstein B. APP peptides stimulate lymphocyte proliferation in normals, but not in patients with Alzheimer's disease. *Neurobiol. Aging* 1996;17:541–547.
390. Urakami K, Sato K, Okada A, Mura T, Shimomura T, Takenaka T, Wakutani Y, Oshima T, Adachi Y, Takahashi K, et al. Cu,Zn superoxide dismutase in patients with dementia of the Alzheimer type. *Acta Neurol. Scand.* 1995;91:165–168.
391. Valenti G. Neuropeptide changes in dementia: pathogenetic implications and diagnostic value. *Gerontology* 1996;42:241–256.
392. Van Duijn CM, Clayton DG, Chandra V, Fratiglioni L, Graves AB, Heyman A, Jorm AF, Kokmen E, Kondo K, Mortimer JA, et al. Interaction between genetic and environmental risk factors for Alzheimer's disease: a reanalysis of case-control studies. EURODEM Risk Factors Research Group. *Genet. Epidemiol.* 1994; 11:539–551.
393. Van Landeghem GF, Sikstrom C, Beckman LE, Adolfsson R, Beckman L. Transferrin C2, metal binding and Alzheimer's disease. *NeuroReport* 1998;9: 177–179.
394. van Leeuwen FW, de Kleijn DP, van den Hurk HH, Neubauer A, Sonnemans MA, Sluijs JA, Koycu S, Ramdjielal RDJ, Salehi A, Martens GJM, Grosveld FG, Peter J, Burbach H, Hol EM. Frameshift mutants of beta amyloid precursor protein and ubiquitin-B in Alzheimer's and Down patients. *Science* 1998;279:242–247.

395. Vanmechelen K, Blennow K, Davidsson P, Cras P, Van de Voorde A. Combination of tau/phospho-tau with other intracellular proteins as diagnostic markers for neurodegeneration. In Iqbal K, Winblad B, Nishimura T, Takeda M, Wisniewski HM, editors *Alzheimer's Disease: Biology, Diagnosis and Therapeutics.* New York: Wiley, 1997;197–203.

396. Van Rensburg SJ, Carstens ME, Potocnik FC, Aucamp AK, Taljaard JJ. Increased frequency of the transferrin C2 subtype in Alzheimer's disease. *NeuroReport* 1993;4:1269–1271.

397. Vogel G. Tau protein mutations confirmed as neuron killers. *Science* 1998;280: 1524–1525.

398. Wahlund LO. Biological markers and diagnostic investigators in Alzheimer's disease. *Acta Neurol. Scand. Suppl.* 1996;165:85–91.

399. Wakutani Y, Urakami K, Shimomura T, Takashi K. Heat shock protein 70 mRNA levels in mononuclear blood cells from patients with dementia of the Alzheimer type. *Dementia* 1995;6:301–305.

400. Wallace DC. Mitochondrial DNA sequence variation in human evolution and disease. *Proc. Natl. Acad. Sci. U.S.A.* 1994;91:8739–8746.

401. Wallace DC, Brown MD, Melov S, Graham B, Lott B. Mitochondrial biology, degenerative diseases and aging. *Biofactors* 1998;7:187–190.

402. Wallin A, Blennow K. Clinical subgroups of the Alzheimer syndrome. *Acta Neurol. Scand.* (Suppl)165:51–57.

403. Walter H, Widen KE. Differential electrophoretic behavior in aqueous polymer solutions of red blood cells from Alzheimer patients and from normal individuals. *Biochem. Biophys. Acta* 1995;1234:184–190.

404. Wang SJ, Liao KK,Fuh JL, Lin KN, Wu ZA, Liu CY, Liu HC. Cardiovascular autonomic functions in Alzheimer's disease. *Age Ageing* 1994;23:400–404.

405. Wang X, DeKosky ST, Wisniewski S, Aston, Kamboh MI. Genetic association of two chromosome 14 genes (presenilin 1 and alpha 1-antichymotrypsin) with Alzheimer disease. *Ann. Neurol.* 1998;44:387–390.

406. Wang X, Luebbe P, Gruenstein E, Zemlan F. Apolipoprotein E (ApoE) peptide regulates tau phosphorylation via two different signaling pathways. *J. Neurosci. Res.* 1998;51:658–665.

407. Weidemann A, Paliga K, Durrwang U, Czech C, Evin G, Masters CL, Beyreuther K. Formation of stable complexes between two Alzheimer's disease gene products: presenilin-2 and beta-amyloid precursor protein. *Nature Med.* 1997;3:328–332.

408. Weitkamp LR, Nee L, Keats B, Polinsky RJ, Guttormsen S. Alzheimer disease: evidence for susceptibility loci on chromosomes 6 and 14. *Am. J. Hum. Genet.* 1983;35:443–453.

409. Welch WJ. Mammalian stress response: cell physiology, structural/function of stress proteins, and implications for medicine and disease. *Physiol. Rev.* 1992; 72:1063–1081.

410. Wetterling T, Tegtmeyer KF. Serum alpha 1-antitrypsin and alpha 2-macroglobulin in Alzheimer's and Bismanger's disease. *Clin. Invest.* 1994;72:196–199.

411. WHO Expert Committee on Biological Standardization. Forty-fifth report. *W.H.O. Tech. Rep. Ser.* 1995;858:1–101.

412. Wilder RL. Neuroendocrine-immune system interactions and autoimmunity. *Annu. Rev. Immunol.* 1995;13:307–338.

413. Wisniewski T, Castano E, Ghiso J, Frangione B. Cerebrospinal fluid inhibits Alzheimer beta-amyloid fibril formation in vitro. *Ann. Neurol.* 1993;34: 631–633.

414. Wisniewski T, Castano EM, Golabek A, Vogel T, Frangione B. Acceleration of Alzheimer's fibril formation by apolipoprotein E in vitro. *Am. J. Pathol* 1994;145:1030–1035.

415. Wood JA, Wood PL, Ryan R, Grraff-Radford NR, Pilapil C, Robitaille Y, Quirion R. Cytokine indices in Alzheimer's temporal cortex: no changes in mature IL-1 beta or IL-1R but increases in the associated acute phase proteins IL-6, alpha 2-macroglobulin and C-reactive protein. *Brain Res.* 1993;629:245–252.

416. Xu S, Gaskin F. Increased incidence of anti-beta-amyloid autoantibodies secreted by Epstein-Barr virus transformed B cell lines from patients with Alzheimer's disease. *Mech. Ageing Dev.* 1997;94:213–222.

417. Yamada K, Kono K, Umegaki H, Yamada K, Iguchi A, Fukatsu T, Nakashima N, Nishiwaki H, Shimada Y, Sugita Y, et al. Decreased interleukin-6 level in the cerebrospinal fluid of patients with Alzheimer-type dementia. *Neurosci. Lett.* 1995;186:219–221.

418. Yan SD, Fu J, Soto C, Chen X, Zhu H, Al-Mohanna F, Collison K, Zhu A, Stern E, Saido T, Tohyama M, Ogawa S, Roher A, Stern D. An intracellular protein that binds amyloid-beta peptide and mediates neurotoxicity in Alzheimer's disease. *Nature* 1997;389:689–695.

419. Yanase T, Fukahori M, Taniguchi S, Nishi Y, Sakai Y, Takayanagi R, Haji M, Nawata H. Serum dehydroepiandrosterone (DHEA) and DHEA-sulfate (DHEA-S) in Alzheimer's disease and in cerebrovascular dementia. *Endocr. J.* 1996;43:119–123.

420. Yankner BA, Duffy LK, Kirschner DA. Neurotrophic and neurotoxic effects of amyloid beta protein: reversal by tachykinin neuropeptides. *Science* 1990;250: 279–282.

421. Yoshida H, Yoshimasu F. Alzheimer's disease and trace elements. *Nippon Rinsho* 1996;54:111–116.

422. Zapatero MD, Garcia de Jalon A, Pascual F, Calvo ML, Escanero J, Marro A. Serum aluminum levels in Alzheimer's disease and other senile dementias. *Biol. Trace Elem. Res.* 1995;47:235–240.

423. Zhou D, Kusnecov AW, Shurin MR, De Paoli M, Rabin BS. Exposure to physical and psychological stressors elevates plasma interleukin 6: relationship to the activation of hypothalamic-pituitary-adrenal axis. *Endocrinology* 1993;133: 2523–2530.

424. Zubenko GS. Endoplasmic reticulum abnormality in Alzheimer's disease: selective alteration in platelet NADH-cytochrome c reductase activity. *J. Geriatr. Psychiatry Neurol.* 1989;2:3–10.

425. Zubenko GS, Teply I, Winwood E, Huff FJ, Moossy J, Sunderland T, Martinez AJ. Prospective study of increased platelet membrane fluidity as a risk factor for Alzheimer's disease: results at 5 years. *Am. J. Psychiatry* 1996;153:420–423.

426. Zubenko GS, Hughes HB, Stiffler JS, Hurtt MR, Kaplan BB. A genome survey for novel Alzheimer disease risk loci: results at 10 cM resolution. *Genomics* 1998;50:121–128.

10

Pupillary Response as a Possible Early Biological Marker for Alzheimer's Disease

Leonard F. M. Scinto

Introduction

Despite the growing understanding of the basic pathological cascade of Alzheimer's disease (AD) over the past decade, there is yet no definitive marker or diagnostic test for this condition. Recent evidence *(1,2)* points to the fact that the disease, and by disease we mean the pathology of AD, may be present many years before there are any clinical manifestations of the disease. AD exists on two planes: the clinical and the pathological. Unfortunately this distinction is often blurred or lost. The clinical manifestation of the disease is temporally subordinate to the presence of pathology. This suggests that the earliest marker for the disease will not be found in identifying clinical symptoms, by which time the pathological process has already done significant damage, but in identifying a biological marker for the disease that is detectable well before frank or even subtle clinical symptoms are apparent.

Recent work *(3)* has shown that 50% of neurons in some layers of the entorhinal cortex may be lost in individuals who would be rated a 0.5 on the Clinical Dementia Rating (CDR) scale. Studies by Morris and others *(1,2)* suggest that the pathology of AD may be present for many years before the onset of even subtle clinical symptoms of dementia. Another recent pathological study *(4)* that autopsied the brains of 98 individuals 65 and older involved in fatal car crashes has shown that some 50% of victims had clear evidence of AD pathology suggesting that the prevalence of the disease might be much higher than expected. Such work confirms the need for diagnostic tests that can detect the presence of the disease well before clinical symptoms become evident.

From: *Early Diagnosis of Alzheimer's Disease*
Edited by L. F. M. Scinto & K. R. Daffner © Humana Press, Inc., Totowa, NJ

Pupil Assay

One intriguing candidate as a potential early marker for AD is a relatively noninvasive pupil assay being developed in our laboratory. In late 1994 we published a finding *(5)* that patients with probable AD (PrAD) could be distinguished from age-matched, healthy controls on the basis of an exaggerated pupil dilation response to a very dilute solution of tropicamide (a cholinergic antagonist). The insight for this observation was suggested in the first instance by the work of Sacks and Smith *(6)* who demonstrated the subjects with Down syndrome had a hypersensitive pupil dilation response to a dilute cholinergic antagonist applied to the eye. Given the known pathological links between the dementia that develops in older individuals with Down syndrome and that of AD *(7)*, it was a simple leap to ask if patients with PrAD might also exhibit a similar hypersensitivity to tropicamide. The possibility was especially compelling, as the pathology of AD is known to particularly affect cholinergic neurons in the brain. Pupillary dilation is in part controlled by structures in the midbrain that are composed of cholinergic neurons *(8)*.

In our original study, the assessment of hypersensitivity to tropicamide using the pupil assay consisted of three basic components:

1. Determination of a stable resting pupil diameter from both eyes
2. Instillation of approximately 33 μL of dilute tropicamide (i.e., 0.01%) to one eye arbitrarily chosen and a control solution to the other eye
3. Measurement of pupil diameter in each eye at seven preselected intervals over approximately 1 hour

In periods between measurements, all subjects and patients were shown segments from the videotape *Fantasia* to help ensure consistent intermeasurement stimulation. Pupil diameter was measured with a video-based, pupil center to corneal reflection, system capable of measuring eye position and pupil diameter (Applied Science Laboratories, Bedford, MA). We measured baseline pupil diameter in each eye for 1 minute (60 times per second) after subjects had accommodated to a dimly lighted environment and before any pharmacological intervention. Data sampling yielded 3600 samples of pupil diameter, which were averaged to compute a baseline diameter for each eye. The baseline diameter in the treated eye was used to determine percentage change in pupil diameter after pharmacological intervention with dilute tropicamide. At each measurement occasion, after instillation of dilute tropicamide, we measured pupil diameter for 30 seconds, which yielded approximately 1800 data samples that were averaged to calculate the mean pupil diameter. We deliberately oversampled to ensure as stable a measure of resting pupil diameter as possible. The pupil is never perfectly at rest but is subject to both minor and more significant variation in size due to both physiological and psychological influences. Oversampling ensures that pupil diameter is not a reflection of a momentary fluctuation in physiological or psychological input to the system.

The calculation of pupil diameter change in the treated eye is expressed as a percentage change over baseline diameter. This calculation is: $(DTE_x - DTE_B) / DTE_B$, where DTE_x is the measured diameter of the treated eye at a time point x after instillation of drug, DTE_B is the baseline diameter of the treated eye.

While we recorded the diameter of the nontreated eye as part of the assay, we choose not to use this eye as the control for determining response to the drug in the treated eye for several compelling reasons. With the equipment in our laboratory, it is not possible to record the diameter of both pupils simultaneously. The delay between measurement of the two pupils can possibly introduce factors that render the two measurements nonequivalent in terms of other influences acting on pupil diameter (e.g., arousal or fatigue). We usually observe some degree of initial anisocoria between the diameters of the two pupils. This initial anisocoria needs to be factored out of any subsequent calculation if an anisocoria calculation were to be used. Other work has shown that as the treated eye responds to the influence of the drug, the nontreated eye, as part of the consensual response, tends to constrict thus magnifying the response in the treated eye if we were to use the untreated pupil diameter as a control. The diameter of the untreated eye is always measured and used to evaluate the overall performance of pupils in the assay. If significant fatigue is encountered and found to influence pupil response during pupil recording an anisocoria calculation, taking into account the initial anisocoria at baseline, could be used to determine response to drug.

As predicted, in our original study *(5)*, we found that the treated pupils of the normal elders showed a minimal increase in pupil diameter over the course of the hour (Fig. 1, lower curve). In contrast, the patients with probable Alzheimer's disease displayed a pronounced response to the pupil dilating effects of tropicamide (Fig. 1, upper curve). Overall the results indicated that at minute 29 there was on average a 23.4% change in the pupil diameter of patients with probable AD compared to an average 5% change for normal elderly subjects. We found that we could distinguish AD patients from a sample of normal community dwelling elders with a sensitivity of 95% and a specificity of 94%. We defined hypersensitivity as pupil dilation that was $\geq 13\%$ over baseline diameter.

Subsequent to our original report, some 29 publications have appeared evaluating the use of the pupil assay. Results from most of the 29 published accounts *(9–37)* strongly suggest that the pupil assay using dilute tropicamide

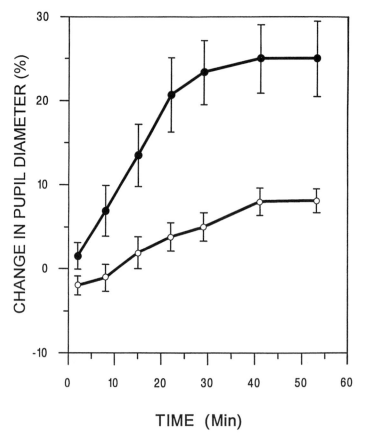

Fig. 1. Mean percentage change in pupil diameter over baseline diameter in treated eye in response to dilute (0.01%) tropicamide at 30 minutes posttreatment for AD patients *(upper curve)* and community dwelling elderly controls *(lower curve)*.

is reflecting the underlying biology of the disease. Despite a bewildering array of measurement techniques, drugs, and experimental conditions (none of which completely replicated our procedures) 16 *(9–22,30)* of 24 *(9–31)* reports comparing PrAD patients with normal controls found that, as a group, PrAD patients dilated more rapidly and/or to a greater extent than normal controls. Nine of these publications *(9–17)* have demonstrated that group differences were statistically significant. Two *(20,21)* found statistically significant differences under certain conditions. Two *(9,22)* found differences that were not statistically significant and one *(10)* showed a trend toward significance. One study found that their PrAD patients dilated more than normal controls, but no statistics were given *(30)*. Two studies *(13,19)* found that ApoE4 positively influences the degree of dilation. Another study *(38)*, in both young and older normal controls, found that individuals with an E4 allele dilated to a greater degree than those without the E4 allele. This suggests that a hypersensitive pupil dilation response is already present in cognitively normal individuals who are considered to be at higher risk for AD. Another study *(12)* examining individuals with PrAD and vascular dementia (VaD) showed 90% sensitivity and 58% specificity for AD, with many VaD patients dilating. This would be predicted if the assay were a marker of AD pathology, since pathological reports suggest greater than 50% of patients with a clinical diagnosis of VaD have underlying AD pathology *(39,40)*. Five studies *(9,41–44)* used either 0.0625% or 0.125% pilocarpine (a cholinergic agonist) rather than 0.01% tropicamide and all found that Alzheimer patients, as a group, exhibited significantly increased meiosis compared to normal controls.

On balance, these reports suggest that the pupil assay is in fact tapping a real phenomenon associated with the pathological process of AD. They confirm, with remarkably few exceptions, given the variety of methodologies employed, that patients with a diagnosis of probable AD exhibit an exaggerated response to tropicamide. The majority of these studies also suggest that there is greater overlap in the response of patients and nondemented elderly controls than suggested by our original report *(5)*. However, this should not surprise us. This is in fact what we should expect from a marker that is tapping the underlying pathological process before the emergence of symptoms of a clinical dementia. As we will discuss below, there is evidence that the pupil assay is sensitive to early pathology and that many purported "normal" controls may have a sufficient burden of AD lesions to give rise to a positive response in the pupil assay.

Ongoing Studies

Since the report of our original observation we have concentrated on assessing several key aspects of this phenomenon of a hypersensitive pupillary response in AD. We have examined the test–retest reliability of the assay and its potential as a preclinical marker of pathology. We have also looked for a possible mechanism to explain our finding by pursuing neuropathological study of AD and control brains. In the following sections we review the results from this work.

Test–Retest Reliability of the Pupil Assay

Any potential assay must meet the criterion of consistency or repeatability *(45,46)*. At a minimum this means that on each occasion that the assay is administered it should give the same or reasonably similar results for a given individual, assuming that no mediating factors have changed enough to alter the biological variable being measured. Without such repeatability, the value and utility of any diagnostic test or screen is compromised. This is a particularly important characteristic to establish for biological assays that measure what are by definition inherently unstable physiological phenomena.

We studied the repeatability of the assay in 29 community dwelling elderly subjects. The mean age of the sample was 71 ± 6 years and consisted of 20 females and 9 males. Of the 29 subjects, 10, who were part of our original report, were retested at least 1 year later (14.6 ± 3.2 months). Of the 29 subjects, 19 were tested on two occasions separated by a minimum of 1 full day (4.89 ± 2.38 days) to allow for drug washout. All subjects entered the study as volunteers responding to advertisements in the local community or from a pool of subjects from the Harvard Cooperative Project on Aging. They were living independently in the community. Subjects were excluded from the study if they were taking medications with known pupil effects or had a history of ophthalmological disease.

All subjects were given a neuropsychological battery of tests that assessed estimated IQ, language, memory, attention, and visuospatial ability. Although many of our subjects had abnormal test scores, none was excluded from the study of test–retest reliability based on neuropsychological performance. They also received a neurological examination and an ophthalmological screen by a neuroophthalmologist who evaluated subjects for a narrow anterior chamber, adequate tear lakes, corneal opacity, rapid tear buildup time, filaments, and mucus in the tear film. No significant ocular pathology or sensorimotor abnormalities were detected in any of the subjects.

Pupil measurements from both eyes were made as described above. Data consisted of percentage change in pupil diameter over baseline (calculated by the method described above). Subjects' dilation responses were coded "+" if by minute 29, the fifth measurement of pupil diameter after instillation of eye drops, they had a percentage increase in pupil diameter over baseline of $\geq 13\%$ or "−" if the percentage change over baseline was $<13\%$. These criteria were based on the finding in our original study *(6)*.

To assess test–retest reliability, we employed the following measures:

1. Simple percentage agreement between dilation values for test–retest occasions
2. Spearman's correlation analysis
3. The kappa statistic, a measure of agreement excluding chance
4. Cronbach's alpha, a measure of test reliability

All statistics were based on the pupil diameter at the fifth measurement (approximately 29 minutes after instillation). Figure 2 illustrates the performance of subjects with a dilation response of $<13\%$ on both occasions and

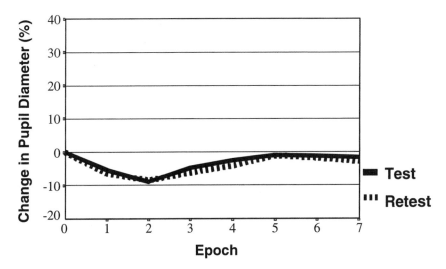

Fig. 2. Pupil response curve for all measurement epochs for all subjects with a dilation response of <13% for occasion 1 and 2.

Figure 3 illustrates the performance of subjects with a response of ≥13% on both occasions. Again, the responses for test–retest closely parallel each other in both cases.

Our analysis revealed that:

1. There was 86% agreement between the pupil response in test 1 and test 2 when we looked at measurement 5 for all subjects irrespective of response magnitude. The percentage agreement for subjects retested within a few days was 89% and for those tested a year or more apart it was 80%.
2. There was a significant correlation (.73, $P <.0005$) between measurement 5 for test 1 and test 2 using Spearman's technique. When we separated the sample into two groups, those that had been retested <1 year apart and those that were tested ≥1 year apart, we found that for measurement 5 there was a correlation of .79 for those subjects tested <1 year apart ($P <.0005$) and a correlation of .66 for subjects tested ≥1 year apart ($P = .04$).
3. Calculating the kappa statistic, we found 72% agreement between dilation responses at measurement 5 for test and retest occasions.
4. Cronbach's alpha showed 84% agreement for dilation responses for test 1 and test 2 at measurement 5.

Based on data from 29 subjects tested on two occasions (some of whom were tested 1 or more years apart) we found significant agreement between the data on pupil response from both test occasions. The results confirm the more than satisfactory test–retest reliability of the assay and its stability in determining cholinergic sensitivity.

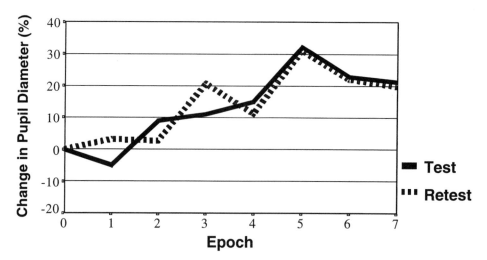

Fig. 3. Pupil response curve for all measurement epochs for all subjects with a dilation response of ≥13% for occasion 1 and 2.

Of the four subjects out of 29 who did not repeat their initial pupil dilation performance on second occasion testing, two had been tested 1 year previously. During their initial evaluation, these subjects performed normally on the neuropsychological battery used in this study and exhibited a nonhypersensitive pupil response. In year 2, neuropsychological testing revealed that these subjects had declined cognitively, with specific deficits in the realm of memory. While not demented by standard clinical criteria, these subjects nonetheless had begun to exhibit difficulties in the storage and retrieval aspects of memory. Subsequent follow-up of these two subjects in our longitudinal study (see below) show that they continue to exhibit additional decline in memory. Declines in memory have been shown to often precede the onset of a clinical dementia *(47–49)*. Coincident with the development of the memory deficit, by the second testing occasion these subjects were also found to exhibit an exaggerated pupil response. The implications of such "conversion" in pupil response are addressed later in this chapter in our discussion of our longitudinal work. Excluding these subjects from consideration for test–retest evaluation, the percentage agreement between the two test occasions would change from 86% to 93% agreement.

Of the two remaining subjects who did not repeat their initial pupil response, factors such as fatigue (depressing the pupil response on a given occasion) or anxiety (enhancing the pupil response) may have in part influenced the result on one of the occasions. It is possible that variations in dosing (the inadvertent administration of a greater or lesser amount of tropicamide) will have introduced more or less active agent into the tear film thus causing a magnified or dampened response in the pupil. Changes in corneal permeability or tear film thickness between the two test occasions may also account for the differences in pupil response.

The data from this aspect of our continued investigation of the pupil assay as a possible marker for AD support the premise that the pupil assay, done under carefully controlled experimental conditions, is a reliable measure of cholinergic sensitivity in elderly subjects. Overall, the consistency of the pupil assay in assessing pupil sensitivity is excellent given the weak solution used and the inherent variability of the pupillary response in which multiple inputs may affect pupil dilation. When administered on two occasions, separated by either a few days or a year, and assuming no significant differences in subject cognitive status or pupil physiology, the assay will give similar findings on cholinergic hypersensitivity.

Longitudinal Findings With the Pupil Assay

As noted in Chapter 2, in major medical centers the accuracy with which we can diagnose AD is impressive. Diagnostic accuracy often approaches 80% to 90%. However, such diagnosis is made after patients exhibit notable symptoms of memory impairment and difficulty with daily living activities. The search for an early presymptomatic marker for AD has yet to be successful. The need for such an early diagnostic test for AD is undisputed. With an early presymptomatic test the search for successful therapies to slow the progress of the disease will be greatly facilitated (see Chapter 11).

The failure of some studies, using the pupil assay (see above), to find significant differences between patients with probable AD and community dwelling elders may in part be due to contamination of the control sample with individuals who are at presymptomatic or preclinical stages of the disease. We need a means to determine if this contention is accurate or if the pupil assay is in fact incapable of distinguishing between patients with probable AD and healthy control subjects.

The main dilemma that confronts us is against what standard are we to judge the accuracy of an early diagnostic marker to detect pathology in the absence of clinical symptoms. How can we judge the predictive power of two tests for the early diagnosis of AD that give contradictory findings? It is unlikely that we will be able to obtain in vivo biopsies as confirmatory data on the accuracy of a given diagnostic test. Autopsy series are also likely to prove either difficult to obtain or problematic in their interpretation given the temporal lag between the administration of an early diagnostic procedure (presymptomatically) and autopsy confirmed AD perhaps many years later.

In order to test the accuracy of such tests to diagnose AD early, longitudinal data may be the best evidence we can bring to bear on this question. The convergence over time of a positive test finding and the development of a cognitive compromise with the eventual emergence of classic clinical symptoms of AD can serve as strong evidence of the power of a given assay to predict the development of probable AD. Such data also allow us to assess the interval over which we can expect to be able to predict the development of clinical symptoms of dementia.

We conducted a prospective longitudinal study of community dwelling elderly subjects' response to dilute tropicamide to determine if the "false positives" in some studies was reflective of a lack of specificity in the assay or rather a measure of the assay's sensitivity to the presence of early AD pathology in the absence of clinical symptoms. The goal of this work was to determine whether a hypersensitive pupil response in asymptomatic individuals was predictive of subsequent cognitive decline suggestive of preclinical AD.

We have evaluated a sample of 55 community dwelling elders for up to 4 years. They are all self-referred volunteers from the Boston area. All lived independently in the community and responded to local advertisements for an Aging and Alzheimer's disease study at Brigham and Women's Hospital. We carefully screened subjects for a history of alcoholism, drug abuse, serious current neurological, medical or psychiatric illness, ocular pathology, and medications with known anticholinergic effects. All subjects have been well characterized with CDR rating scores, neurological examination, psychiatric interview, medical history, ApoE genotyping, pupil assay, and a comprehensive battery of neuropsychological tests selected from the literature to be sensitive to preclinical Alzheimer's disease. Of the 55 individuals in our longitudinal sample, all have 2 years of data; 19 have 3 years of data and 7 have 4 years of data. Demographics for the 55 subjects in the final analysis are given in Table 1.

We used a prospective longitudinal design to assess the predictive power of the pupil assay to identify individuals who would over time progress to exhibit

Table 1
Demographics Longitudinal Subjects

	Minimum	Maximum	Mean	Std. Deviation
AGE	57	87	69.62	6.09
EIQ	106	131	122.78	5.58
IMC	0	4	.87	1.06
Years of education	12	20	15.60	2.51

measurable cognitive decline in the areas of memory and attention in a pattern consistent with an early dementing process. Subjects were assessed yearly with a neuropsychological battery of tests sensitive to preclinical and early AD. At each yearly evaluation subjects received a neurological as well as neuroophthalmological examination. Medical history was updated yearly. At their initial evaluation, subjects were screened for cognition and mood that included the Blessed Dementia Scale (BDS) *(50)*, the American modification of the National Adult Reading Test (AmNART) *(51,52)*, and the Geriatric Depression Scale (GDS) *(53)*. The Blessed Dementia Scale was chosen because it has been widely used to identify the presence and severity of dementia. The American modification of the National Adult Reading Test (AmNART) was chosen to provide an estimate of premorbid IQ. The AmNART is reported as a more reliable indicator of premorbid ability because it capitalizes on the subject's premorbid familiarity with words and controls for the lack of formal education in the elderly *(54)*. The Geriatric Depression Scale was chosen as a measure for depression. Lower scores (0–10) indicate a normal range of functioning. Higher scores are indicative of mild (11–20) to moderate/severe (21–30) ranges of depression. Subjects were also screened for ApoE allele type and pupillary reaction to dilute tropicamide (a cholinergic antagonist) was determined using the pupil assay *(5)*.

Subjects underwent an experimental battery of neuropsychological tests known from the literature to be sensitive to preclinical Alzheimer's disease. The tests measured the following cognitive domains:

Attention: Digit Span from the Wechsler Adult Intelligence Scale-Revised *(55)*; FAS *(56)*; Category Generation Test (i.e., animals, vegetables, and fruit) *(57)*; Recitation of Months Forward and Months Backward;
Memory: Bushke Selective Reminding Test-6 trial *(58)*;
Language: Boston Naming Test *(59)*;
Visuospatial: Benton Form Discrimination Test *(56)*.

The literature reports memory loss as the earliest symptom of "at risk populations" *(47–49)*. The additional measures were chosen because demonstrable impairments in word fluency, naming and complex attention improve the power of prediction with respect to which elders go on to develop a frank dementia state *(51,60–63)*.

The average estimated IQ of our sample was in the superior range (mean: 123). Therefore, we were concerned that the detection of preclinical or presymptomatic AD in intellectually higher functioning individuals would be masked by use of conventionally published neuropsychological test norms *(63,64)*. We estimated premorbid IQ for subjects in our sample based on their performance in the AmNART. This was used as a means of assessing decline from an estimated premorbid baseline capacity. Despite individual diversity in functional laterality and brain organization, it is generally accepted in the psychometric literature on "deficit measurement" that most normal adults show a consistent performance on neuropsychological tests across a broad range of cognitive skills and domains for their expected level of performance (65,66). If an individual had an estimated IQ in the superior range (120–130), which is 1.7 standard deviations above a mean of 100, we would expect a similar level of performance on tests of cognition and memory. By contrast, if a superior functioning individual performed in the average range on tests of memory, such a performance would suggest a significant decline from premorbid functioning (66). To determine decline from baseline we adjusted the norms in which the revised "mean" value of the standardized published norms was defined (64) in the following manner:

- If the Estimated AmNART IQ was <120, standard norms were used based on the published literature
- If the Estimated AmNART IQ was ≥120 but ≤130, standard cutoff scores were derived from an adjusted mean based on 1.7 SD above the normative mean where the mean IQ = 100.
- If the Estimated AmNART IQ was ≥131, standard cutoff scores were derived from an adjusted mean based on 2 SD above the normative mean where the mean IQ = 100.

Test scores that fell 2 standard deviations below the adjusted mean were considered abnormal. This method adjusts for any age associated memory loss as suggested by NIMH proposed standards of ≥1 standard deviation below the mean for young adults (40,41). Based on their cognitive performance in the experimental battery, subjects were classified as falling into one of four status categories defined as follows:

Category 0: Normal: no test abnormalities.
Category 1: Mild cognitive impairment but no dementia (abnormalities in one cognitive realm: a) memory, b) nonmemory, or c) IMC ≥2).
Category 2: Questionable Dementia (abnormalities in 2 or more realms, one being memory).
Category 3: Possible preclinical AD (scores on tests of memory and word fluency that fall substantially greater than 2 SD below the adjusted mean*).
Category 4: Meets DSM-IV and ADRDA criteria for PrAD.

---

*Scores used in determining Category 3 status included: Categories <37; one of the following Buschke subtest scores ≤ to the following − TR 30, LTS 16, LTR 12, Delay 2, MC 9, 30'MC 9.

Subjects received a pupil assay each year. Retesting allowed us to see if subjects with a nonexaggerated response in a given year would maintain that response or "convert" to a positive exaggerated response in light of developing pathology (see below).

We used logistic regression for a discrete-time survival analysis (DTSA) to estimate the relative risk of a predictor variable in detecting a pattern of cognitive decline. DTSA provides information about target event occurrence patterns among members of a predictor group. These models are conceptually similar to multiple regression models and can be used to determine the effect of multiple predictors on the conditional probabilities that an event will occur in a given time period. As with multiple regression, DTSA modeling can determine whether the inclusion of a predictor variable in the model contributes statistically significant information to the prediction of a given outcome marker. This model yields an odds ratio for each predictor variable which estimates the magnitude of the effect *(67)*.

A discrete time survival model was used because it has distinct advantages over traditional methods for handling methodological and analytical difficulties. Discrete time survival analysis has the feature of incorporating repeatable dichotomous predictors, outcome variables and time-varying covariates into analysis. Unlike other methods that require traditional temporal ordering, this model allows predictors to precede an outcome event and does not require that all subjects experience the target event within the discrete-time framework. Such a model can account for the censoring of cases (subjects who do not meet the terminal event in the model during the time of evaluation).

We hypothesized that subjects with a positive pupil response would experience greater cognitive decline compared to subjects with a negative pupil response. We tested this hypothesis by including pupil response as a time dependent predictor variable in the model that has as events the category neuropsychological classification (early dementing pattern/no early dementing pattern, i.e., $\geq$Category 2).

Pupillary response (dichotomous: $\geq$13% or <13% over baseline diameter) was used as the primary predictor in the model. Cognitive status $\geq$2 (see above) was defined as the terminal event in the model. The goal of the analysis was to determine whether the risk of early dementia differed among the hypersensitive pupillary responders (positive dilators) and nonhyperresponders (negative nondilators). Multivariate evaluation incorporated other covariates that were, based on literature in the field and considered associated with increased risk for dementia.

A person–period data set was created for our sample. This data set contained 55 subjects with repeated data points for each predictor and outcome variable (i.e., pupil response and cognitive status). A chronological baseline model of risk probability was estimated by using logistic regression with time as an independent predictor. Having established the baseline model, a series of hierarchical models were fitted by adding variables of substantive interest in particular, age and ApoE allele to control for the effects of each of these risk factors.

Pupillary response was examined as the primary predictor of outcome events. Multivariate control was achieved by adding age into the model. A hypersensitive pupillary response of 13% or greater emerged as a significant, independent predictor of eventual cognitive decline (OR = 3.0; p = 0.017; CI: 1.22–7.80). The overall model was significant at p = 0.02.

We added ApoE allele status as a covariate to the baseline model. Allele type was defined as having as least one 4 allele or no 4 allele. With ApoE as a covariate we found that pupil was still the most significant predictor (OR = 4.0; p = 0.01; CI: 1.37–12.13).

The results of this pilot study strongly suggest an exaggerated pupil response ($\geq$13% over baseline diameter) is a significant independent risk factor for developing a pattern of cognitive decline consistent with an early dementing process. Additional years of data will be required before we can more precisely assess the relative risk associated with an exaggerated pupil response. The relative risk based on the models in this pilot analysis suggests that the risk of early stage dementia is increased by about fourfold. This is a significant increase in risk when compared to risks associated with hypercholesterolemia for death from HID or a family history of breast cancer for death form breast cancer. This analysis also helps explain why cross-sectional studies may show varying degrees of overlap in the pupil response of diagnosed patients with probable AD and nondemented community dwelling elderly.

Underlying Mechanism for Pupillary Sensitivity

Our search for a mechanism to explain the exaggerated dilation response of AD patients led us to consider the possibility that this hypersensitivity might be a consequence of pathology at the level of the Edinger-Westphal nucleus, a known center for the control of pupillary function. In light of the clinical nosology of Alzheimer's disease and the known patterns of the distribution of pathology in AD *(68)* the finding of a peripheral hypersensitivity to tropicamide seemed puzzling. However, a review of the available literature revealed that reports of AD pathology in the brainstem suggested that the deposition and distribution of such pathology is relatively more extensive in rostral regions of the brainstem within which the neurons that contribute to pupillary function are located *(69–71)*. We suspected that the Edinger-Westphal nucleus (EW), which is documented to play a role in various aspects of pupillary control (e.g., constriction and accommodation) *(8)*, might be a target for early pathological changes that could lead to the observed hypersensitivity of patients with PrAD *(1)*.

Animal studies *(72,73)* have demonstrated that the parasympathetic preganglionic efferent output for pupillary response originates in the EW, the small-celled autonomic division of the oculomotor complex. This nucleus lies medial and dorsal to the main oculomotor nuclei in the midbrain. It is located ventral to the periaqueductal gray matter (PAG) and extends from the level of the caudal pole of the red nucleus to the region of the nucleus interstitialis, a distance of approximately 5–7 mm. The EW receives input from the retina via the pretectum *(72–76)*, and in turn sends its axons through the oculomotor nerve to the ciliary ganglion. In animals, injections of cholinergic agents into this region have been shown to affect pupil size *(77)*.

Most studies of midbrain pathology in AD *(78)* have shown that the PAG is the region with the heaviest deposition of lesions. A recent study *(79)* of the PAG region showed very robust correlations between the pathological burden in this area and pathology in the entorhinal cortex. Since the entorhinal cortex is markedly affected by AD pathology early in the course of the disease, the PAG and EW might also be early targets for pathology. There have been contradictory reports in the literature with respect to pathology in the oculomotor complex *(80,81)*.

Eight brains from clinically and pathologically confirmed (CERAD criteria) *(82)* cases of Alzheimer's disease, seven brains from community dwelling, neurologically normal individuals, three brains from age-matched, neurologically normal community dwelling elderly with cortical AD pathology and one brain from a case of clinically and pathologically confirmed progressive supranuclear palsy (PSP) were used in this study *(71a)*. Neither age nor postmortem interval were different for the patient and control groups (Age: Jonckheere-Terpstra Test:: J-T = −.083, P = .934; PMI: J-T = −.332, P = .740).

The brainstem of each case was separated by a cut placed rostral to substantia nigra, into the thalamus, to preserve the oculomotor (and EW) nucleus. Fixed tissue was sectioned at 40 μm on a freezing microtome into 0.1 M phosphate buffer containing 0.02% sodium azide. Series of 1 in 4 sections from each brainstem were stained for Nissl using cresyl violet and used for anatomical localization and morphological characterization of the EW and adjacent structures.

Immunohistochemistry was performed using the avidin–biotin–peroxidase complex (ABC) method employing the vectastain Elite ABC kit (Vector Laboratories, Burlingame, CA). Free-floating sections were rinsed three times in 0.1 M phosphate-buffered saline (PBS), at pH 7.4. This rinse was repeated after every incubation step. Sections were treated with 0.4% triton X-100 in PBS for 30 minutes at room temperature and then soaked for 1 hour in the carrier medium consisting of 10% normal goat serum and 0.1% triton X-100 in PBS. Tissue was incubated in the primary antibody at appropriate dilutions for 24 hours at 4°C. Sections were then incubated in biotinylated goat secondary IgG (1/500) for 15 hours, followed by the ABC complex (1/100) for 2 hours. The resultant peroxidase labeling was visualized by incubating the sections in 0.005% diaminobenzidine and 0.01% H_2O_2 in 50 mM Tris-Hcl (pH 7.6) for 10–20 minutes. Following termination of the reaction by rinsing in the Tris-Hcl buffer, sections were mounted on slides, air-dried, dehydrated in graded alcohols, cleared in xylene and coverslipped under permount. Control sections were processed using nonspecific IgG in place of the primary antibody or by omitting the primary antibody.

The polyclonal antibody 1282, which recognizes Aβ (kindly supplied by Dr. Dennis Selkoe, Center for Neurologic Diseases, Brigham and Women's Hospital, Boston, MA), a monoclonal antibody (PHF1) which specifically recognizes tau phosphorylated at Ser396/Ser404 and the monoclonal antibody Alz-50 which recognizes epitopes associated with the cytoskeletal pathology of Alzheimer's disease (generous gift of Dr. Peter Davies, Albert Einstein College of Medicine, Bronx, New York) were used to assess pathology. To ascertain specificity of staining, some sections were processed in the presence of nonspecific IgG in place of the antibody. Thioflavin-S staining was used to visualize compact plaques, dystrophic neurites, neuropil threads, and tangles. All stained sections were subjected to careful microscopic examination and the presence of AD-type lesions in the EW noted. The specificity of such pathology was ascertained by comparing the EW with the somatic portion of CN3 and other neighboring structures.

To obtain a quantitative measure of the extent of tangle and dystrophic neurite/neuropil thread (NT/DN) formation, we counted the number of PHF1-positive lesions in the EW of 3 AD cases, 3 normal controls, and the 3 cases that were clinically silent but exhibited cortical pathology. Counting was carried out at ×40 magnification using an ocular grid placed in the eyepiece of the microscope. Sections through the anterior, intermediate and posterior regions of the EW, matched across all cases, were used for counting. The mean numbers of tangles and DN/NT in the three groups were analyzed for significant effects using nonparametric tests (i.e., Kruskal-Wallis and Kolmogrov-Smirnov).

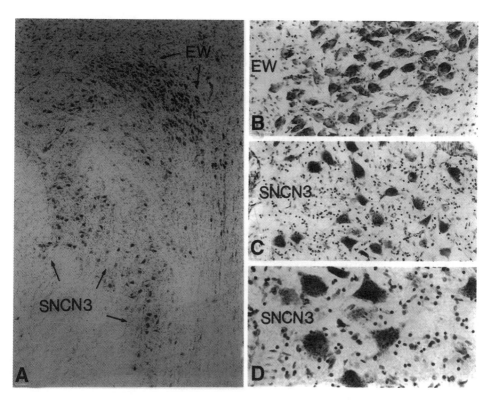

Fig. 4. Morphological characteristics of neurons within the oculomotor complex in Nissl stained sections from normal subjects. (**A**) The neurons of the somatic component of the nucleus of the third cranial nerve (SNCN3) are diffusely scattered, while the neurons of the Edinger-Westphal (EW) nucleus are grouped together in a compact region dorsal and medial to the SNCN3. (**B**) Neurons within the EW are fusiform or oval in shape and the Nissl substance is diffusely scattered throughout the cell. (**C**) Neurons within the SNCN3 are larger than EW neurons, have multipolar morphology and stain darkly for Nissl. (**D**) At high magnification, the Nissl substance within the SNCN3 has a granular and clumped appearance. Panel A: ×215; Panels B and C: ×560; Panel D: ×1120. Reproduced with permission from ref. *71a.*

Anatomical identification of the EW in this study was guided by the brainstem atlas of Olszewski *(83)* that remains the standard anatomic characterization for this nucleus. The EW could be identified within the oculomotor complex by the morphological characteristics of its cells (Fig. 4a,b,c). The neurons of this nucleus were densely arranged, small to medium in size and fusiform, oval, or triangular in shape (Fig. 4b). They had a prominent nucleus and the Nissl substance was diffusely distributed throughout the cytoplasm. By contrast, neurons of the somatic portion of the nucleus of the third cranial nerve (SNCN3) (Fig. 4c) were large, multipolar, and stained darker than cells in the EW. The Nissl substance in SNCN3 neurons was granular and clumped in appearance (Fig. 4d). Morphological characterization of the oculomotor nucleus in our sample of normal subjects, using Nissl-stained sections revealed numerous densely packed neurons throughout the EW (Fig. 4a). The EW could be divided into three divisions, an anterior unpaired portion lying in the midline, a paired central portion lying dorsal and medial to the SNCN3 and a posterior paired portion lying on either side of the midline.

We used PHF1 and Alz-50 immunoreactivity to study the distribution of tangles and neuropil threads/dystrophic neurites (NT/DN) within the oculomotor complex and adjacent regions. In normal control cases, virtually no PHF1- or Alz-50-positive tangles or NT/DN were observed within the oculomotor complex (Fig. 5f). Unlike the control cases, PHF1 and Alz-50 staining revealed a dense accumulation of structures with the morphology of tangles and NT/DN in the EW of all AD cases (Fig. 5b). Adjacent sections stained with thioflavin S confirmed the presence of tangles and NT/DN in the EW. In striking contrast, the SNCN3 was almost completely free of tangles and NT/DNs (Fig. 6b). Some adjacent areas, such as the dorsal raphe nucleus and the PAG, exhibited heavy burdens of pathology (data not shown). Examination of the cerebral cortex revealed that AD cases with the greatest number of cortical tangles and NT/DN, also exhibited the heaviest deposition of pathology in the EW.

Next, we determined the presence of tangles and NT/DN in the EW of the three cases that had been clinically silent, but displayed an accumulation of these lesions within the cerebral cortex. Cortical pathology in one case was relatively mild while there was sufficient pathology present in the second and third cases to satisfy a classification of possible AD by CERAD criteria *(82)*. A moderate density of PHF1- and Alz-50-positive neurons and NT/DN were observed in the EW (Fig. 5d) of all three cases. Thioflavin-S-stained sections showed occasional tangles and a moderate density of NT/DN (data not shown). Again, the SNCN3 was completely free of pathology. In all cases, tangles and NT/DN were also observed in some adjacent areas.

The results of the quantitative assessment of tangles and NT/DNs are presented in Figures 7 and 8. The three groups differed significantly in the numbers of tangles ($p = 0$, 2-tailed) and NT/DN ($p = 0.016$, 2-tailed) at all levels of the EW studied. The EW of the AD group and the control group with AD pathology had significantly higher numbers of tangles and NT/DN as compared with the normal control group ($p = 0.015$, 2-tailed). There was also a trend toward significant differences in the numbers of tangles and NT/DN in the EW of the AD sample and controls with cortical pathology ($p = 0.065$). Tangle counts in posterior sectors of EW did not show such a trend ($p = 0.290$, 2-tailed).

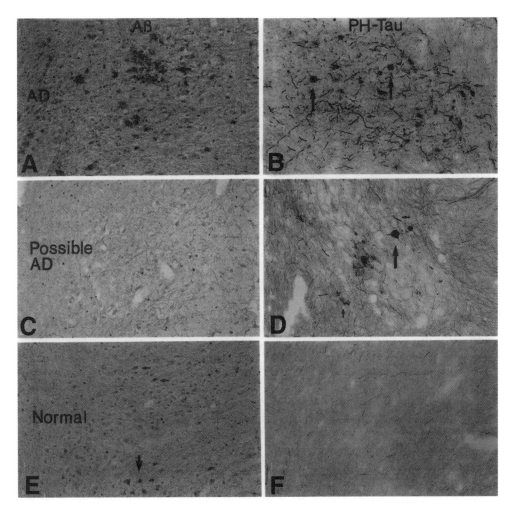

Fig. 5. β-Amyloid (Aβ) stained plaques and hyperphosphorylated tau (PH-Tau, PHF1)-stained tangles and neuropil threads/dystrophic neurites (NT/DN) in the EW of AD and normal brains. **(A)** Many Aβ-positive plaques *(arrow)* are observed within the EW of AD brains. **(B)** Staining with the PHF1 antibody visualizes a large number of PH-Tau-positive structures with the morphology of tangles *(large arrows)* and NT/DNs *(small arrows)* within the EW of AD brains. Virtually the same results are obtained using the Alz-50 antibody. **(C)** Staining for Aβ in a clinically nondemented case with the pathological diagnosis of possible AD fails to visualize any plaques in the EW. **(D)** In the same case as in panel C, a number of structures with the morphology of tangles *(large arrow)* and NT/DN *(small arrows)* are PH-tau-positive. **(E)** No Aβ-positive plaques are found in the EW of normal cases. In some normal and AD cases, weak Aβ staining is observed within the neurons of the EW *(small arrows),* and darker staining in the neurons of the SNCN3 *(large arrow).* This staining is entirely due to recognition of high contents of the amyloid precursor protein (APP) within these neurons by the Aβ antibodies (Geula and Scinto, unpublished observations). **(F)** No PH-tau staining is present within the EW of normal cases. Virtually identical results were obtained using the thioflavin S stain. Panels A–F: ×280. Reproduced with permission from ref. *71a.*

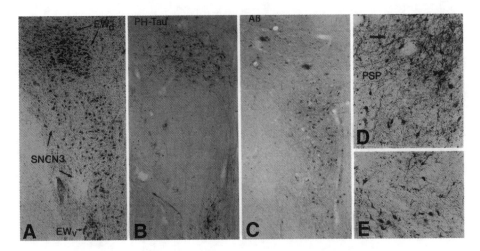

Fig. 6. Regional specificity of Alzheimer pathology within the oculomotor complex of AD brains. (**A**) Nissl-stained sections through the intermediate aspect of the oculomotor complex visualize neurons within the dorsal and ventral portions of EW (EWd and EWv, respectively) and the SNCN3. (**B**) A high density of PH-Tau-positive tangles and NT/DN is found within the EW of AD cases. The SNCN3, however, is almost completely free of pathology. (**C**) Aβ-positive plaques are found within the EW in AD. No plaques are observed within the SNCN3. Aβ staining in neurons within the oculomotor complex is entirely due to high cellular content of APP (Fig. 2). (**D**) PHF1 staining in the oculomotor complex from a patient suffering from progressive supranuclear palsy (PSP) reveals PH-tau-positive neurons, tangles, and NT/DN within the EW *(large arrow)* as well as the SNCN3 *(small arrows)*. (**E**) In the PSP case, tangles are found throughout the SNCN3 *(small arrows),* consistent with clinical oculomotor abnormalities in this disorder. Panels A–C: ×180; panels D and E: ×360. Reproduced with permission from ref. *71a.*

We also investigated the presence of plaques using β amyloid (Aβ) immunohistochemistry. In the normal control cases, no Aβ-positive plaques were observed in the EW (Fig. 5e) or the SNCN3. A relatively small number of diffuse Aβ deposits were observed in the cerebral cortex and PAG of some normal cases. By contrast, many Aβ-positive plaques were distributed throughout the EW of all AD cases (Figs. 5a and 6c). Thioflavin S-stained sections revealed that most of these Aβ-positive plaques were of the diffuse type. Very rare diffuse plaques were observed within the SNCN3 in AD cases. All of the AD brains contained a high density of Aβ- and thioflavin S-positive plaques within the cerebral cortex and the PAG. The EW of the three clinically silent cases with cortical pathology contained no plaques (Fig. 5c). The cerebral cortex of these cases, however, exhibited a density of plaques between those of normal control and definite cases of AD.

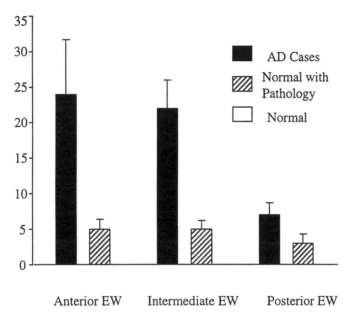

Fig. 7. Bar graph of the mean number of tangles in anterior, intermediate, and posterior sectors of the EW of ADs, controls with cortical pathology, and normal control cases without cortical pathology. AD cases exhibited the highest counts in all sections. Normal control cases without cortical pathology exhibited no tangles in any sections. Reproduced with permission from ref. *71a.*

We studied the distribution of AD-type pathology within the oculomotor complex of the brain from a patient who suffered from progressive supranuclear palsy (PSP), a disorder known to present with clinical oculomotor abnormalities. Numerous Alz-50- and PHF1-positive tangles, neurons and NT/DN were observed in both the EW and SNCN3 in this case (Fig. 6d,e). This distribution is in sharp contrast to that observed in AD cases in which the SNCN3 was virtually spared (Fig. 6b,c).

Our observations confirmed our speculation and demonstrated that the EW is a specific target of pathology, unlike the somatic portion of NCN3, which is spared. In contrast, PSP patients appear to exhibit more general pathology throughout the oculomotor complex. Of particular note is the finding of pathology in the EW in three of out 10 control cases. The presence of pathology in the EW of these individuals, who were clinically silent and one of who does not meet pathological criteria for AD, suggests that the deposition of pathology in the EW may constitute a relatively early event in the pathological cascade. More recent pilot work in our laboratory on cell loss in the EW shows that both AD patients and "normals" with EW pathology show significant cell loss in the EW compared to normals without pathology in this structure.

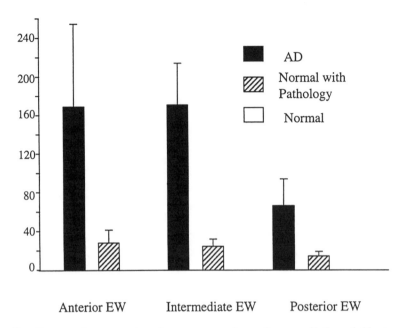

Fig. 8. Bar graph comparing the mean number of neuropil threads/dystrophic neurites (NT/DN) in the anterior, intermediate, and posterior sectors of EW for ADs, controls with cortical pathology and normal control cases without cortical pathology. NT/DN counts were highest for AD cases in all sections. Normal controls exhibited no NT/DN in any sections. Reproduced with permission from ref. *71a.*

The failure of some clinical studies of the pupil assay, to find significant group differences in the response of patients and control subjects to dilute tropicamide, is in large part due to a number of methodological variations (e.g., recording methodology and testing conditions, screening procedures for controls, simultaneous use of a dilating agent and corneal stain, and inadequate testing of drug concentration). However, our pathological work suggests an additional explanation for such results. The presence of AD pathology in the EW of some of our elderly control cases who did not meet clinical criteria for AD could lead to a hypersensitive response to tropicamide. Since AD pathology appears to be present in the EW early in the course of the disease, a hypersensitive pupil response may serve as a marker for the disease process long before patients have sufficient pathology to either exhibit clinical symptoms or qualify for a clinical diagnosis of probable AD. The findings from our initial analysis of longitudinal data (see above) are consistent with the hypothesis that pathology in the EW is a relatively early event leading to a positive response to the pupil challenge.

Pathology within the EW, a known center for pupillary control, leading to neuronal loss, likely initiates a cascade of events leading to the hypersensitivity that we have observed in the exaggerated mydriatic response of the pupil of AD patients to cholinergic agents such as the antagonist, tropicamide. The finding of mild but selective pathology in the EW in normal brains further suggests that a hypersensitive pupil response may be present in some community dwelling elderly subjects who are otherwise clinically silent.

Future Directions

Will the pupil assay prove useful as an early clinical marker for AD? To date, data on the assay do not permit us to answer this question definitively. Does the assay reflect a biological phenomenon associated with AD? Here the data suggest that the assay is in fact linked to an early aspect of the pathological cascade of the disease. Additional longitudinal work will ultimately sort out whether an exaggerated response to dilute tropicamide can be used as a predictor of the eventual development of dementia and how early such a predictor will be useful as a marker. Further work on specificity, with appropriate control populations such as patients with frontotemporal dementia will be required to determine to what extent the pupil assay is a specific marker of AD.

If future research continues to be supportive and the pupil assay as a marker of early pathology is confirmed, the clinical utility of the assay will have to be determined. Can it be formalized into a "test" that is easily administered in a primary care setting? Can it be administered quickly and inexpensively enough to serve as a screen? How early should such a test be used? It is likely that in the first instance, if the pupil assay is useful, its chief use will be in selecting appropriate subjects for clinical trials of new agents aimed at stemming disease progression.

It is possible and perhaps likely that the pupil assay will be but one of many possible markers for AD. There may be a succession of markers that turn positive along some time line of disease progression. Therapeutic intervention may be deemed appropriate (depending on the toxicity of agents) when some number of these markers turn positive and before others turn positive. As for other potential biological markers for AD, longitudinal studies will be required to assess their relationship (temporal and pathological) to the clinical manifestation of the disease. Their utility will depend on how early they mark a process that ultimately leads to clinical dementia. In summary, preliminary data suggest that the pupil assay is related to the pathological cascade of AD, is a stable marker, and most importantly appears to be associated with a significantly increased risk for developing clinical dementia.

References

1. Morris JC, McKeel DW, Storandt M, et al. Very mild Alzheimer's disease: informant-based clinical, psychometric, and pathologic distinction from normal aging. *Neurology* 1991;41:469–478.
2. Morris JC, Storandt M, McKeel DW, et al. Cerebral amyloid deposition and diffuse plaques in "normal" aging: evidence for presymptomatic and very mild Alzheimer's disease. *Neurology* 1996;46:707–719.
3. Hyman BT, Van Hoesen GW, Damasio AR, Barnes CL. Alzheimer's disease: cell-specific pathology isolates the hippocampal formation. *Science* 1984;225: 1168–1170.
4. Johansson K, Bogdanovic N, Kalimo H, Winblad B, Viitanen M. Alzheimer's disease and apolipoprotein E ε4 allele in older drivers who died in automobile accidents. *Lancet* 1997;349:1143–1144.
5. Scinto LFM, Daffner KR, Dressler D, et al. A potential noninvasive neurobiological test for Alzheimer's disease. *Science* 1994;226:1051–1054.
6. Sacks B, Smith S. People with Down's syndrome can be distinguished on the basis of cholinergic dysfunction. *J. Neurol. Neurosurg. Psychiatry* 1989;52:1294–1295.
7. Coyle JT, Oster-Granite ML, Gearhart JD. The neurobiologic consequences of Down syndrome. *Brain Res. Bull.* 1986;16,773–787.
8. Gamlin PD, Reiner A. The Edinger-Westphal nucleus: sources of input influencing accommodation, pupilloconstriction, and choroidal flow. *J. Comp. Neurol.* 1991; 306:425–438.
9. Kaneyuki H, Mitsuno S, Nishida T, Yamada M. Enhanced miotic response to topical dilute pilocarpine in patients with Alzheimer's disease. *Neurology* 1998;50: 802–804.
10. Graff-Radford N, Lin SC, Brazis P, et al. Tropicamide eye drops cannot be used for reliable diagnosis of Alzheimer's disease. *Mayo Clin. Proc.* 1997;72:495–504.
11. Higuchi S, Matsushita S, Hasegawa Y, Muramatsu T, Arai H. Pupillary response to tropicamide in Japanese patients with alcoholic dementia, Alzheimer's disease, and vascular dementia. *Exp. Neurol.* 1997;144:199–201.
12. Kalman J, Kanka A, Magloczky E, Szoke A, Jardanhazy T, Janka Z. Increased mydriatic response to tropicamide is a sign of cholinergic hypersensitivity but not specific to late-onset sporadic type of Alzheimer's disease. *Biol. Psychiatry* 1997; 41:909–911.
13. Arai H, Terajima M, Nakagawa T, Higuchi S, Mochizuki H, Sasaki H. Pupil dilation assay by tropicamide is modulated by apolipoprotein E ε4 allele dosage in Alzheimer's disease. *NeuroReport* 1996;7:918–920.
14. Gomez-Tortosa E, del Barrio A, Jimenez-Alfaro I. Pupil response to tropicamide in Alzheimer's disease and other neurodegenerative disorders. *Acta Neurol. Scand.* 1996;94:104–109.
15. Kono K, Miyao M, Ishihara S, et al. Do Alzheimer's patients have a hypersensitive pupil dilation response to a cholinergic antagonist? *Neurobiol. Aging* 1996;17: S165.
16. Robles A, Tourino R, Sesar A, Suarez P, Noya M. Experiencia con el test pupilar de tropicamida en la enfermedad de Alzheimer. *Rev. Neurol. (Barc.)* 1996;24:65–68.

17. Woodruf-Pak DS, Romano SJ, Hinchliffe M. Detection of Alzheimer's disease with eyeblink classical conditioning and the pupil dilation response. *Alzheimer Res.* 1996;2:173–180.

18. Imamura Y, Kojima H, Haraoka K. Pupil dilation response to the acetylcholine receptor antagonist tropicamide in normal aged and senile dementia subjects. *Neurobiol. Aging* 1996;17:S165.

19. Matsushita S, Arai H, Hasegawa Y, et al. Apolipoprotein Eϵ4 allele and pupillary response to tropicamide in Alzheimer's disease and cognitively normal subjects. *Neurobiol. Aging* 1996;17:S164.

20. Loupe DN, Newman NJ, Green RC, et al. Pupillary response to tropicamide in patients with Alzheimer's disease. *Ophthalmology* 1995;103:495–503.

21. Reitner A, Baumgartner I, Thuile C, et al. The mydriatic effect of tropicamide and its diagnostic use in Alzheimer's disease. *Vis. Res.* 1997;37:165–168.

22. Kurz A, Marquand R, Fremke S, Leipert KP. Pupil dilation response to tropicamide: a biological test for Alzheimer's disease. *Pharmacopsychiatry* 1997;30:12–15.

23. Buque C, Jacob B, Charlier JR, Hache JC, Pasquier F, Petit H. Pupil reactivity in AD: a reappraisal. *Invest. Ophthalmol. Vis. Sci.* 1997;38:S391.

24. Fridh M, Havelius U, Elofsson G, Hindfelt B. The pupillary response to tropicamide in Alzheimer's disease. *Acta Ophthalmol. Scand.* 1996;74:276–279.

25. Growdon JH, Graefe K, Tennis M, Wray SH, Hayden D. Pupillary dilation to tropicamide is not specific for Alzheimer's disease. *Arch. Neurol.* 1997;54:841–844.

26. FitzSimon JS, Waring SC, Kokmen E, McLaren JW, Brubaker RF. Response of the pupil to tropicamide is not a reliable test for Alzheimer's disease. *Arch. Neurol.* 1997;54:155–159.

27. Hasegawa NA, Collin C, Hosein CA, Chertkow H, Overbury O. Evaluation of tropicamide in the diagnosis of early Alzheimer's disease. *Invest. Ophthalmol. Vis. Sci.* 1997;38:S392.

28. Tourino R, Robles A, Santos L, Capeans C, Sanchez-Salorio M. Diagnosis of the Alzheimer's disease by using the tropicamide test. *Invest. Ophthalmol. Vis. Sci.* 1997;38:S391.

29. Nuzzi R, Bogetto C, Ferrario E, Molaschi L, Villa L, Varetto O, Grignolo FM. Alzheimer's disease and computerized pupillography. *Neurobiol. Aging* 1996;17:S165.

30. Schweitzer I, Chang V, Kabov J, Ames D, Vingrys A, Tuckwell V. Anticholinergic eye drops in differentiating Alzheimer's disease and depression. *Biol. Psychiatry* 1996;39:662.

31. Ferrario E, Molaschi M, Villa L, Varetto O, Bogetto C, Nuzzi R. Is videopupillography useful in the diagnosis of Alzheimer's disease? *Neurology* 1998;50:642–644.

32. Marx JL, Kumar SR, Thach AB, Kiat-Winarko T, Frambach DA. Detecting Alzheimer's disease [Letter]. *Science* 1995;267:1577–1581.

33. Wilhelm B, Wilhelm H, Wormstall H, Kircher T, Kriegbaum C. *Nervenheilkunde* 1997;16:458–463.

34. Litvan I, FitzGibbon E. Can tropicamide eye drop response differentiate patients with progressive supranuclear palsy and Alzheimer's disease from healthy control subjects? *Neurology* 1996;47:1324–1326.

35. Treolar A, Assin M, MacDonald A. Pupillary response to topical tropicamide as a marker for Alzheimer's disease. *Br. J. Clin. Pharmacol.* 1996;41:256–257.

36. Fieler V, Inzelberg R, Korczyn AD. Cholinergic sensitivity of the pupil of demented Parkinson's patients. *Neurology* 1996;46:A162.

37. Leszek J, Gasiorowski K, Wojtowicz B. Pupil dilation by tropicamide in Alzheimer's disease patients and probands. *Neurobiol. Aging* 1996;17:S164.

38. Higuchi S, Matsushita S, Hasegawa Y, Muramatsu T, Arai H. Apolipoprotein E ε4 allele and pupillary response to tropicamide. *Am. J. Psychiatry* 1997;154:694–696.

39. Victoroff J, Mack WJ, Lyness SA, Chui HC. Multicenter clinicopathological correlation in dementia. *Am. J. Psychiatry* 1995;152:1476–1484.

40. Hulette C, Nochlin D, McKeel D, Morris JC, Mirra SS, Sumi SM, Heyman A. Clinical-neuropathologic findings in multi-infarct dementia: a report of six autopsied cases. *Neurology* 1997;48:668–672.

41. Hannannel M, Feiler-Ofry V, Kushnir M, Korczyn A. Parasympathetic function of the eye in dementia of the Alzheimer's type (DAT). *Neurology* 1995;45:A356.

42. Idiaquez J, Alvarez G, Villagra R, San Martin RA. Cholinergic supersensitivity of the iris in Alzheimer's disease. [Letter]. *J. Neurol. Neurosurg. Psychiatry* 1994;57: 1544–1550.

43. Katz B. Detecting Alzheimer's disease. [Letter]. *Science* 1995;67:1577–1581.

44. Sitaram N, Pomara P. Increased pupillary miotic response to pilocarpine in cognitively impaired elderly subjects. *IRCS Med. Sci.* 1981;9:409–410.

45. Goroll AH, May LA, Mulley AG. *Primary Care Medicine.* Philadelphia: Lippincott, 1981.

46. Kraemer HC. *Evaluating Medical Tests.* Newbury Park, Sage Publications, 1992.

47. Petersen R, Smith G, Ivnik R, Kokmen E, Tangelos E. Memory function in very early Alzheimer's disease. *Neurology* 1994;44:867–872.

48. Flicker C, Ferris SH, Reisberg B. A two-year longitudinal study of cognitive function in normal aging and Alzheimer's disease. *J. Geriatr. Psychiatry Neurol.* 1993;34:294–295.

49. Linn RT, Wolf PA, Backman DL, et al. The "preclinical phase" of probable Alzheimer's disease. *Arch. Neurol.* 1995;52:485–490.

50. Blessed G, Tomlinson BE, Roth M. The association between quantitative measures of dementia and of senile change in the cerebral grey matter of elderly subjects. *Br. J. Psychiatry* 1968;114:797–811.

51. Nelson HE, McKenna P. The use of reading ability in the assessment of dementia. *Br. J. Soc. Clin. Psychol.* 1975;14:259–267.

52. Grober E, Sliwinski M. Development and validation of a model for estimating premorbid verbal intelligence in the elderly. *J. Clin. Exp. Neuropsychol.* 1991;13: 933–949.

53. Yesavage JA, Brink TL, Rose TL, et al. Development and validation of a geriatric depression screening scale. *J. Psychiatr. Res.* 1983;17:37–49.

54. Katzman R. Education and the prevalence of dementia and Alzheimer's disease. *Neurology* 1993;43:13–20.

55. Wechsler D. *Wechsler Adult Intelligence Scale—Revised.* New York: The Psychological Corporation, 1981.

56. Benton AL, DeS.Hamsher K, Varney NR, Spreen O. *Contributions to Neuropsychological Assessment.* Oxford: Oxford University Press, 1983.

57. Monsch AU, Bondi MW, Butters N, Salmon D, Katzman R, Thal LJ. Comparisons of verbal fluency tasks in the detection of dementia of the Alzheimer's type. *Arch. Neurol.* 1992;49:1253–1258.

58. Masur DM, Fuld PA, Blau AD, Thal LJ, Levin HS, Aronson MK. Distinguishing normal and demented elderly with the Selective Reminding Test. *J. Clin. Exp. Neuropsychol.* 1989;11:615–630.

59. Kaplan E, Goodglass H, Weintraub S. *The Boston Naming Test: Assessment of Aphasia and Related Disorders,* 2nd ed. Philadelphia:Lea & Febiger, 1983.

60. Hart S, Smith CM, Swash M. Word fluency in patients with early dementia of the Alzheimer's type. *Br. J. Clin. Psychol.* 1988;27:115–124.

61. Martin A, Fedio P. Word production and comprehension in Alzheimer's disease. *Brain Lang.* 1983;19:124–141.

62. Jacobs DM, Sano M, Dooneief G, Marder K, Bell KL, Stern Y. Neuropsychological detection and characterization of preclinical Alzheimer's disease. *Neurology* 1995;45:957–962.

63. Sliwinski M, Lipton RB, Bushke H, Stewart W. The effects of preclinical dementia on estimates of normal cognitive functioning in aging. *J. Gerontol.* 1996;51B:217–225.

64. Rentz DM, Calvo VL, Scinto LFM, Sperling RA, Budson AE, Daffner KR. Detecting early cognitive decline in high functioning elders. *J. Geriatr. Psych.* In press.

65. Lezak MD. *Neuropsychological Assessment.* New York: Oxford University Press, 1995.

66. Filskov SB, Leli DA. Assessment of the individual in neuropsychological practice. In: Filskov SB, Boll TJ, editors. *Handbook of Clinical Neuropsychology.* New York: John Wiley & Sons, 1981:545–576.

67. Miller TQ. Statistical methods for describing temporal order in longitudinal research. *J. Clin. Epidemiol.* 1997;50:1155–1168.

68. Pearson RCA, Esiri MM, Hierns RW, Wilcock GK, Powell TPS. Anatomical correlates of the distribution of the pathological changes in the neocortex in Alzheimer's disease. *Proc. Natl. Acad. Sci. U.S.A.* 1985;81:4531–4534.

69. Brilliant M, Elble RJ, Ghobrial M, Struble RG. Distribution of amyloid in the brainstem of patients with Alzheimer's disease. *Neurosci. Lett.* 1992;148:23–26.

70. Iseki E, Matsushita M, Kosaka K, Kondo H, Ishii T, Amano N. Distribution and morphology of brain stem plaques in Alzheimer's disease. *Acta Neuropathol.* 1989;78:131–136.

71. Ishino H, Otsuki S. Frequency of Alzheimer's neurofibrillary tangles in the basal ganglia and brain-stem in Alzheimer's disease, senile dementia and the aged. *Folia Psychiatr. Neurol. Jpn.* 1975;29:279–287.

71a. Scinto LFM, Wu CK, Firla KM, Daffner KR, Saroff D, Geula C. Focal pathology in the Edinger-Westphal nucleus explains pupillary hypersensitivity in Alzheimer's disease. *Acta Neuropathol.* 1999:97:557–564.

72. Kourouyan HD, Horton JC. Transneuronal retinal input to the primate Edinger-Westphal nucleus. *J. Comp. Neurol.* 1997;381:68–80.

73. Loewy AD, Saper CB, Yamodis ND. Re-evaluation of the efferent projections of the Edinger-Westphal nucleus in the cat. *Brain Res.* 1978;141:153–159.

74. Klooster J, Beckers HJM, Vrensen GFJM, van der Want JJL. The peripheral and

central projections of the Edinger-Westphal nucleus in the rat: a light and electron microscopic study. *Brain Res.* 1993;632:260–273.

75. Loewy AD, Saper CB. Edinger-Westphal nucleus: projections to the brain stem and spinal cord in the cat. *Brain Res.* 1978;150:1–27.

76. Loewy AD, Saper CB, Yamodis ND. Re-evaluation of the efferent projections of the Edinger-Westphal nucleus in the cat. *Brain Res.* 1978;141:153–159.

77. Sharpe LG, Pickworth WB, Martin WR. Pupillary changes following microinjections of opioids, sympathomimetics and cholinomimetics into the oculomotor nucleus in the dog. *Soc. Neurosci.* 1977;3:967

78. Giess R, Scholte W. Localisation and association of pathomorphological changes at the brainstem in Alzheimer's disease. *Mech. Ageing Dev.* 1995;84:209–226.

79. Wu GF, Solodkin A, Van Hoesen GW. Compartmental periaqueductal gray pathology in Alzheimer's disease. [Abstract]. *Soc. Neurosci.* 1996;83:4.

80. Arima K, Murayama S, Oyanagi S, Akashi T, Inose T. Presenile dementia with progressive supranuclear palsy tangles and Pick bodies: an unusual degenerative disorder involving the cerebral cortex, cerebral nuclei, and brain stem nuclei. *Acta Neuropathol.* 1992;84:128–134.

81. Jellinger K, Riederer P, Tomonaga M. Progressive supranuclear palsy: clinicopathological and biochemical studies. *J. Neural. Trans. [Suppl]* 1980;16:111–128.

82. Mirra SS, Heyman A, McKeel D, Sumi SM, Crain BJ, Brownlee LM, Vogel FS, Hughes JP, Van Belle G, Berg L. The consortium to establish a registry for Alzheimer's disease (CERAD). Part II. Standardization of the neuropathologic assessment of Alzheimer's disease. *Neurology* 1991;41:479–486.

83. Olszewski J, Baxter D. *Cytoarchitecture of the Human Brain Stem,* 2nd ed. Basel: S. Karger, 1982.

11

Implications of Early Diagnosis for the Development of Therapeutics for Alzheimer's Disease

David S. Knopman

Successful development of treatments for Alzheimer's disease (AD) and early and more accurate diagnoses of AD are complementary. One reinforces the necessity of the other. Assessment of treatment effects will be improved by earlier and more accurate diagnoses. In turn, the better the treatments, the more motivation and justification there is to pursue diagnostic methods for presymptomatic at-risk individuals and for earlier diagnoses in symptomatic persons. With improved diagnostic methods, research in new treatments will be facilitated by access to more diagnostically homogeneous populations. When treatments are ready to enter general practice, early diagnosis will allow treatment to be initiated earlier. This chapter reviews present and future scenarios of treatments for AD, and the diagnostic requirements of these treatment options.

Range of Potential Pharmacological Treatment Options

Treatment of AD might take one or more of the following forms. Different diagnostic issues arise depending upon how early the diagnosis can be made, what kinds of treatments are available, and what specificity the treatments have for specific forms of AD (if subtypes exist). The state of our diagnostic acumen has a major bearing on the feasibility of treatment under the more optimal scenarios. To be sure, at the present time, only palliative therapies exist, but an explicit goal of AD research is to find treatments that are preventive, arrestive, or curative. Consider first, different treatments as a function of stage of disease at the time of diagnosis and the effectiveness of the therapy.

From: *Early Diagnosis of Alzheimer's Disease*
Edited by L. F. M. Scinto & K. R. Daffner © Humana Press, Inc., Totowa, NJ

Palliative Treatments

Palliative therapies are those that affect the symptomatic expression of AD, but have no effect on the underlying biology of the disease. With potent palliative therapy, early diagnosis of symptomatic disease is of value because it is at this point in the illness when the greatest benefits of palliative therapy are likely to occur. At the point where the patient is closest to functioning at a pre-morbid level, treatment will be likely to result in greater independence and quality of life than later treatment. Outcomes such as allowing patients to live in their own homes for a longer period of time is of great value to caregivers and to the patients. By contrast, if diagnosis were delayed and treatment not initiated until later when home residence was already marginally difficult, there would be less value to all parties. Regardless of when palliative treatment was initiated, benefits would gradually diminish over time. Eventually the patient would decline to severe levels of disability with only palliative therapy.

If available pharmacological agents offer only palliation, presymptomatic diagnosis would be of less value than if the treatment had some potential to slow the underlying pathological progression. Politically and economically, if palliative therapies alone were available, it would be hard to make a strong case for diagnosing at-risk but symptom-free individuals. Thus, with only a palliative therapy in the armamentarium, the diagnostic challenge would be to diagnose the disease as early as possible in the symptomatic course. If the degree of palliation were only modest, some critics might even question the need for early diagnosis.

If palliative therapy resulted in some tangible change in the patient's symptomatic disease, it would be far more successful politically than if the therapy merely stabilized the patient clinically. Reduction in the rate of worsening is very difficult for treating physicians and caregivers to perceive, and consequently can result in a return of nihilism and doubt about the treatment.

Preventive Treatments

The appearance of clinical disease is almost certainly a relatively late event in the course of AD. There is growing evidence that the pathology of AD develops over decades *(1)*. Neuronal and synaptic loss may begin initially in the years (or decades) preceding clinical manifestations. Preventive treatments would be aimed at the initiating events in the preclinical disease.

A preventive treatment would be feasible only if the therapy could be economically applied to an entire population or if presymptomatic diagnosis were possible. Because treatment of the entire middle-aged and elderly population would almost certainly be prohibitively expensive and logistically impossible, the existence of a preventive therapy would certainly require diagnostic methods for identification of at-risk presymptomatic disease in order to limit the number of individuals to be treated. As will be discussed later, the primitive state of identification of at-risk individuals currently makes it very difficult to conduct primary prevention trials. Progress in the diagnosis of at-risk individuals is virtually a prerequisite for finding preventive treatments.

Arrestive Therapies

Arrestive therapies are those that slow down or possibly even cause the symptoms of memory loss or impaired function to improve, but do not result in a complete remission of symptoms. Arrestive therapies would have to have some effect on the underlying tempo of the biochemistry of the disease. Preventive and arrestive treatments could be thought of as similar, differing only in the state of available diagnostic tools, and consequently, in the point at which treatment can be initiated. Arrestive therapy would apply in the context where diagnostic procedures existed only for symptomatic diagnosis. The political and economic case for early symptomatic diagnosis would be far stronger with the existence of an arresting therapy than it is for a palliative therapy. Furthermore, evidence for arrest of the disease would be a powerful impetus to extend the therapy to presymptomatic at-risk individuals. Still, arrestive therapy is of value to patients and families only if diagnosis occurs early in the clinical course.

Some of the caveats regarding the detection of the effects of palliative treatment also apply to arrestive therapies as well. An arrestive therapy that truly stopped the disease in its tracks but resulted only in lack of progression rather than improvement might still leave us with a major struggle to justify early diagnosis, compared to an arrestive therapy that produced obvious improvements, at least temporarily.

Curative Therapies

The least plausible scenario for the next several decades, curative therapy, seems highly unlikely if applied only when the disease becomes symptomatic. The only effective "curative" therapy for AD is likely to be that of primary prevention.

Different Treatments for Different Etiologies

It is plausible that AD is a syndrome due to different causes, and treatments could emerge for some but not all of the causes. For example, among the sequence of events between altered cellular homeostasis, overproduction or altered production of β-amyloid deposition and neuron death (assuming that β-amyloid is pathogenetically important), there may be steps at one point in the sequence where the disease is initiated in some, but not all, patients. By analogy, consider the clotting cascade or disorders leading to hyperammonemia. If AD proved to have different biochemical initiators, diagnosis of the "etiological type" of AD would be critical first at the stage of therapy development and then later in using it in practice. Diagnostic methods for this circumstance would almost undoubtedly have to be biochemical or molecular, rather than symptomatic or clinical, in nature.

Biological Effects Are Variable Across Individuals

There is good evidence for heterogeneity among individuals with AD on almost any parameter of the disease one wishes to consider. The variable expression of classical neurotransmitter deficits, and especially the variability of the cholinergic deficit, are particularly relevant examples in the present era of cholinomimetic therapies (2). The ability to diagnose patients with the treatable variants would be of great value for development and widespread use of targeted treatments.

Treatment Since 1996

Prior studies of drugs to treat dementia using lecithin (3), ergot alkaloids (4,5), and other agents failed to show obvious benefits. These earlier antidementia clinical trials were plagued by numerous methodological difficulties, some of which will be discussed later. Diagnostic problems were certainly a big problem for studies before the 1980s. Definition of what constitutes benefit or efficacy also was a major problem with earlier studies. Studies over the past 10 years and especially in the past 2–3 years have established that cholinesterase inhibitors have efficacy in treating AD. Consensus on methodology helped considerably in bringing about progress.

So far, the cholinesterase inhibitors appear to be purely palliative in effect. There is considerable controversy over the magnitude of the benefit, but the evidence is quite consistent now that enhancement of cholinergic transmission has a salutory effect on the disease. Other cholinomimetic approaches, such as muscarinic and nicotinic cholinergic agonists, are also under investigation.

Tacrine

Several well-designed studies have shown that tacrine has beneficial effects on cognition (6,7); these effects can also be detected by physicians performing clinical interviews, and give an important lesson about the complexities of anti-AD drug development *(8)*. Tacrine originally gained notice on the basis of a short-duration study in which dramatic effects were claimed *(9)*. The original report was followed by a number of trials of varying lengths, varying dosages, and varying sample sizes *(10–15)*. Diagnostic issues did not play an explicit role in the controversy over tacrine, but, to the extent that AD cholinergic deficits or genetic factors are of variable symptomatic importance across patients, our failure to recognize AD subtypes might have greatly hampered our appreciation of the effects of tacrine.

There are many reasons why some early studies with tacrine were reported as negative. The reasons relate to failures in understanding of its dose requirements, its side effects and consequent attrition rates, and its effect size. It appears that tacrine's effects are most consistently seen when the daily dose exceeds 80 mg/day. Some of the earlier negative studies used that dose or lower doses. When the dose range of the drug was finally explored, 80 mg/day proved to be too low. The dose of 80 mg/day may have a positive effect in a few patients, but it may be short-lived.

A number of the early studies *(10,12,13)* began with rather small numbers of subjects. Even without attrition, power to detect tacrine's modest effects was low. However, attrition was a large issue, as over half of patients begun on tacrine are unable to tolerate the medication due to gastrointestinal or hepatic side effects.

Comparing the tacrine-treated to the placebo-treated patients, the short-term beneficial cognitive effects over 30 weeks *(7)* at the highest doses were in the range of about 2.5 points on the Mini-Mental State Examination (MMSE) *(16)* or about 4 points on the Alzheimer's Disease Assessment scale-cognitive (ADAS-cog) *(17)*. The variability in response to tacrine across subjects is immense, mirroring the placebo group's variability. In the tacrine (160 mg/day)-treated patients who completed the 30 week trial, the improvement in the MMSE was 2 points, but the standard deviation was 3.6 points. The magnitude of the treatment effect and its degree of variability requires sample sizes much larger than most of the negative studies. The duration of the trials is another issue related to effect size that has generated much concern regarding the conduct of clinical trials and benefits of tacrine. Given the high short-term variability of tests such as the MMSE, including placebo effects, trials of at least 6 months were necessary to show beneficial drug effects against the background of variability of the disease. The clearest picture of the likely effects of tacrine on an individual patient comes from the cumulative distribution plots of cognitive test scores such as the MMSE or the ADAS-cog (see Figure 2 in ref. *7)*. Compared to the placebo group, patients who titrated up to 160 mg/day of tacrine and remained on the drug through the course of the 30-

week study were more likely to have improved performance compared to the placebo group patients. Among those improving ≥4 points on the ADAS-cog, 40% of those treated with high-dose tacrine experienced such a change over 30 weeks compared to 25% of placebo patients.

Questions about the effect size and the clinical significance of tacrine were raised as soon as positive results began to emerge. Neither the research community, the lay advocates or the FDA had a clear sense of what "clinically important" benefits really were. It will take years of experience before a consensus emerges on the definition of a clinically important benefit of an anti-AD drug. A recent assessment of tacrine's long-term benefits suggested that multiyear, high-dose tacrine use was associated with reductions in nursing home placement *(18)*. In this study, nursing home placement was used as a proxy for the development of severe dementia, an assumption that may not be entirely valid. The reduction in nursing home placement was of the magnitude of about 400 days for the point at which 25% of low-dose patients entered nursing homes versus the time point at which the higher dose patients entered nursing homes (see Figure 2 in ref. *18*). The reduction in the odds ratio of nursing home placement was about 2.7. From a clinical point of view, a reduction in nursing home placement of this magnitude seems clinically important both for individual patients and for populations. This study was not controlled, and hence there remains uncertainty over the causal role of tacrine on outcome.

The side effects and dosing regimen of tacrine have been an impediment to the drug's acceptance. The gastrointestinal (GI) side effects have been a major reason for tacrine discontinuation in ordinary practice, to the same extent as was seen in clinical trials. The alanine transaminase (ALT) elevations have proved to be more benign than originally thought *(19)*, but 29% experience a threefold elevation of ALT and 6% of patients experience elevations in levels of ALT more than 10 times the upper limit of normal. The current package insert for tacrine states that the drug should be discontinued when ALT levels reach five times ULN. To my knowledge, no instances of chronic hepatitis have been documented as due to tacrine therapy.

One of the other barriers to widespread use of tacrine has been the need for laboratory monitoring. Mobility may be a problem for some patients and caregivers—making trips to a clinic for blood tests may be a burden. Its four times a day dosing requirements also pose substantial logistical problems for the typical dementia patient. It may be impossible to ensure compliance among AD patients who live alone, or whose caregiver sees them only some of the day.

The variable response to tacrine is an area in which diagnostic advances are needed. It would be very surprising if the same issue does not affect all of the pending cholinomimetic drugs. The distribution of responses to tacrine was gaussian, implying that there are not distinct subsets of responders and non-responders. The fact that there were no subsets of responders does not mean that different patients have differing pathology in cholinergic and noncholinergic pathways. The wide differences strongly suggests that characterization of the biological substrate for tacrine's effect might lead to selective use of tacrine and other cholinomimetic drugs only in selected AD patients. For example, neuropathological and neurochemical data show that 1) some patients, mainly older ones have a biochemical profile in which noncholinergic deficits are modest or nonexistent and cholinergic deficits are marked *(20)*, 2) some patients appear to have primarily septal-derived deafferentation of the hippocampus whereas other patients have primary entorhinal-derived deafferentation *(21)*, and 3) ApoE effects on response to tacrine, while complex, suggest different responses between €4 and non-€4 carriers *(22)*. Diagnostically, it is important to try to develop methods for predicting which patients are likely to respond to cholinesterase therapy.

The experience with tacrine has proved to be a valuable in identifying impediments to treatment in AD patients. Ease of administration and lack of toxicity proved to be more tangible problems than concerns about efficacy. It seems to have been easier to convince a caregiver to allow the patient to try an anti-AD drug by noting that "it might do something, but it doesn't have any side effects," as compared to saying "it definitely has benefits but it does have some side effects." As of late 1997, it is probably unlikely that many new prescriptions are being written for tacrine because of the availability of donepezil.

Donepezil

The second cholinesterase inhibitor to be approved by the FDA was donepezil. It was given final approval by the FDA on November 26, 1996. Donepezil entered the market in mid-January 1997. Although there are no published data on the number of prescriptions written since its introduction, anecdotal evidence suggests that donepezil is being widely prescribed to patients with AD.

In two 12-week studies *(23,23a),* and a 24-week study *(24)*, donepezil produced statistically significant beneficial effects in cognition and clinician's global assessments. Donepezil rapidly replaced tacrine as the first-line drug for AD. No unexpected adverse effects have occurred in postmarketing experience.

It is difficult to compare the treatment effects between tacrine and donepezil due to differences in analytic methods and other factors, but the effects appear quite similar. The cognitive assessment instrument was the same between the 30-week tacrine trial and the 24-week donepezil trial, but the global assessment instruments were somewhat different in their methodologies. In addition, the donepezil study used an intent-to-treat analysis, capturing all patients who took double-blind study medication and had at least one follow-up assessment, in the setting where nearly 70% of high-dose-treated donepezil patients completed the study. By contrast, an intent-to-treat analysis of the 30-week tacrine study captured only ~30% of high-dose tacrine subjects with complete 30-week data. Comparison of mean scores on the ADAS-cog between intent-to-treat populations shows an slight advantage for donepezil. While some might criticize the comparison as biased, at the least, donepezil appears to be as effective as tacrine.

In contrast to tacrine, donepezil is given as a once a day dose, and it does not require laboratory monitoring. Furthermore, donepezil treatment is not associated with high attrition rates: cholinergic-GI toxicity appears to be much less intense than tacrine. The lower rate of peripheral cholinergic effects is thought to be due to the selective acetylcholinesterase inhibition produced by donepezil. Donepezil has much less activity for butyrylcholinesterase inhibition *(27,28)*. Inhibition of peripheral butyrylcholinesterases is thought to mediate many of the cholinergic side effects of cholinomimetic drugs.

It is not yet clear whether donepezil's availability in routine clinical practice has had an impact on the probability of early diagnosis of AD. A treatment that is perceived as effective and free of side effects might spur primary physicians, neurologists, and psychiatrists to make earlier diagnoses of AD than they were willing to do in the tacrine era or the no-treatment era. On the other hand, if the efficacy of donepezil is similar to that of tacrine, its perception as a palliative therapy may fail to spark enthusiasm in the primary care community. Obvious demonstrations of benefit are infrequent with purely palliative therapies, and without personal experience with seeing improvement with donepezil, tacrine, or the other agents to be discussed next, the motivation may still not be there to seek diagnoses of AD aggressively.

New Cholinesterase Inhibitors and Muscarinic Agonists

A controlled release form of physostigmine has also been shown to have efficacy in AD. Thal and colleagues *(25)* have reported positive results that are very similar in magnitude to those observed with tacrine and donepezil in a study of similar design and length. While physostigmine can be administered as a twice-a-day dosage, it is associated with a moderate amount of nausea and vomiting. It has been subsequently withdrawn from further development.

Rivastigmine a cholinesterase inhibitor, has effects that appear very similar to tacrine and donepezil in terms of efficacy parameters *(26,27)*. Its side-effect profile is quite favorable, with only GI side effects common. The GI side effects are a function of dose, as with other cholinesterase inhibitors. It is administered as a bid dose, making it more convenient than tacrine but less than donepezil. It was approved by the US FDA in May 1999.

Metrifonate *(28,29)* also has efficacy in mild to moderate AD. It is dosed once per day. Concerns about somatic muscle weakness leave metrifonate's future uncertain.

Galantamine, another cholinesterase inhibitor with possible nicotinic modulating properties, is under active investigation and has recently been submitted for approval to the FDA. Possible future trials of this drug with mildly cognitively impaired subjects are under discussion.

There are several muscarinic agonists that had been subjected to clinical trials. Neither xanomeline *(30)* nor SB202026 *(31)* showed improvement on both objective mental status examinations and clinician's global assessments.

Other agents

Evidence supporting a role for antioxidants in AD has come from a large-scale clinical trial using the antioxidants selegiline and alpha-tocopherol (vitamin E) published in 1997 *(32)*. In this trial from the Alzheimer's Disease Cooperative Study (ADCS) Group, therapy with selegiline and tocopherol each (but not in combination) resulted in a delay of about 8 months in reaching the endpoints associated with severe dementia, in comparison with the placebo group. These findings, coupled with the very favorable safety and cost profile of vitamin E, suggest that it can be recommended to most patients with AD. The implications of these findings for treatment of mild or incipient AD are not clear, but are to be the focus of subsequent investigations. If the mechanism of action of vitamin E in moderately severe dementia involved interruption of oxidative injury, it is plausible, but by no means assured, that such a mechanism would also be beneficial earlier in the disease.

For the other therapeutic classes of potential anti-AD drugs, there is no definitive data from adequately powered clinical trials. Based on epidemiological evidence, most recently a prospective study *(33)*, and neuropathological evidence (reviewed in Ref. *34)*, antiinflammatory agents are a particularly exciting class of potential anti-AD therapies. One placebo-controlled trial with an antiinflammatory drug, indomethacin, has been reported to date *(35)*. Interpretation of an effect for the drug was hampered by a high attrition rate due to its gastrointestinal toxicity. A multicenter trial of prednisone in AD under the auspices of the ADCS will be presented shortly. While prednisone is unlikely to be the agent of the future for AD, a positive outcome would provide proof of the concept. Nonsteroidal antiinflammatory drugs such as celecoxib with far less gastrointestinal toxicity however, are in clinical trials *(34)*.

There is considerable interest in the protective action of estrogen, but the evidence so far comes from epidemiological studies *(36–38b)* and small clinical trials *(39,39a)*. Investigation of the potential value of estrogen in symptomatic AD is being carried out by the ADCS and other groups *(39b,39c)*. A large prospective study by the Women's Health Initiative of nondemented subjects is ongoing *(40)*, but its conclusion is years away.

There has been growing anticipation about clinical trials using a γ-secretase inhibitor. The purpose of such an agent would be to reduce the production of Aβ by altering the cleavage of the amyloid precursor protein (APP) *(41,41a)*. As reviewed in Chapter 4, Aβ has been strongly implicated in the pathological cascade of AD. Recently, researchers at Elan Pharmaceuticals reported that in a transgenic mouse model of Alzheimer's disease, immunization with Aβ prevented the development of amyloid plaques and dystrophic neurons in young animals, and slowed and partially reversed the progression of existing pathology in older animals *(41b)*. Additional research is planned to determine the clinical significance of these findings *(41c)*.

Methodology of Clinical Trials as it Relates to Diagnosis

The formulation of diagnostic criteria for AD ("probable AD") *(42)* by a panel appointed by the National Institute of Neurological and Communicative Disorders and Stroke and the Alzheimer's Disease and Related Disorders Association (NINCDS-ADRDA) antedated the current era of clinical trials. The NINCDS-ADRDA criteria for probable AD have proved to be one of the least controversial areas in clinical trials methodology recently. This is due to thoughtfulness of their construction but also to their very conservative nature. Very little modification of diagnostic criteria for probable AD for clinical trials has occurred over the past 10 years, even while major changes have come about in other areas of trial design. Recently, ApoE genotyping has been added to allow subtyping of enrolled patients (e.g. Ref. *22)*, although its value remains unclear.

Despite the success of the current criteria for probable AD, there are notable deficiencies. At least 13% of patients included in clinical trials can be assumed to have non-AD pathology primarily based on the experience of the Consortium to Establish a Registry for Alzheimer's Disease *(43)*. The presence of such patients with non-AD dementias must increase the variance associated with the treatment effect. Even if non-AD patients are evenly distributed across treatment groups, and assuming that non-AD patients derive no benefit from a truly effective treatment, the effective sample size will have to be that much larger than if diagnostic certainty were higher. Thus, a diagnostic test that reduces the number of non-AD patients in clinical trial samples could increase the efficiency of clinical trials. The diagnostic method would have to be at least as sensitive as current methods, so as not to eliminate true AD patients, and it would have to be substantially more specific than current clinical criteria, so as to reduce the number of non-AD patients who enter trials.

A nearly uniform practice in current clinical trials is to employ a restricted range of scores on the MMSE *(16)* as an inclusion criteria. The upper limit is our concern here: patients with MMSE scores of >26 are excluded from trials. The rationale for excluding probable AD patients who score >26 on the MMSE is twofold. First, the criteria is intended to eliminate individuals whose cognitive impairment may be due to something other than dementia. Patients with low educational achievement and patients with lifelong, static cognitive deficits may score 26 or below. The other argument that is used to justify excluding mild patients is their slower rate of decline on cognitive tests compared to patients with lower baseline MMSE scores. Several studies have shown that rate of decline exhibits an inverted U-shaped function *(44,45)*, such that milder patients decline less than patients in the mid range of mental status. For efficiency in terms of sample size and trial duration, inclusion of mild patients poses a burden on the research program in terms of misdiagnosis and an increased likelihood of no decline among placebo-treated subjects.

The unfortunate effect of the exclusion of very mild AD patients from clinical trials is to reduce the demand for early diagnosis at the present time. If a diagnostic test were to become available that allowed patients with mild disease to be diagnosed with AD with higher certainty, the issue of raising the maximal entry score on the MMSE could be revisited. Unfortunately, the issue of slower rate of decline would remain and might be a reason for continuing to exclude such patients. The additional capability of identifying patients likely to experience rapid decline would be very useful here.

It is possible that an improved diagnostic method for AD would reduce the number of patients excluded from clinical trials due to the presence of other illnesses that are possibly contributory to the dementia. Among the common nonneurological illnesses that may coexist with AD are concurrent use of psychoactive medications, depression, vitamin B_{12} deficiency, and hypothyroidism. The two most common neurological diseases that overlap with AD are Parkinson's disease and vascular dementia. It is becoming increasingly clear that dementia due to pure Lewy body pathology *(46)* or pure vascular pathology *(47)* in the absence of AD pathology is quite rare. On the other hand, the extent to which both types pathological lesions coexist and amplify the dementia of AD is probably underestimated at present (46,48). Thus, if one of the nonneurological conditions, stroke or some element of Parkinsonism were present clinically in a demented patient, a positive diagnostic test for AD might allow that patient to be included in a trial. It is possible that patients with other disorders, if included in clinical trials, would increase treatment response heterogeneity. However, if AD is the dominant driving force of the dementia, then broadening access by using a diagnostic test for AD might not increase variance.

Clinical Trials for Early Alzheimer's Disease and At-Risk Individuals

Until recently, there have been no trials aimed at prevention of AD in previously nondemented individuals, or in patients at risk for AD. Formidable methodological problems stand in the way of a primary prevention trial. Diagnostic identification of at-risk individuals is a major component of the methodological challenge of successful development of drugs to prevent AD. There are two diagnostic issues: identifying at-risk individuals and diagnosing incident dementia in the course of the trial.

Without the use of a diagnostic method for identifying at-risk individuals, prevention trials must be large, long or both. The incidence rate of AD in the general population over age 65 is low enough (49–51) that studies of a minimum of 3 years duration that include several thousand individuals are required. The Women's Health Initiative Memory Study (40) has enrolled 8000 women and will take 7–10 years to complete, for example. Alternatively, there would be a cost to reduce the size of the study population, because the number of individuals screened to participate would have to be quite large. Still, the added costs of screening would likely be less than the costs of following a much larger cohort for twice as long, for example.

In a clinical trial of an agent intended to prevent AD among at risk individuals, there will be different demands on the diagnostic methods depending upon whether they are clinical or biological. The clinical method is to look for individuals with some evidence of cognitive impairment. For example, suppose that criteria were used in which older individuals who were at risk were identified by performance on a battery of psychometric testing (see Chapter 8) (52–56). It is critical when using such criteria to ensure that potential participants who were identified by the cognitive screen had normal function in daily living. The diagnostic challenge would be to exclude patients who were actually demented at the time of entry. Exclusion criteria would be required that used methods to identify functional impairment or deficits in areas other than memory. Ironically, it appears that improvements in the most traditional and conceptually simple of methods of the diagnosis of dementia, relating to decline in daily function from a previously higher level, is necessary to solve this problem. These challenges are being addressed in a recently initiated study of patients with mild cognitive impairment.

The alternative to clinical diagnostic methods would be to use some sort of biological marker many of which are discussed in this book. A biological test that identified at-risk patients (that turned positive with "presymptomatic" disease or was inherited) would be of value here only if it predicted that the clinical disease would begin within the time frame of the study. Practically speaking, for a biological marker to be useful in identifying at-risk individuals for clinical trials, the test would have to predict AD to appear clinically within 2 to 3 years. Alternatively, a biological marker could be coupled with a clinical marker of incipient dementia. As an example, Petersen and colleagues *(54)* found that ApoE genotyping was a strong predictor of incident AD among individuals who at entry into the study had isolated memory impairment.

Determining the outcome measure in a prevention trial presents different problems. There are two choices of outcome. One would be a clinical diagnosis of AD, with the attendant difficulties alluded to above. To make a diagnosis of incident dementia in a clinical trial with credibility, the research program would have to present unimpeachable evidence for the absence of dementia at baseline. The alternative approach that provides greater objectivity of baseline versus endpoint differences would be psychometric testing. Exceeding some relative or absolute difference between baseline and follow-up would serve as the endpoint. A psychometric endpoint has advantages in that reliability is much higher. On the other hand, minimizing a psychometric change would not be as convincing (to the interested parties: lay people, insurers, FDA) as prevention of dementia itself.

Effect of Diagnostic Certainty and Earliness of Diagnosis on the Use of anti-AD Drugs in Clinical Practice

In current clinical practice, it is well-known that patients with AD are not diagnosed until several years of symptoms have been present *(57,58)*. At present, the interplay between treatment options and diagnosis is poorly understood. There are few data on whether or not practicing physicians require a diagnosis of probable AD before using tacrine, for example. The uncertainty surrounding tacrine made it difficult to know if the extant nihilism about early diagnosis and treatment of AD among primary care physicians was due to tacrine's reputation or to negative perceptions about AD. As other therapies enter the market, will interest in diagnostic precision for AD increase, decrease or remain at the present low level? Once a treatment gains the popular perception that it is effective, there will be created a rather dramatic paradigm shift in how clinicians, family members and health plan administrators view dementing illness. With appropriate physician education on the benefits of early treatment and on improved methods of early diagnosis, one would hope physicians would be motivated to diagnose and treat AD more aggressively.

The reality is that major changes in clinical practice are slow in achieving widespread penetration. Diagnostic and treatment issues that those in the academic and research communities take for granted may sound like obscure jargon to primary physicians, simply because such issues have had little relevance in actual practice up to now. New methods of diagnosis will be helpful, but increasing skill levels for using current clinical criteria must also occur. For example, treatment of AD associated with other illnesses might be appropriate in the clinical practice setting, whereas it was not in the research setting. Physicians will have to understand the definition of dementia and how it differs from delirium and depression, above and beyond possessing an accurate laboratory marker for AD. Physicians also will have to understand the different stages of AD if they are going to understand the effects of treatment over time.

If an effective preventive agent against AD were discovered, there would be strong motivation to begin population screening for at-risk individuals. Efficient methods for population screening similar to those described above will need to be developed. This will be the only way to circumvent the problems of poor detection of AD in routine practice. As more patients come under managed care, and if managed care organizations begin to assume risks for long-term care, it could become cost-effective for health care delivery systems to attempt to prevent the onset of dementia and the subsequent need for long-term care. The cost-effectiveness will depend upon the balance between costs of screening, costs of treatment, and costs of long-term care. Looking into the future, the efficacy of treatments for AD will determine how aggressively health-care systems will mandate early diagnosis, in effect shifting the responsibility for diagnosis from patient and physician to the health system. Mandated early diagnosis of AD would raise many ethical questions, which are discussed in Chapter 12.

Benefits of Early Diagnosis for Nonpharmacological Treatments

Informal observation of practice patterns relating to AD at the present time suggests that nonpharmacological interventions in AD are not perceived as sufficiently valuable to justify early diagnosis. That reality is unfortunate because there are a number of nonpharmacological interventions that are important at an early stage of the symptomatic illness. Interventions in patients with incipient or very mild AD can enhance present safety and facilitate future planning. Employment decisions could be of critical importance in the case of patients who might still be working. Or, consider the case of driving. While there may be many instances in which patients with mild AD can still drive *(59)*, there probably are some patients who should not drive, and there are some instances where and when otherwise safe drivers should have a "copilot" *(60)*.

Financial planning could be an important issue, especially when there is a spouse involved or there are substantial assets. Patients who have responsibility for checking accounts, etc need to involve others to avoid financial missteps. Planning for future care should be an increasingly important aspect of geriatric management. Patients should be given choices about future care; being cognitively intact when making the decisions is an obvious necessity.

Prevention or reduction of the risk of delirium could be another important benefit of early diagnosis. Delirium is a complication of acute illness that occurs in a minimum of 10% to 20% of hospitalized elderly *(61,62)*. Patients with delirium have nearly double the length of stay compared to those who do not experience delirium *(62)*. Cognitive impairment that antedates the hospitalization is a recognized risk factor for the development of delirium *(61,62)*. It is likely that most of the preexisting cognitive impairment represented AD. Clinical trials that have attempted to reduce the incidence of delirium itself or the rate of complications of delirium have not so far been successful, but perhaps that is because recognition of prior cognitive impairment needs to begin at the hospital door, not 24 hours into an ICU stay *(63)*.

Cognitive impairment contributes to the risk of events such as falls in the elderly and medication misuse. Early recognition of cognitive impairment might also play a role in preventing misadventures with medications. Imagine the scenario of an elderly individual being instructed in the use of a new medication, to be taken several times per day, possibly with various restrictions on what to take it with. It seems highly likely that the medication will be incorrectly used, leading either to iatrogenic complications or to undertreatment of the underlying disease. There is no data on how often this might occur in undiagnosed AD, but it is hard to believe that such events don't occur.

Summary

Early diagnosis of AD coupled with effective early treatment may dramatically change the current approach to the disease. With some luck and the conviction that we can change our society's generally nihilistic view of geriatric illnesses, early diagnosis and treatment of AD can improve the quality of life for many elders in the years ahead.

References

1. Ohm TG, Muller H, Braak H Bohl J. Close-meshed prevalence rates of different stages as a tool to uncover the rate of Alzheimer's disease-related neurofibrillary changes. *Neuroscience* 1995;64:209–217.
2. Bondareff W, Mountjoy CQ, Roth M, et al. Age and histopathologic heterogeneity in Alzheimer's disease: evidence for subtypes. *Arch. Gen. Psychiat.* 1987;44:412–417.
3. Little A, Levy R, Chuaqui-Kidd P, Hand D. A double-blind, placebo controlled trial of higher-dose lecithin in Alzheimer's disease. *J. Neurol. Neurosurg. Psychiat.* 1985;48:736–742.
4. Thompson TL, Filley CM, Mitchell WD, et al. Lack of efficacy of hydergine in patients with Alzheimer's disease. *N. Engl. J. Med.* 1990;323:445–448.
5. Schneider LS, Olin JT. Overview of clinical trials of Hydergine in dementia. *Arch. Neurol.* 1994;51:787–798.
6. Farlow M, Gracon SI, Hershey LA, Lewis KW, Sadowsky CH, Dolan-Ureno J. A controlled trial of tacrine in Alzheimer's disease. *JAMA* 1992;268:2523–2529.
7. Knapp MJ, Knopman DS, Solomon PR, Pendlebury WW, Davis CS, Gracon SI. A 30-week randomized controlled trial of high-dose tacrine in patients with Alzheimer's disease. *JAMA* 1994;271:985–991.
8. Knopman D. Tacrine in Alzheimer's disease: a promising first step. *Neurologist* 1995;1:86–94.
9. Summers WK, Majovski LV, Marsh GM, Tachiki K, Kling A. Oral tetrahydroaminoacridine in long-term treatment of senile dementia, Alzheimer-type. *N. Engl. J. Med.* 1986;315:1241–1245.
10. Chatellier G, Lacomblez L et al. Tacrine and lecithin in senile dementia of the Alzheimer type: a multicentre trial. *BMJ* 1990;300:495–499
11. Davis K, Thal LJ, Gamzu ER, Davis CS, Woolson RF, Gracon SI et al. A double-blind, placebo-controlled multicenter study of tacrine for Alzheimer's disease. *N. Engl. J. Med.* 1992;327:1253–1259.
12. Gauthier S, Bouchard R, Lamontagne A, Bailey P, Bergman H, Ratner J, et al. Tetrahydroaminoacridine-lecithin combination treatment in patients with intermediate-stage Alzheimer's disease. *N. Engl. J. Med.* 1990;322:1272–1276.
13. Maltby N, Broe GA, Creasey H, Jorm AF, Christensen H, Brooks WS. Efficacy of tacrine and lecithin in mild to moderate Alzheimer's disease: double blind trial. *BMJ* 1994;308:879–883.
14. Wilcock GK, Surmon DJ, Scott M, Boyle M, Mulligan K, Neubauer KA, et al. An evaluation of the efficacy and safety of tetrahydroaminoacridine (THA) without lecithin in the treatment of Alzheimer's disease. *Age Aging* 1993;22:316–324.
15. Eagger SA, Levy R, Sahakian B. Tacrine in Alzheimer's disease. Lancet 1991;337:989–992.
16. Folstein MF, Folstein SE, McHugh PR. "Mini-mental state": a practical method for

grading the cognitive state of patients for the clinician. *J. Psychiat. Res.* 1975; 12:189–98.

17. Rosen WG, Mohs RC, Davis KL. A new rating scale for Alzheimer's disease. *Am. J. Psychiatry* 1984;141:1356–1364.

18. Knopman D, Schneider L, Davis K, et al. Long-term tacrine (Cognex) treatment: effects on nursing home placement and mortality. *Neurology* 1996;47:166–177.

19. Watkins PB, Zimmerman HJ, Knapp MJ, Gracon SI, Lewis KW. Hepatotoxic effects of tacrine administration in patients with Alzheimer's disease. *JAMA* 1994; 271:992–998.

20. Rossor MN, Iversen LL, Reynolds GP, Mountjoy CQ, Roth M. Neurochemical characteristics of early and late onset types of Alzheimer's disease. *BMJ* 1984;288:961–964.

21. Hyman BT, Kromer LJ, Van Hoesen GW. Reinnervation of the hippocampal perforant pathway zone in Alzheimer's disease. *Ann. Neurol.* 1987;21:259–267.

22. Farlow MR, Lahiri DK, Poirier J, Davignon J, Schneider L, Hui SL. Treatment outcome of tacrine therapy depends on apolipoprotein genotype and gender of the subjects with Alzheimer's disease. *Neurology* 1998;50:669–677.

23. Rogers SL, Friedhoff LT. The efficacy and safety of donepezil in patients with Alzheimer's disease: results of a US Multicentre, Randomized, Double-Blind, Placebo-Controlled Trial. The Donepezil Study Group. *Dementia* 1996;7:293–303.

23a. Rogers SL, Doody RS, Mohs RS, Mohs R, Friedhoff LT. Donepezil improves cognition and global function in Alzheimer disease: a 15-week, double-blind, placebo-controlled study. Donepezil Study Group. *Arch. Intern. Med.* 1998;158:1021–1031.

24. Rogers SL, Farlow MR, Doody RS, Mohs R, Friedhoff LT. A 24-week, double-blind, placebo-controlled trial of donepezil in patients with Alzheimer's disease. Donepezil Study Group. *Neurology* 1998; 50:136–145.

25. Thal LJ, Ferguson JM, Mintzer J, Raskin A, Targum SD. A 24-week randomized trial of controlled-release physostigmine in patients with Alzheimer's disease. *Neurology* 1999;52:1146–1152.

26. Rosler M, Anand R, Cicin-Sain A, Gauthier S, Agid Y, Dal-Bianco P, Stahelin HB, et al. Efficacy and safety of rivastigmine in patients with Alzheimer's disease: international randomised controlled trial. *BMJ* 1999;318:633–640.

27. Corey-Bloom J, Anand R, Veach J, for the ENA 713 B352 Study Group. A randomized trial evaluating the efficacy and safety of ENA 713 (rivastigmine tartrate), a new acetylcholinesterase inhibitor, in patients with mild to moderately severe Alzheimer's disease. *Int. J. Geriatric. Psychopharmacol.* 1998; 1:55–65.

28. Morris JC, Cyrus PA, Orazem J, Mas J, Bieber F, Ruzicka BB, Gulanski B. Metrifonate benefits cognitive, behavioral, and global function in patients with Alzheimer's disease. *Neurology* 1998;50:1222–1230.

29. Cummings JL, Cyrus PA, Bieber F, Mas J, Orazem J, Gulanski B. Metrifonate treatment of the cognitive deficits of Alzheimer's disease. Metrifonate Study Group. *Neurology* 1998;50:1214–1221.

30. Bodick N, Offen W, Levey AI, et al. Effects of xanomeline, a selective muscarinic receptor agonist, on cognitive function and behavioral symptoms in Alzheimer disease. *Arch. Neurol.* 1997;54:465–473.

31. Kumar R. on behalf of the SmithKline Beecham Alzheimer's Disease Study Group.

Efficacy and safety of SB202026 as a symptomatic treatment for Alzheimer's disease. [Abstract]. *Ann. Neurol.* 1996;40:504.

32. Sano M, Ernesto C, Thomas RG, et al. A controlled trial of selegiline, alpha-tocopherol, or both as treatment for Alzheimer's disease. *N. Engl. J. Med.* 1997;336:1216–1222.

33. Stewart WF, Kawas C, Corrada M, Metter EJ. Risk of Alzheimer's disease and duration of NSAID use. *Neurology* 1997;48:626–632.

34. Aisen PS, Davis KL. The search for disease-modifying treatment for Alzheimer's disease. *Neurology* 1997;48(Suppl 6):S35–S41.

35. Rogers J, Kirby LC, Hempelman SR, et al. Clinical trial of indomethacin in Alzheimer's disease. *Neurology* 1993;43:1609–1611.

36. Paganini-Hill A, Henderson VW. Estrogen deficiency and risk of Alzheimer's disease. *Am. J. Epidemoil.* 1994;140:256–261.

37. Tang MX, Jacobs D, Stern Y, et al. Effect of estrogen during menopause on risk and age at onset of Alzheimer's disease. *Lancet* 1996;348:429–432.

38. Kawas C, Resnick S, Morrison A, et al. A prospective study of estrogen replacement therapy and the risk of developing Alzheimer's disease. *Neurology* 1997;48:1517–1521.

38a. Waring SC, Rocca WA, Petersen RC, et al. Postmenopausal estrogen replacement therapy and risk of AD. *Neurology* 1999;52:965–970.

38b. Baldershi M, DiCarlo A, Lepore V, et al. Estrogen-replacement therapy and Alzheimer's disease in the Italian longitudinal study on aging. *Neurology* 1998;50:996–1002.

39. Asthana S, Craft S, Baker LD, et al. Transdermal estrogen improves memory in women with Alzheimer's disease. *Soc. Neurosci. Abstr.* 1996;22:200

39a. Ohkura T, Isse K, Akazawa K, et al. Evaluation of estrogen treatment in female patients with dementia of the Alzheimer type. *Endocrine J.* 1994;41:361–371.

39b. Simpkins JW, Singh M, Bishop J. The potential role for estrogen replacement therapy in the treatment of cognitive decline associated with Alzheimer's disease. *Neurobiology of Aging* (Suppl 2) 1994;15:S195–S197.

39c. Finch CE. Therapeutic targets for Alzheimer's disease: suggestions for the NIA. *Neurobiology of Aging* (Suppl 2) 1994;15:S183–S185.

40. Shumaker S, Rapp S. Hormone therapy in dementia prevention: the Women's Health Initiative memory study. *Neurobiol. Aging* 1996;17(Suppl 4s):S9.

41. Selkoe DJ. Translating cell biology into therapeutic advances in Alzheimer's disease. *Nature* 1999; 399 Supp A23–A31.

41a. Wolfe MS, Xia W, Ostaszewski BL, Diehl TS, Kimberly WT, Selkoe DJ. Two transmembrane aspartates in presenilin-1 required for presenilin endoproteolysis and γ-secretase activity. *Nature* 1999;398:513–517.

41b. Schenk D, Barbour R, Dunn W, et al. Immunization with amyloid-β attenuates Alzheimer-disease-like pathology in the PDAPP mouse. *Nature* 1999;400:173–177.

41c. St George-Hyslop PH, Westaway DA. Antibody clears senile plaques. Nature 1999;400:116–117.

42. McKhann G, Drachman D, Folstein M, Katzman R, Price D, Stadlan EM. Clinical diagnosis of Alzheimer's disease: report of the NINCDS-ADRDA work group

under the auspices of Department of Health and Human Services task force on Alzheimer's disease. *Neurology* 1984;34:939–944.

43. Gearing M, Mirra SS, Hedreen JC, Sumi SM, Hansen LA, Heyman A. The consortium to establish a registry for Alzheimer's disease (CERAD). *Neurology* 1995;45: 461–466

44. Morris JC, Edland S, Clark C, Galasko D, Koss E, Mohs R, et al. The consortium to establish a registry for Alzheimer's disease (CERAD). Part IV. Rates of cognitive change in the longitudinal assessment of probable Alzheimer's disease. *Neurology* 1993;43:2457–2465.

45. Stern RG, Mohs RC, Davidson M, et al. A longitudinal study of Alzheimer's disease: measurement, rate and predictors of cognitive deterioration. *Am. J. Psychiatry* 1994;151:390–396.

46. Hansen LA, Samuel W. Criteria for Alzheimer's disease and the nosology of dementia with Lewy bodies. *Neurology* 1997;48:126–132.

47. Hulutte C, Nochlin D, McKeel D, et al. Clinical-neuropathological findings in multi-infarct dementia: a report of six autopsied cases. *Neurology* 1997;48: 668–672.

48. Snowdon DA, Greiner LH, Mortimer JA, Riley KP, Greiner PA, Markesbery WR. Brain infarction and the clinical expression of Alzheimer Disease. *JAMA* 1997;277: 813–817.

49. Bachman DL, Wolf PA, Linn RT, et al. Incidence of dementia and probable Alzheimer's disease in a general population: the Framingham study. *Neurology* 1993;43:515–519.

50. Hebert LE, Scherr PA, Beckett LA, et al. Age-specific incidence of Alzheimer's disease in a community population. *JAMA* 1995;273:1354–1359.

51. Kokmen E, Chandra V, Schoenberg BS. Trends in incidence of dementing illness in Rochester, Minnesota in three quinquennial periods, 1960–1974. *Neurology* 1988; 38:975–980.

52. Katzman R, Aronson M, Fuld P, et al. Development of dementing illnesses in an 80-year-old volunteer cohort. *Ann. Neurol.* 1989;25:317–324.

53. Masur DM, Sliwinski M, Lipton RB, Blau AD, et al. Neuropsychological prediction of dementia and the absence of dementia in healthy elderly persons. *Neurology* 1994;44:1427–1432.

54. Petersen RC, Smith GE, Ivnik RJ, Tangalos KG, Schaid DJ, Thibodeau SN, et al. Apolipoprotein E status as a predictor of the development of Alzheimer's disease in memory-impaired individuals. *JAMA* 1995;273:1274–1278.

55. Tierney MC, Szalai JP, Snow WG, Fisher RH, Nores A, Nadon G, et al. Prediction of probable Alzheimer's disease in memory impaired patients: a prospective longitudinal study. *Neurology* 1996;46:661–665.

56. Jacobs DM, Sano M, Dooneief G, Marder K, Bell KL, Stern Y. Neuropsychological detection and characterization of preclinical Alzheimer's disease. *Neurology* 1995;45:957–962.

57. Callahan CM, Hendrie JC, Tierney WM. Documentation and evelution of cognitive impairment in elderly primary care patients. *Ann. Intern. Med.* 1995;422:429.

58. Ross GW, Abbott RD, Petrovitch H, et al. Frequency and characteristics of silent dementia among elderly Japanese-American men. *JAMA* 1997;277:800–805.

59. Drachman DA, Swearer JM, for the Collaborative Study Group. Driving and Alzheimer's disease: the risk of crashes. *Neurology* 1993;43:2448–2456.
60. Shua-Haim JR, Gross JS. The "co-pilot" driver syndrome. *J. Am. Geriatr. Soc.* 1996;44:815–817.
61. Francis J, Martin D, Kapoor WN. A prospective study of delirium in hospitalized elderly. *JAMA* 1990;263:1097–1101.
62. Schor JD, Levkoff SE, Lipsitz LA, et al. Risk factors for delirium in hospitalized elderly. *JAMA* 1992;267:827–831.
63. Cole MG, Primeau FJ, Bailey RF, et al. Systematic intervention for elderly inpatients with delirium: a randomized trial. *Can. Med. Assoc. J.* 1994;151:965–970.

12

An Ethical Context For Presymptomatic Testing in Alzheimer's Disease

Kenneth S. Kosik, Stephen G. Post, and Kimberly A. Quaid

Shall it be male or female? say the fingers
That chalk the walls with green girls and their men.
I would not fear the muscling-in of love
If I were tickled by the urchin hungers
Rehearsing heat upon a raw-edged nerve.
I would not fear the devil in the loin
Nor the outspoken grave.

—Dylan Thomas

Introduction

Myths—from Adam eating the forbidden fruit to Faust exchanging his soul to the Devil—teach us that profound knowledge can be a dangerous thing. The danger lies in knowing the future. Among the modern temptations toward a knowledge that may hold dangers as well as rewards is the genetic code. Although increasingly detailed probing of our own genomes seems inevitable, the appropriate uses of this information are much debated. The Faustian myth teaches us that a quest for knowledge, despite its price, is part of human nature. What is the price of knowing our genes?

If we learn that lying quietly within our genome is a mutation that will cause a disease when we reach our third, fourth, or fifth decade, then this knowledge can be the source of overriding despair. In a relatively small, but heuristically vital group of patients, Alzheimer's disease (AD) is caused by any of several mutations. Current estimates suggest that 1–3% of all cases of AD are caused by known genetic mutations. These scientific advances have forcefully put the issue of genetic testing before us. The ease with which genetic testing is done

From: *Early Diagnosis of Alzheimer's Disease*
Edited by L. F. M. Scinto & K. R. Daffner © Humana Press, Inc., Totowa, NJ

leads to pressure on patients from many directions, including the physician who is enthusiastic about the new technology, but has not considered the profound personal and psychosocial implications of genetic testing, particularly the potential consequences for education, employment, and insurance. Ideally, an individual should have the right to know his or her genetic profile without the burden this knowledge creates in the hands of others. In a recent editorial President Clinton stated: ". . . none of our discoveries should be used to label or discriminate against any group or individual. With stunning speed, scientists are now moving to unlock the secrets of our genetic code. Genetic testing has the potential to identify hidden inherited tendencies toward disease and to spur early treatment. But that information could also be used, for example, by insurance companies and others to discriminate and stigmatize people" *(1).*

Genetic Markers for the Presymptomatic Diagnosis of Alzheimer's Disease

There are three known genetic loci where mutations cause a fully penetrant form of AD most distinctly characterized by an early age of onset. These loci are the presenilin 1 (PS-1) gene on chromosome 14 *(2),* the presenilin 2 (PS-2) gene on chromosome 1 *(3),* and the amyloid precursor protein (APP) gene on chromosome 21 *(4).* Five mutations have been described in APP, which lead to AD and a sixth mutation (A692G) that can lead to AD or cerebral hemorrhages *(5).* At this time approximately 45 different mutations in PS-1 have been described, and all but one of these are missense mutations. The single exception is an in-frame deletion of exon 9 *(6).* Among the families that harbor mutations in PS-1 is the extended Colombian family, which represents the largest kindred in the world with familial AD *(7).* In PS-2, two different mutations have been described, one of which is found in another very large kindred known as the Volga Germans. All of these mutations cause an inherited form of AD that is clinically and pathologically indistinguishable from sporadic disease except for the early age of onset. Although specific cases vary greatly, the disease onset with APP and PS-2 is about a decade later than PS-1 mutations, which often have an onset in the 40s. However, even within families that carry the same mutation there may be more than a 20-year span in age at onset, and therefore it is not possible to predict when the individual carrying a mutation will develop the disease. All of these mutations are fully penetrant autosomal dominant, and therefore, if the individual lives long enough, the disease will inexorably develop. (There are exceedingly rare anecdotal reports of individuals with an Alzheimer-type mutation who escape the disease and therefore a more conservative estimation of disease occurrence with a mutation is probably higher than 99%, but less than 100%.)

The determination of genetic risk factors represents an entirely different genetic approach. In contrast to the fully penetrant mutations described above, having a genetic risk factor increases the odds of getting the disease. Among the many examples are mutations in the breast and ovarian cancer susceptibility genes *BRCA1* and *BRCA2*, or mutations in the *APC* gene that increase the likelihood of developing colon cancer. There are data suggesting that the presence of one or two apolipoprotein E (ApoE) ε4 alleles increase the risk of developing Alzheimer's disease (reviewed in refs. *8* and *9* and Chapter 5). Key to interpreting this information is knowing how much of an increased risk an ApoE ε4 allele confers. While many studies have attempted to calculate the increased risk, there remains a lack of consensus about the significance of ApoE, particularly in distinct ethnic groups. Certainly risk factor information has clear health implications for breast or colon cancer, diseases in which screening may detect early-stage tumors and be life-saving. In Alzheimer's disease, preventive strategies do not now exist. This unfortunate fact leaves ApoE risk testing with no clear discernible clinical use and great potential for misuse.

Like many genetic tests that assess risk, an ApoE4-positive test does not imply that the individual will get Alzheimer's disease and a test with negative results does not imply the individual will avoid the disease. In fact, ApoE status changes the likelihood of AD by a very small degree *(10.)* Other factors, such as gender or occurrence of the disease among relatives, also modestly influence the risk of AD. For example, the theoretical 90-year lifetime risk for AD among first-degree relatives (parents, siblings, and children) of rigorously diagnosed probands is about 50%, a figure that does not differ from the autosomal inheritance patterns observed in early-onset probands. However, competing mortality associated with late-onset disease results in the expression of Alzheimer symptoms within relatives' actual lifetimes in only about one-third the number of those who carry a theoretical risk. Therefore, the actual lifetime risk of Alzheimer-like illness is not 50%, but instead about 19% for first-degree relatives of probands, 10% for second-degree relatives, and 5% for population controls. At any given age, first-degree relatives of AD probands appear to have three to four times the risk of progressive dementia observed in population controls *(11)*.

For insurance companies whose livelihood is based on the accurate measurement of risk in populations, the ApoE test is potentially very useful despite its lack of sensitivity or specificity. The widespread use of ApoE testing and the difficulties in keeping medical information invisible to third-party payers only means that ApoE testing may further erode our protections in obtaining health insurance and will certainly affect actuarial calculations used to establish policy in long-term care and life insurance. Because there is still an incomplete understanding of exactly what the risks of a positive ApoE test are in different populations and because the distribution of the ApoE alleles differs significantly among various ethnic groups, the test is rife with the potential for misinterpretation and the drawing of false conclusions with serious repercussions.

In addition to ApoE several other polymorphisms have been to reported to confer an increased risk of AD. Although the data to support an enhanced risk has not been reproducibly substantiated for any of these genes, the likelihood that such genes exist is high. The wide age range of disease onsets among patients that carry an identical mutation and share a similar environment strongly suggests a genetic modifier effect. Although the ApoE genotype may influence age of onset among patients with APP mutations, the ApoE allele distribution in patients with PS-1 mutations does not correlate with age of onset. A second recently described modifier gene is the HLA-A2 allele *(12)*. Collectively, these findings indicate that genetic factors modulate age of onset.

Nongenetic Markers for Presymptomatic Diagnosis and Their Significance

One of the most promising types of nongenetic presymptomatic testing currently on the horizon for AD is brain imaging. Most of the more recent imaging studies utilize MRI scans to determine the volume of key brain regions known to be targeted by the disease process. Using MRI techniques, with their emphasis on anatomical detail, the regions that appear most affected in early dementia are the hippocampus and neighboring medial temporal structures *(13–21)*. Although few studies begin with an asymptomatic group, the reported results in a longitudinal study *(22)* suggest that elderly individuals destined to become demented have smaller hippocampi when first scanned and have a more rapidly progressive atrophy of the temporal lobe. Metabolic labeling techniques such as [^{18}F]fluorodeoxyglucose positron emission tomography have also shown some tentative success in presymptomatic diagnosis *(23–26)*. Mostly metabolic alterations in the temporal and parietal cortices have been described, although, more recently, hypoperfusion in the posterior cingulate cortex was also noted *(26,27)*. SPECT scans, a technique that usually uses [^{99m}Tc]HMPAO, provides similar metabolic information for a considerably lower cost than PET scans. Eventually, direct imaging of the amyloid burden in living individuals is likely to become the diagnostic modality of choice because there is a lengthy interval of more than a decade between the first appearance of plaques and the onset of symptoms. Other surrogate markers are also being explored, including mitochondrial abnormalities *(28),* pupillary dysfunction *(29),* and more powerful neuropsychological instruments, including controlled and standardized simulations of real life situations using virtual reality.

Entangled within the problem of a presymptomatic test is defining the point of disease onset. In the case of cancer diagnosis there are clear histological criteria for what constitutes a precancerous lesion. For AD, the clinical diagnosis is based on cognitive impairment, and the definitive diagnosis is based on the presence of senile plaques and neurofibrillary tangles in the brain *(30).* It is well-established that senile plaques, and probably neurofibrillary tangles, precede the onset of clinical AD by many years. We therefore are presented with a quandary: do we diagnose AD in an asymptomatic individual with plaques and tangles or do these lesions in the absence of dementia represent a presymptomatic marker? Caution is imperative in applying the Alzheimer label even in the presence of plaques and tangles because cognitively normal individuals with these lesions are known *(31).* While the possibility of having histological data on a non-demented individual may seem remote, it is possible. For example, an asymptomatic patient may have a meningioma removed, and AD changes are found at the tumor margin. More germane to the argument here is whether the presence of any brain changes might be construed as disease in an asymptomatic patient. An abnormal brain scan in an asymptomatic individual probably does affect some neuropsychological function even in those who test normal with current instruments.

Another more common setting in which the meaning of presymptomatic diagnosis may be ambiguous is in individuals who complain of a cognitive impairment, but who perform normally on neuropsychological tests. This problem usually affects those who perform in the superior range, perhaps because current neuropsychological instruments are insensitive to small decrements at the higher range of function. In these cases the individual is symptomatic, and, if the complaint is coupled with an abnormal brain scan suggestive of AD, some clinicians might be inclined to diagnose AD.

Distinguishing between a positive presymptomatic test and the diagnosis of AD carries important ethical implications because a positive result in either a genetic or nongenetic presymptomatic test is not tantamount to having the disease. In fact, "presymptomatic" by definition, means the tested individual whether with or without a mutation does not have the disease as defined by the presence of clinical dementia. The importance of this rule is that it leaves no basis for discrimination against a person based upon his or her genetic fate; on the other hand, individuals who carry a mutation are not entitled to special benefits or disability. AD begins when there is detectable cognitive impairment. Other presymptomatic tests, such as the findings detected using pupillary dilatation techniques, presumably represent the effects of the disease on body physiology that occur before dementia becomes apparent. For all such nongenetic tests it will be necessary to know the interval between the time when the test results turn positive and the first appearance of dementia. The detection of PS-1, PS-2, or APP point mutations in those rare cases of familial AD is possible in affected individuals, unaffected family members, and even the unborn fetus of a pregnant women. Thus, the detection of mutations represents the earliest form of presymptomatic diagnosis; other means to diagnose AD all rely on steps in the disease process that occur well after the formation of the zygote.

Who Gets Tested

By far the most salient reason that presymptomatic testing for AD poses such ethical problems is the absence of a treatment. If an effective treatment that carried little risk were available, presymptomatic screening would be used widely the way blood pressure measurements are for the detection of hypertension as a risk for heart disease and stroke. Family members of patients who harbor one of these mutations are all candidates for presymptomatic testing; however, a strong note of caution regarding the premature introduction of genetic testing for AD was struck in a recent consensus statement *(32)* and in an experience with early-onset familial AD in Sweden *(33)*. Presymptomatic genetic tests entail many additional considerations because of the implications, not only for the tested individual, but also for members of the family. Predictive genetic testing should not be undertaken without the expressed permission of the patient, the assurance of confidentiality, the protection of the information from access by anyone other than the patient, and the availability of counseling services both before and after the testing. An approach to genetic counseling with several pre- and post-test visits to the counselor has been defined for unaffected members in families with Huntington's disease *(34,35)* and has been modified for use in AD *(36)*.

Because the mutations that cause AD are rare and only account for about half of all early-onset inherited AD, screening of individuals who lack a family history is not indicated. Another type of pitfall applies to families in which AD is inherited, but the affected members have not been tested. If a member of such a family requests testing for the known mutations and the result is negative, the patient still has a significant chance of getting AD. The counselor must not convey false assurances in this setting. Once the counseling support services are in place, the use of genetic testing in symptomatic individuals is a more accepted practice. However, in this circumstance the tested individual must understand that the results imply genetic information about family members who may not care to know their genetic status.

Although in those 1–3% of families that carry an AD mutation, it is possible to predict whether one will get the disease, the age of onset cannot be predicted. Often people say they want genetic testing for planning purposes, but because onset can vary more 20 years, even among individuals who carry the same mutation, planning may be difficult. Some of the youngest ages of onset occur in PS-1 mutations that range from 29 to 62 years, a span that is skewed somewhat earlier than patients with APP mutations, which range from 37 to 65 years *(37)*. The greatest range of onsets is seen in the Volga German families with a mutation in the PS-2 gene and range of onsets from 40 to 82 years. On the other hand, there are some small families and even unrelated kindreds who share a common mutation, such as the His163Arg mutation found in American, Canadian, French, and Japanese families, all of whom have similar ages of onset. Some studies suggest that the ApoE allele may modify the age of onset in patients with APP mutations *(38,39)*, but not with PS-1 mutations *(40–42)*.

An important guideline is that children should not be tested. By 8 to 10 years of age, children in families that harbor a mutation may be acutely aware of their risk. Nevertheless, there are numerous reasons why testing should not be done. Among the reasons are that the child could be stigmatized by the parents and others, and the knowledge represents a burden no child should bear. Further, our views evolve greatly throughout life, and therefore the child's wishes with regard to testing may differ greatly upon reaching maturity.

Prenatal testing for AD raises a number of serious ethical issues. When screening in utero for childhood diseases, there is often agreement that the burden of a genetic disease present at birth is unacceptable. In such cases the parents assume the well-accepted role of making a decision for an unborn child. More problematic is the burden of a genetic disease that begins in adulthood. Can the parents responsibly make a decision for a future adult? A first approximation toward the solution of many ethical dilemmas is introspection—to imagine ourselves in such a situation and examine our own feelings concerning the various options. But the decision may remain difficult, and this issue has been specifically treated by Post and coworkers *(43)*. The guideline against testing children implies that prenatal testing be done only if the parents agree to abort the fetus if the test results are positive. Furthermore, the detection in the fetus of a dominant AD mutation (PS-1, PS-2, APP), implies that either the mother or father also carries the gene and will get the disease. Therefore, testing of the at-risk parent should be done first, and counseling must be available.

Disclosure

Once the evaluation is complete for any individual, whether symptomatic or presymptomatic, there is an obligation on the part of the physician to inform the affected individual of the results. Usually the rationale for withholding the diagnosis is presented as in the patient's interest because the news would be devastating. On the other hand, the right to know is a matter of human dignity. Informing the person enables him or her to

1. plan for optimal life experiences in the remaining years of intact capacities.
2. prepare a durable power of attorney for health-care decisions to be implemented upon eventual incompetence.
3. consider possible enrollment in AD research programs based on comprehended choices and decide about taking new antidementia compounds.
4. participate actively in support groups.

A final and most difficult solution that must cross the mind of everyone faced with the diagnosis of AD is the issue of suicide, either assisted or unassisted. Clearly the desirability of suicide will increase if we cannot offer assurance to these individuals that their rights and decisions concerning their own health care will be respected *(44)*.

Confidentiality

Repeatedly stressed in all considerations regarding patient genetic information is confidentiality. There is widespread, but not universal, agreement around this fundamental necessity. The most vocal opponents to strict patient confidentiality are the insurance industry representatives who have said publicly that they would classify the positive results of a gene test as a preexisting condition. They maintain that limits on their access to genetic information is an assault upon fundamental underwriting practices *(45)*. Despite widespread objections to this view from many sectors of the public and the medical community, the legal protections that would truly prevent genetic information from going beyond the patient record are not in place. Discriminatory practices based on genetic makeup are a real and urgent issue.

While assurances of confidentiality may seem like a desirable goal, even in this area with so much unanimity of thinking, there are circumstances that cloud the issue. For example, is confidentiality required from family members? Because the significance of this information goes beyond the individual, there might be differences of opinion among siblings or between parents and grown children regarding whether to obtain a predictive test? Might a spouse, when considering to have children, need to know the genetic status of the partner? Might a fiancé(e), when considering marriage, need to know the genetic status of the intended? Should investors know the genetic status of the individual they select as a CEO? Should Congress know the genetic status of Supreme Court appointees? Should the public know the genetic status of presidential candidates? Among these provocative questions, issues of genetic knowledge within the family may be the most pressing. Part of the burden of knowing one's genetic status is the perceived obligation to inform others who may be directly affected by the eventual expression of the disease. When another individual learns about the mutation, then even the "best kept secrets" can spread and ultimately result in stigmatization. Labeling members of a family as genetic misfits is particularly damaging in small communities where there is little anonymity.

Forecasting a disease in an asymptomatic individual may evoke desperate responses when there is little or no hope of treatment. On the other hand, this knowledge becomes crucially important, but less dangerous and less explosive when a treatment is available. For AD we believe the next decade represents a window of time when genetic information will be increasingly available, but treatments will remain only minimally effective. For this reason, the issue of genetic testing for AD should be approached cautiously and with appropriate concern for the impact of testing on patients and their families.

References

1. Clinton W. Science in the 21st century. *Science* 1997;276:1951.
2. Sherrington R, Rogaev EI, Liang Y, Rogaeva EA, et al. Cloning of a novel gene bearing missense mutations in early onset familial Alzheimer disease. *Nature* 1995;375:754–760.
3. Levy-Lahad E, Wasco W, Poorkaj P, Romano DM, et al. Candidate gene for the chromosome 1 familial Alzheimer's disease locus. *Science* 1995;269:973–977.
4. Goate A, Chartier-Harlin M-C, Mullan M, Brown J, et al. Segregation of a missense mutation in the amyloid precursor protein gene with familial Alzheimer's disease. *Nature* 1991;349:704–706.
5. Hardy J. New insights into the genetics of Alzheimer's disease. *Ann. Med.* 1996; 28:255–258.
6. Prihar G, Fuldner RA, Perez-Tur J, Lincoln S, et al. Structure and alternative splicing of the presenilin-2 gene. *NeuroReport* 1996;7:1680–1684.
7. Lopera F, Ardilla A, Martinez A, Madrigal L, et al. Clinical features of early-onset Alzheimer disease in a large kindred with an E280A presenilin-1 mutation. *JAMA* 1997;277:793–799.
8. Corder EH, Saunders AM, Risch NJ, Strittmatter WJ, et al. Protective effect of apolipoprotein E type 2 allele for late onset Alzheimer's disease. *Nature Genet.* 1994;7:180–184.
9. Roses AD. Apolipoprotein E alleles as risk factors in Alzheimer's disease. *Ann. Rev. Med.* 1996;47:387–400.

10. Kosik KS, Gifford DR, Greenberg SM, Morris JC, et al. Dementia Care in *Continuum. Am. Acad. Neurol.* 1996.
11. Breitner JCS. Clinical genetics and counseling in Alzheimer's disease. *Ann. Intern. Med.* 1991;115:601–606.
12. Payami H, Schellenberg GD, Zareparsi S, Kaye J, et al. Evidence for association of HLA-A2 allele with onset age of Alzheimer's disease. *Neurology* 1997;49:512–518.
13. Seab JP, Jagust WJ, Wong ST, Roos MS, et al. Quantitative NMR measurement of hippocampal atrophy in Alzheimer's disease. *Magn. Reson. Med.* 1988;8:200–208.
14. Kesslak JP, Nalcioglu O, Cotman C. Quantification of magnetic resonance scans for hippocampal and parahippocampal atrophy in Alzheimer's disease. *Neurology* 1991;41:51–54.
15. Jack C, Petersen RC, O'Brien P, Tangalos E. MR-based hippocampal volumetry in the diagnosis of Alzheimer's disease. *Neurology* 1992;42:183–188.
16. Pearlson GD, Harris GJ, Powers RE, Barta PE, et al. Quantitative changes in mesial temporal volume regional cerebral blood flow, and cognition in Alzheimer's disease. *Arch. Gen. Psychiatry* 1992;49:402–408.
17. Killiany RJ, Moss MB, Albert MS, Tamas S. Temporal lobe regions on magnetic resonance imaging identify patients with early Alzheimer's disease. *Arch. Neurol.* 1993;50:949–954.
18. Lehericy S, Baulac M, Chiras J, Pierot L, et al. Amydgalohippocampal MR volume measurements in the early states of Alzheimer disease. *AJNR* 1994;15:929–937.
19. Laakso M, Partanen K, Riekkinen P, Lehtovirta M, et al. Hippocampal volumes in Alzheimer's disease, Parkinson's disease with and without dementia, and in vascular dementia: an MRI study. *Neurology* 1996;46:678–681.
20. Rusinek H, deLeon MJ, George AE, Stylopoulos LA, et al. Alzheimer disease: measuring loss of cerebral gray matter with MR imaging. *Radiology* 1991;178:109–114.
21. Murphy DG, DeCarli CD, Daly E, Gillette JA, et al. Volumetric magnetic resonance imaging in men with dementia of the Alzheimer type: correlations with disease severity. *Biol. Psychiatry* 1993;34:612–621.
22. Kaye JA, Swihart T, Howieson D, Dame A, et al. Volume loss of the hippocampus and temporal lobe in healthy elderly persons destined to develop dementia. *Neurology* 1997;48:1297–1304.
23. Haxby JV, Grady CL, Duara R, Schageter N, et al. Neocortical metabolic abnormalities precede nonmemory cognitive defects in early Alzheimer's-type dementia. *Arch. Neurol.* 1986;43:882–885.
24. Kennedy AM, Frackowiak RS, Newman S, Bloomfield PM, et al. Deficits in cerebral glucose metabolism demonstrated by positron emission tomography in individuals at risk of familial Alzheimer's disease. *Neurosci. Lett.* 1995;186:17–20.
25. Small GW, Mazziotta JC, Collins MT, Baxter LR, et al. Apolipoprotein E type 4 allele and cereberal glucose metabolism in relatives at risk for familial Alzheimer's disease. *JAMA* 1995;273:942–947.
26. Reiman EM, Caselli RJ, Yun LS, Chen K, et al. Preclinical evidence of Alzheimer's disease in persons homozygous for the epsilon 4 allele for apolipoprotein E. *N. Engl. J. Med.* 1996;334:752–758.
27. Minoshima S, Giordani B, Berent S, Frey KA, et al. Metabolic reduction in the posterior cingulate cortex in very early Alzheimer's disease. *Ann. Neurol.* 1997;42:85–94.

28. Davis RE, Miller S, Herrnstadt C, Ghosh SS, et al. Mutations in mitochondrial cytochrome c oxidase genes segregate with late-onset Alzheimer disease. *Proc. Natl. Acad. Sci. U.S.A.* 1997;94:4526–4531.

29. Scinto LFM, R DK, Dressler D, Ransil BJ, et al. A potential noninvasive neurobiological test for Alzheimer's disease. *Science* 1994;266:1051–1054.

30. Hyman BT, Trojanowski JQ. Editorial on consensus recommendations for the postmortem diagnosis of Alzheimer disease from the National Institute on Aging and the Reagan Institute Working Group on Diagnostic Criteria for the neuropathological assessment of Alzheimer's disease. *J. Neuropathol. Exp. Neurol.* 1997;56:1095–1097.

31. Snowdon DA. Aging and Alzheimer's disease: lessons from the Nun study. *Gerontologist* 1997;37:150–156.

32. Post SG, Whitehouse PJ, Binstock RH, Bird TD, et al. The clinical introduction of genetic testing for Alzheimer's disease: an ethical perspective. *JAMA* 1997;277: 832–836.

33. Lannfelt L, Axelman K, Lilius L, Basun H. Genetic counseling in a Swedish Alzheimer family with amyloid precursor protein mutation. *Am. J. Hum. Genet.* 1995;56:332–335.

34. Quaid KA. Presymptomatic testing for Huntington's disease: recommendations for counseling. *J. Genet. Counsel.* 1992;1:277–302.

35. Went L. Guidelines for the molecular genetics predictive test in Huntington's disease. *Neurology* 1994;44:1533–1536.

36. Lennox A, Karlinsky H, Meschino W, Buchanan JA, et al. Molecular genetic predictive testing for Alzheimer's disease: deliberations and preliminary recommendations. *Alz. Dis. Assoc. Disord.* 1994;8:126–147.

37. Farrer LA, Cupples LA, Kukull WA, Volicer L, et al. Risk of Alzheimer disease is associated with parental age among apolipoprotein E ε4 heterozygotes. *Alz. Res.*

38. St. George-Hyslop P, McLachlan P, Tsuda DC, Rogaev T. Alzheimer's disease and possible gene interaction. *Science* 1994;263:537.

39. Sorbi S, Nacmias B, Forleo P, Piacentini S, et al. Epistatic effect of APP717 mutation and apolipoprotein E genotype in familial Alzheimer's disease. *Ann. Neurol.* 1995;38:124–127.

40. Lendon CL, Martinez A, Behrens IM, Kosik KS, et al. The E280A PS-1 mutation causes Alzheimer's, but age of disease onset is not determined by ApoE alleles. *Hum. Mutat.* 1997;10:186–195.

41. Van Broeckhoven C, Backhovens H, Crust M, Martin JJ, et al. APOE genotype does not modulate age of onset in families with chromosome 14 encoded Alzheimer's disease. *Neurosci. Lett.* 1994;169:179–180.

42. Levy-Lahad E, Lahad A, Wijsman E, Bird TD, Schellenberg GD. Apolipoprotein E genotypes and age at onset in early-onset familial Alzheimer's disease. *Ann. Neurol.* 1995;38:678–680.

43. Post SG, Botkin JR, Whitehouse P. Selective abortion for familial Alzheimer's disease? *Obstet. Gynecol.* 1992;79:794–798.

44. Post SG. Physician-assisted suicide in Alzheimer's disease. *J. Am. Geriatr. Soc.* 1997;45:647–651.

45. Pokorski RJ. Insurance underwriting in the genetic era. *Am. J. Hum. Genet.* 1997;60: 205–216.

APPENDIX

Consensus Report of the Working Group on: "Molecular and Biochemical Markers of Alzheimer's Disease"

THE RONALD AND NANCY REAGAN RESEARCH INSTITUTE OF THE ALZHEIMER'S ASSOCIATION AND THE NATIONAL INSTITUTE ON AGING WORKING GROUP[1,2,3,4]

The Ronald and Nancy Reagan Research Institute of the Alzheimer's Association, Chicago, IL and the National Institute on Aging, Bethesda, MD

The ideal biomarker for Alzheimer's disease (AD) should detect a fundamental feature of neuropathology and be validated in neuropathologically-confirmed cases; it should have a sensitivity >80% for detecting AD and a specificity of >80% for distinguishing other dementias; it should be reliable, reproducible, non-invasive, simple to perform, and inexpensive. Recommended steps to establish a biomarker include confirmation by at least two independent studies conducted by qualified investigators with the results published in peer-reviewed journals. Our review of current candidate markers indicates that for suspected early-onset familial AD, it is appropriate to search for mutations in the presenilin 1, presenilin 2, and amyloid precursor protein genes. Individuals with these mutations typically have increased levels of the amyloid $A\beta_{42}$ peptide in plasma and decreased levels of APPs in cerebrospinal fluid. In late-onset and sporadic AD, these measures are not useful, but detecting an apolipoprotein E e4 allele can add confidence to the clinical diagnosis. Among the other proposed molecular and biochemical markers for sporadic AD, cerebrospinal fluid assays showing low levels of $A\beta_{42}$ and high levels of tau come closest to fulfilling criteria for a useful biomarker. © 1998 Elsevier Science Inc.

---

[1]The names of the Working Group Members and the names of the Working Group Advisory Committee Members are listed in the Appendix (section VI).

[2]Address correspondence to: John H. Growdon, Chair of the Working Group Advisory Committee, WACC 830, Massachusetts General Hospital, Boston, MA 02114.

[3]The Reagan Institute Working Groups are planned and organized by Z.S. Khachaturian and T.S. Radebaugh; Fax: 301-879-2023; E-mail: zaven@idt.net.

[4]Reprinted from *Neurobiology of Aging,* Vol 19, 1998, pp. 109-116, with permission from Elsevier Science.

The Working Group on Molecular and Biochemical Markers of Alzheimer's Disease was convened to examine the relative merits of biological markers proposed for the early diagnosis of Alzheimer's disease (AD). At present, diagnosing AD and distinguishing it from other dementias depend primarily on clinical evaluation, and ultimately on clinical judgment. Based on this approach, a great deal has been learned about the genetics, age of onset, duration, clinical course, neurological and psychiatric manifestations, response to treatment, and neuropathological lesions of AD. Having molecular and biochemical markers of AD would complement clinical approaches, and further the goals of early and accurate diagnosis. Building on recent information concerning the genetic factors and molecular causes of AD, the Working Group sought to assess the status of various antemortem markers. The Working Group had three goals:

1. define the characteristics of ideal biological markers;
2. outline the process whereby a biological marker gains acceptance in the medical and scientific communities; and
3. review the current status of all proposed biomarkers for AD.

Early in 1997, on the basis of a comprehensive literature search, a general call for papers was sent to all investigators who had published in the field, inviting them to submit a brief position paper on the current state of knowledge concerning antemortem diagnosis of AD. These papers were to address the clinical and scientific issues that need to be resolved in order to improve the accuracy, sensitivity, reliability, and validity of biochemical and molecular diagnostic measures. Fifty-five invitations were sent and thirty position papers were submitted. The titles, authors, and their affiliations are noted in Appendix I. Their contributions reflect the diverse perspectives among the international community of investigators engaged in research on the diagnosis of AD. In September 1997, the Advisory Committee of the Working Group (the Appendix lists the committee members) met to review these papers and develop the accompanying consensus statement on Molecular and Biochemical Markers of Alzheimer's Disease. Some of the position papers, selected by the Advisory Committee, are published along with the consensus statement.

The Ronald and Nancy Reagan Research Institute of the Alzheimer's Association and the National Institute on Aging, the sponsors of this Working Group, have begun to convene a series of working groups focused on important topics in dementing disorders such as AD. The mission of each working group is to develop a position paper and, if possible, a consensus statement to help:

1. identify scientific opportunities or new research directions;
2. determine the need for additional research resources;
3. evaluate barriers that impede the progress of research; and
4. guide public policy on research.

The first Working Group, on Neuropathological Criteria, completed its task in 1997 and published a consensus paper that established new pathological guidelines for the diagnosis of AD (Neurobiol.Aging 4S: 1997). The deliberations and conclusions of the second Working Group, on Molecular and Biochemical Markers, are published here.

Criteria For Defining, Developing, and Assessing Biomarkers

All future publications describing any putative diagnostic marker or its use in a study should include detailed information on target populations, uses, and accuracy of the marker. Target population refers to the distinction between early-onset familial AD (FAD) and sporadic disease and emphasizes the fact that markers that are useful in FAD may not all be useful in sporadic disease. A biomarker has at least five different uses: confirming diagnosis, epidemiological screening, predictive testing, monitoring progression and response to treatment, and studying brain-behavior relationships. The value of a marker will vary across these uses. For example, a biomarker may be well-suited as an aid to clinical diagnosis but have little value in monitoring changes over time in dementia.

Proposed markers for AD should include as many features of an ideal diagnostic test as possible (see Kennard; Klunk). Ideally, the marker should be:

1. able to detect a fundamental feature of Alzheimer's neuropathology;
2. validated in neuropathologically confirmed AD cases;
3. precise (able to detect AD early in its course and distinguish it from other dementias);
4. reliable;
5. non-invasive;
6. simple to perform; and
7. inexpensive.

Among the many proposed molecular and biochemical markers (see below), none has yet achieved universal acceptance, nor fully met the proposed criteria for an ideal biomarker. Nonetheless, there has been sufficient progress toward this goal so that this review and consensus statement are warranted.

Molecular and biochemical markers should be validated in neuropathologically confirmed (definite) AD cases whenever possible. Because most biomarkers will be tested and later used for diagnosing patients who are still living, it will not be possible to have a diagnosis of Definite AD for judging most biomarkers (molecular genetic tests are an exception to this generalization). It is therefore recommended that testing of biomarkers be carried out on patients with the diagnosis of Probable AD, and not in people with Possible AD, to ensure that diagnostic accuracy is as high as possible (see Litvan).

Characteristics of a Useful Biomarker

The setting in which a biomarker will be used should be carefully defined. The utility of various biomarkers will vary depending upon the purpose for which they are used. For example, biomarkers useful for establishing prevalence in epidemiological studies may be less useful in monitoring individual patients over time to evaluate the efficacy of a particular medication. Hence, different criteria for usefulness may be needed for different applications of a biomarker.

Criteria for Evaluating Biomarkers

Molecular and biochemical markers for AD require evaluation based upon their sensitivity, specificity, prior probability, positive predictive value, and negative predictive value (see Mayeu; Robles). Sensitivity refers to the capacity of a biomarker to identify a substantial percentage of patients with the disease. A sensitivity of 100% would indicate a marker that can identify 100% of patients with AD. The mathematical expression of sensitivity is true positive cases of AD divided by true positive cases plus false negative cases. Because the currently used clinical criteria for AD in patients with Probable AD provide a sensitivity of approximately 85% when compared to autopsy-confirmed cases, an excellent biomarker should have a sensitivity approaching or exceeding this value. The biomarker would then be applied to patients with Possible AD, or possibly in testing asymptomatic subjects who may have preclinical disease.

Specificity refers to the capacity of a test to distinguish AD from normal aging, other causes of cognitive disorders, and other dementias. A test with 100% specificity would be capable of differentiating AD from other causes of dementia in every case. Mathematically, specificity represents the true negative instances of AD divided by the true negative cases plus the false positive cases. For a biomarker to have sufficient specificity to be useful in the diagnosis of AD, it should have a specificity of approximately 75–85% or greater.

Prior probability is defined as the frequency of occurrence of a disease in a particular group. If the group under study includes a large number of affected individuals, prior probability is equivalent to prevalence. The mathematical representation of prior probability is the true positives plus the false negatives divided by the total population. A perfect biomarker would detect only true positives and no false negatives and thus would reflect accurately the prevalence of the disease in the population.

Positive predictive value is a measure of the percentage of people who have a positive test who can be shown at subsequent autopsy examination to have the disease. The mathematical representation of positive predictive value is the number of true positives divided by the number of true positives plus the number of false negatives. A positive predictive value of 100% would indicate that all patients with a positive test actually have the disease. For a biomarker to be useful clinically, it should have a positive predictive value of approximately 80% or more.

Negative predictive value represents the percentage of people with a negative test who subsequently at autopsy prove not to have the disease. Mathematically it is represented as the number of true negatives divided by the number of true negatives plus the number of false negatives. A negative predictive value of 100% indicates that the test completely rules out the possibility that the individual has the disease, at least at the time that the individual is tested. A reliable marker with a high negative predictive value would be extremely useful. A test with low negative predictive value might still be useful in some circumstances if it also had a high positive predictive value.

Control Groups

Any diagnostic test must be validated against a control group with a distribution of ages and genders similar to the patient group (see Foster). This requirement presents difficulties because sporadic AD (SAD) principally affects older individuals. Consequently, irrespective of how carefully the control group is screened for cognitive status, some of the group may have preclinical AD. This essentially precludes the possibility that any biomarker would have 100% sensitivity and 100% specificity.

Context

The value of biomarkers will vary depending upon the reason for testing a particular person, group, or population. In a community screening for descriptive epidemiological studies, for example, high sensitivity is important in a biomarker because all patients who truly have the disease should be identified. In this instance, specificity may be low, and the test may still be useful. When applied to a single patient, both specificity and sensitivity of a biomarker become very important. Many physicians and their patients will wish to know whether a positive test with a biological marker indicates that the patient has a high probability of having AD (i.e., a high positive predictive value).

Plausibility

Some diagnostic tests have proven to have high positive predictive value, yet the scientific reason for this was unclear initially. The finding of an association between apolipoprotein E4 and sporadic late-onset AD is a good example of this. Nevertheless, it is useful to seek biomarkers with some plausible connection to the known neuropathological changes in AD.

Qualities of an Biomarker

A useful biomarker should be precise, reliable and inexpensive. It should be convenient to use and not threatening to the patient. The biomarker should be noninvasive or only moderately invasive. Noninvasive tests include studies on blood, urine, saliva, or buccal scrapings. Moderately invasive tests are those that utilize skin or rectal biopsies, bone marrow samples, or cerebrospinal fluid (CSF). Highly invasive tests include those that require sampling of brain tissue. A useful biomarker should be sufficiently simple to be adaptable for routine use in screening the elderly. An ideal biomarker would also be useful in monitoring the progression of the disease and evaluating the effects of treatment on disease progression. Use of biomarkers for evaluation of treatment has two aspects. One is to determine whether the treatment induces a measurable biochemical change. For example, a biomarker may consist of an assay to determine whether an enzyme inhibitor is causing a change in enzymatic activity. The second use is to determine whether treatment changes the progression of the illness, using the biomarker as an index of disease status.

Normalization

Some markers may need to be adjusted or normalized for other variables. Examples of adjustments include the age, gender, and possibly the race of an individual patient. Another adjustment might be the anatomic site from which a patient's sample is taken. For example, a CSF sample removed from the cervical region may show different biomarker levels than CSF taken from the lumbosacral region.

Initial Evaluation of Biomarkers

The initial evaluation of a new biomarker should focus on the distinction between patients with Probable AD and normal control subjects with comparable age distributions. Sample size is important and a power analysis should be performed to determine the size of the sample needed. If covariants, such as age, gender, apolipoprotein genotype, will be included in the analysis, a large series of observations will be needed. Geography may also be important, given likely genetic polymorphisms in different countries and races. The biomarker should be examined in more than one group before generalized to all Alzheimer's patients.

Range of the Marker

It is critical to establish a normal range of values for a biomarker (see Galasko). An ideal effective biomarker will show a clear separation between normal control subjects and patients with AD.

Utility of Multiple Markers

A combination of biomarkers may provide greater diagnostic accuracy than any single one individually. Critical evaluation of multiple simultaneous biomarkers should utilize the same principles outlined above, including sensitivity, specificity, prior probability, positive predictive value, and negative predictive value. Of these, high sensitivity and specificity are most important as they indicate the accuracy of the test.

Follow-up Evaluation of Biomarkers

Proposed biomarkers should be tested in patients with Probable AD to ensure as high a diagnostic accuracy as possible. Ultimately, successful biomarkers will be applied to preclinical subjects at risk for the disease and to people with Possible AD. It is vital to follow the patients with Probable AD initially studied with the biomarker through the full course of their disease and obtain autopsy verification of the disease in as many subjects as possible. This process is the optimal means of testing any biomarker against the most credible and accepted diagnostic standard.

Recommended Steps in the Process of Establishing a Biomarker

1. There should be at least two independent studies that specify the biomarker's sensitivity, specificity, and positive and negative predictive values.
2. Sensitivity and specificity should be no less than 80%; positive predictive value should approach 90%.
3. The studies should be well powered, conducted by investigators with expertise to conduct such studies, and the results published in peer-reviewed journals.

4. The studies should specify type of control subjects, including normal subjects and those with a dementing illness but not AD.
5. Once a marker is accepted, follow-up data should be collected and disseminated to monitor its accuracy and diagnostic value.

Review of Some Putative Molecular and Biochemical Markers

Molecular Genetics

Early-onset autosomal-dominant AD is relatively rare; only 120 families worldwide are currently known that carry deterministic mutations (see St. George-Hyslop). Mutations in the presenilin 1 (PS1) gene on chromosome 14 are the most common causes of autosomal-dominant FAD; these account for 30–50% of all early-onset cases and are the primary causes of FAD with onset before the age of 55 years. Mutations in the amyloid precursor protein (APP) gene on chromosome 21 are very rare, affecting fewer than 25 families worldwide. Like PS1 mutations, APP mutations are found in pedigrees with autosomal-dominant transmission of AD with an age of onset before 65 years. Mutations in the presenilin 2 (PS2) gene have been described in only two pedigrees. Compared to the PS1 and APP mutations, families carrying the PS-2 mutation exhibit a more variable age of onset, ranging between 40 and 80 years, and a suggestion of incomplete penetrance. Mutational analyses of the PS1, PS2, and APP genes as an adjunct to diagnosing dementia in patients with an early age of onset and strong family history is appropriate. Finding a mutation in the PS1 or APP gene has a high predictive value (presumed to be 100%) for the eventual development of AD. Because the age of onset in PS1 and APP families does not vary much within each family, accurate predictions of risk and approximate age of onset can be made. Pre-test and post-test genetic counseling, education, and support should be offered in all cases of molecular genetic screening. A number of pedigrees with the PS1 or the APP mutations have atypical disease phenotypes with cases that include cerebral hemorrhage, spongiform encephalopathy, familial spastic paraparesis and Pick-like inclusions. These observations reinforce the point made in the accompanying paper by St. George-Hyslop that genetic screening for mutations should be limited to early-onset pedigrees where the phenotype aside from age, is typical for a progressive degenerative dementia.

In contrast to deterministic genetic mutations, there are genetic factors that modify the risk of develophig AD. Several of the proposed factors, such as α-antichymotrypsin and HLA A2, are controversial or exert weak effects. Among the proposed genetic modifiers, alleles of apolipoprotein E (APOE) are the most powerful and best documented (2). There is universal agreement that the e4 allele is a strong risk factor for the late-onset and sporadic forms of AD whereas the e2 allele appears to protect against AD or at least delay its onset. Having an e4 allele does not confer AD as many e4 individuals reach old age without developing dementia (see Hyman). Conversely, the absence of an e4 allele does not exclude AD, as many AD patients do not carry an e4 allele. Nevertheless, in autopsy series more than half of the patients with a confirmed diagnosis of AD had an e4 allele. Testing for APOE is appropriate as an adjunct to the suspected clinical diagnosis of AD, where finding an e4 allele has a positive predictive value between 94% and 98% (1,4). The sensitivity and the specificity of the e4 allele alone are low, indicating that this measure cannot be used as the sole diagnostic test for AD. However when used in sequence with conventional clinical assessments early in the course of disease when diagnostic accuracy is least secure, the presence of an e4 allele can add at least 5–10% confidence to the diagnosis of AD (3). Thus, the clinically relevant use of ApoE testing is in patients with early dementia and suspected AD. As with autosomal dominant genetic mutations, APOE genotyping should be linked to adequate pre- and post-test counseling, education, and support. There is unanimous agreement that APOE genotyping should not be conducted in asymptomatic individuals. In line with this view, the commercially available test for APOE genotype is restricted to patients with cognitive impairments.

In summary, searching for PS1, PS2, and APP genetic abnormalities should be limited to probands and families with a pattern of early-onset (<60 years old) FAD. Genetic testing should always be conducted in the framework of genetic counseling. APOE genotyping may be used as an adjunct test in the diagnostic workup of an individual with suspected AD; finding an e4 allele adds a small percentage of confidence to the clinical diagnosis.

Biomarkers Reflecting Neuropathological Changes in Brain

Amyloid Protein Derivatives in Blood and CSF. Numerous studies during the last 5–7 years have examined the possibility that proteolytic derivatives of the β-amyloid precursor protein (APP) are altered in amount in the CSF or plasma of patients with AD compared to age-matched controls. The interest in using APP derivatives as laboratory markers to help confirm a clinical diagnosis of AD arises from evidence that cerebral accumulation of the amyloid β-peptide (Aβ) a fragment of APP, occurs in virtually all cases of AD.

One criterion for a potentially useful diagnostic test is a biologically plausible relationship of the marker to the pathogenesis of the disease. In this regard, all four currently known genetic causes of FAD (missense mutations in the APP, PS1, APP genes, and the e4 polymorphism of the ApoE gene) have been linked to increased production and/or deposition of Aβ, as measured directly in the brains and/or biological fluids of patients harboring each of these AD genetic traits. Moreover, deposits of the $A\beta_{42}$ peptide in the form of so-called diffuse plaques have been shown to be among the earliest detectable neuropathological alterations in the brains of patients with both familial and sporadic forms of AD. As a result, numerous research groups have assayed CSF and/or plasma for the APP metabolities APP_s (the large soluble ectodomain fragment of APP normally secreted by cells) and $A\beta_{42}$ and $A\beta_{40}$, (the 42-residue and 40-residue forms of the Aβ fragment of APP normally secreted by cells).

Aβ Peptides. Studies assaying the amounts of total Aβ peptides ($A\beta_{total}$ = $A\beta_{42}$ + $A\beta_{40}$) in human CSF have shown no definite quantitative correlation with the presence of AD; thus, measuring $A\beta_{total}$ has no clear diagnostic utility. In contrast, several studies of $A\beta_{42}$ concentrations in CSF have shown a decrease in the levels of this peptide in subjects with AD compared to age-matched normal or neurologic disease control subjects (see Galasko; Lannfelt). The probable biological explanation for a decrease in $A\beta_{42}$ levels in AD CSF is that the levels of soluble $A\beta_{42}$ in the brain interstitial fluid decrease as the peptide becomes increasingly insoluble and form deposits in the form of large numbers of diffuse and neuritic plaques. According to this formulation, the drop in soluble $A\beta_{42}$ in the brain is reflected by a decline in the soluble peptide in CSF. To date, at least 3 controlled studies by independent research groups in the United States and Japan have reported statistically significant decreases in CSF $A\beta_{42}$ levels in AD patients compared to controls (5,6,7). In each study, the levels of $A\beta_{42}$ in AD patients were significantly lower than those in controls having other neurological diseases. The mean decrease observed in 37 AD subjects was significant at $p < 0.0001$ when compared to mean levels in 32 neurologically diseased controls or 20 healthy controls (6). Simultaneous measurement of CSF $A\beta_{total}$ levels in the same subjects showed no significant differences, underscoring the specific involvement of $A\beta_{42}$ peptide. In this study, a CSF level of 505 pg/mL of $A\beta_{42}$ was used to separate optimally AD from subjects with other neurological diseases and from normal control subjects. Use of this level as a cutoff led to a calculated sensitivity of 100% and a specificity of 63% for low $A\beta_{42}$ as a marker for the presence of clinical AD.

Simultaneous analysis of $A\beta_{42}$ and tau protein measurements in the same CSF sample demonstrated a correlation of low $A\beta_{42}$ plus high tau levels with a clinical diagnosis of AD. With certain specific cutoffs for $A\beta_{42}$ and tau levels, the presence of elevated tau plus reduced $A\beta_{42}$ levels in a CSF sample showed a specificity of 96% for AD. Conversely, high $A\beta_{42}$ and low tau levels were observed only in control patients in this study. The mean $A\beta_{42}$ level in 20 AD patients was less than half the mean level in 34 control subjects with neurological diseases ($p < 0.0005$) (7). Thus all studies completed to date have shown significant decreases in mean CSF $A\beta_{42}$ levels, usually correlated with significant increases in mean CSF tau levels, in clinically probable AD subjects. Sensitivities for the clinical diagnosis of AD compared to normal nondemented subjects for finding low CSF $A\beta_{42}$/high tau levels have been found to be in the range of 60–94%, and specificities for the clinical diagnosis of AD were in the range of 70–96%. These values are much lower, however, when compared to subjects with non-Alzheimer neurological diseases (5).

Aβ in Plasma. A single published study has reported an increase in plasma $A\beta_{42}$ levels in a small subset (~10–20%) of SAD subjects (8). Elevation of plasma $A\beta_{42}$ levels has also been reported in subjects bearing mutations in the APP or the presenilin genes, including some subjects who were still presymptomatic (see Iwatsubo). Insufficient numbers of well-powered, controlled studies of $A\beta_{42}$ levels in plasma have been completed to allow any firm conclusion about the potential diagnostic utility of plasma Aβ in SAD.

Aβ in Urine. There has been a report of the detection of Aβ peptides in human urine, but no clinical studies of its possible diagnostic utility in AD or control subjects have been completed. *APP$_s$ in CSF.* A number of studies quantitating the APP ectodomain derivative, APP$_s$, in CSF of AD vs. control subjects have been published. Most studies have shown no clear statistically significant difference between these subjects. However, several published studies in which the APP$_s$ levels were assayed by one research group using a particular antibody that recognizes native APP$_s$ provided evidence of deceased levels of APP$_s$ in subjects with clinical AD, including subjects with sporadic or familial forms of the disease (see Lannfelt). Some of the studies utilizing this antibody reported a correlation between low CSF levels of APP$_s$ and poor performance on cognitive tests. One study using the same antibody also found significant decreases in CSF APP$_s$ in four patients with Gerstmann-Straussler-Scheinker disease, leading to the authors' suggestion that low levels of APP$_s$ may not be unique to diseases characterized by β-amyloid deposition, but also occur in other disease processes involving neuritic pathology or neuronal degeneration. Overall, the utility APP$_s$ levels in confirming a clinical diagnosis of AD has not yet been established.

CSF Tau. The known correlation between the abundance of neurofibrillary lesions in the brain and clinical indices of dementia has resulted in a surge of recent studies of CSF levels of tau in AD patients (see Galasko; Hock) (9,11). Using enzyme-linked immunosorbant assays (ELISAs), studies have shown that the levels of CSF tau are significantly elevated in AD patients compared to normal elderly control subjects. However, elevated levels of CSF tau were detected in patients with other acute and chronic neurological diseases, including dementing disorders that resemble AD clinically. Not surprisingly, the sensitivity and specificity of a CSF tau assay will vary depending on the patient population examined. For example, a CSF tau level of 70 pg/mL or greater identified probable AD patients with a sensitivity of 82% and a specificity of 70% when compared to non-demented healthy control subjects (10). However, when patients with a clinical diagnosis of possible AD were compared to control subjects or patients with other non-Alzheimer dementias, it was difficult to determine a CSF tau cutoff level that was diagnostically informative. In addition to their potential as a diagnostic aid, CSF tau assays may become useful as predictors of their progression to AD in individuals with memory impairments but who do not meet clinical criteria for dementia (9). Overall, detecting elevated levels of tau in CSF is a promising antemortem marker for establishing or confirming a diagnosis of AD, and possibly for monitoring progression of disease and response to treatment. Additional research, including development of more specific tau antibodies, might improve measurement of tau (either alone or in combination with other potential protein markers in the CSF such as amyloid fragments, kineses, and proteases) as a reliable, sensitive and specific biomarker of AD.

CSF Neuronal Thread Protein. Neuronal thread proteins (NTP) are a family of molecules that are expressed in the brain, and that are immunologically related to pancreatic thread protein. In a postmortem study, brains from patients with AD contained significantly more NTP-immunoreactivity than brains from patients with other neurological diseases and brains from control subjects without disease (14). Examining CSF, it was reported that levels of NTP were increased in advanced cases of AD, and correlated with progression of dementia and neuronal degeneration (13). The NTP fragment in CSF is a 41-kDa protein; levels above 3 ng/mL identified 62% of patients with clinically diagnosed AD and 84% of neuropathologically verified cases (12). Although measurement of NTP in CSF appears to be a promising biomarker for AD, there is a need to confirm sensitivity and specificity in additional independent studies in living patients.

CSF Neurotransmitters and Neurotransmitter Metabolites. Neurochemical analyses of brain tissue obtained at postmortem examination and with surgical biopsy reveal deficits in multiple neurotransmitter systems. Among neuronal populations affected, those that synthesize and release acetylcholine are most affected, although there are deficits in monoamines and neuropeptides (17). Analyzing CSF for neurotransmitters and their metabolites began shortly after the initial discoveries of these abnormalities in brain. This strategy was based on the fact that CSF bathes the brain and spinal cord and might reflect alterations in the state of activity of adjacent neural tissue. It was therefore anticipated that the neurotransmitter abnormalities in brain would be reflected in the CSF. The initial enthusiasm for this line of investigation quickly faded because all markers had poor sensitivity and specificity (15). Somatostastin is a typical exemple: mean CSF levels were significantly reduced in AD, but the range of individual values overlapped with normal control and neurologic control subjects and precluded diagnostic specificity (16).

In summary, tests directed toward detecting neuropathological features of AD are among the most promising approaches to defining biomarkers. The diagnostic utility of finding increased levels of $A\beta_{42}$ in plasma is mostly limited to FAD, but levels of $A\beta_{42}$ in CSF are significantly decreased in many patients with SAD. A universal finding is that mean CSF levels of tau are increased in AD. CSF measures of $A\beta$ and tau alone have modest sensitivities and specificities, but these indices improve when the two measures are combined. Detecting alterations in other proteins in CSF that are specific to AD, such as NTP, appears promising for early diagnosis and for monitoring change over time or in response to treatment but requires further study prior to clinical use.

Systemic Alterations as Molecular and Biochemical Markers of AD

Skin. The discovery that the $A\beta$ peptide circulated in blood and CSF, coupled with the development of specific antibodies to amyloid fragments, allowed investigators to test the hypothesis that patients with AD would have greater deposits of amyloid in peripheral tissues than those without AD. Although this prediction was true in skin biopsy tissue, there was substantial overlap with nondemented elderly control subjects (24). This lack of specificity precluded testing for amyloid deposits in skin biopsy as a biomarker for AD.

Olfactory Epithelium. AD patients show evidence of olfactory perception deficits early in the course of disease, and the olfactory epithelium is accessible for biopsy during life. Dystrophic neurites in postmortem and in vivo biopsy samples of the olfactory epithelium from patients with AD have been described (29). However, similar lesions have been described in the olfactory epithelium of individuals with other conditions, including those without neurological disease. Thus, examining olfactory epithelium is not a useful biological marker for AD.

Fibroblasts. Electrophysiological and biochemical abnormalities have been identified in fibroblasts that are hypothesized to reflect changes in the central nervous system of patients with AD. (19,23) Dysfunction in potassium channels was described in fibroblasts from AD patients compared to control subjects (19). Changes in protein kinase C activity were identified in AD fibroblasts compared to control subjects (21). These techniques have not gained currency as biological markers for AD, in part because of overlap with non-AD subjects, in part because of the invasive nature of the test (a skin biopsy is required), and in part because of the complexity and sophistication of the assays. Studies with fibroblasts, however, show promise as a method of studying AD-related mechanisms, including APP processing (20).

Platelets. An abnormality of increased platelet membrane fluidity was first described in 1984 (32). This finding was a surprise, as membrane fluidity generally decreases with advancing age. Nonetheless, subsequent investigations confirmed the increased fluidity in AD, although there are the substantial overlaps between AD and control subjects that limits its diagnostic value (31). There is even the proposal that increased membrane fluidity is a risk factor that predicts development of AD (33), but this observation requires independent confirmation. There is increasing evidence of mitochondrial abnormalities in AD that lead to reductions in ATP and increases in oxygen-reactive species that damage neurons (26). Decreased mitochondrial cytochrome C oxidase activity in platelets of AD patients has been described (27). Subsequently, the decrease in cytochrome oxidase activity in AD patients compared to control subjects was confirmed, and it was shown that this deficit corresponded to an increase in reactive oxygen species (18). This finding is controversial however and may reflect a technical artifact (30). Additional studies will be needed to substantiate the role of oxidative stress in the neuronal damage of AD, and the sensitivity and specificity of complex IV abnormalities in AD, before this test can be accepted as a biological marker.

Blood. It has been reported that the soluble form of the iron-binding protein p97 was elevated in AD patients compared to control subjects (25). All AD patients had elevated levels of p97 in their serum compared with controls, and there were no overlaps between these two groups. To date, this report has not been extended by the authors; no reports confirming or repudiating these data have appeared from other groups.

Tropicamide Eye Test. Pupil dilation in response to installation of a dilute solution of tropicamide has been proposed as a non-invasive biological diagnostic test for AD (28). In the original report, the test had a sensitivity of 95% and a specificity of 94%. In subsequent studies, the specificity was lower with much more overlap between AD and control groups; in some reports (22), there was no difference in dilation response between AD and non-demented control subjects.

In summary, none of the systemic alterations proposed as characteristic biological markers of AD can be accepted for widespread use at present. Some of the markers such as amyloid deposits in the skin, detecting dystrophic neurites in olfactory epitheliutn, and measuring pupil dilation in response to a dilute solution of tropicamide, lack sufficient specificity to qualify as useful biological markers. Although serum levels of the p97 protein showed complete separation between AD and control groups in the sole report to date, additional confirmatory studies will be necessary before accepting this test as a biological marker. Studies with fibroblasts provide a method of examining electrophysiological and biochemical changes believed to take place in brains of patients with AD. This potential use outweighs their current clinical value as diagnostic markers.

Acknowledgment

The workshop and the publication of this supplement were sponsored in part by an unrestricted grant to the Alzheimer's Association from Athena Neurosciences, Inc.

References

Genetics
1. Saunders, A. M.; Hulette, C.; Welsh-Bohmer, K. A., et al. Specificity, sensitivity, and predictive value of apolipoprotein E genotyping for sporadic Alzheimer's disease. Lancet 348:90–93; 1996.
2. Saunders, A. M.; Strittmatter, W. J.; Schmechel, D., et al. Association of apolipoprotein E allele e4 with late-onset familial and sporadic Alzheimer's disease. Neurology 43:1467–72; 1993.
3. Mayeux, R.; Saunders, A. M.; Shea, S., et al. Utility of the Apolipoprotein-E Genotype in the diagnosis of Alzheimer's disease. New Engl. J. Med. 338:506–511; 1998.
4. Welsh-Bohmer, K. A.; Gearing, M.; Saunders, A. M., et al. Apolipoprotein E Genotype in a Neuropathological Series from the Consortium to Establish a Registry for Alzheimer's Disease. Ann. Neurol. 42:319–325; 1997.

Amyloid
5. Galasko, D.; Chang, L.; Motter, R., et al. High cerebrospinal fluid tau and low amyloid beta 42 levels in the clinical diagnosis of Alzheimer disease and relation to apolipoprotein ε genotype. Arch. Neurol. (in press).
6. Motter, R.; Vigo-Pillrey, C.; Kholodenko, D.; Barbour, R.; Johnson-Wood, K.; Galasko, D.; Chang, L.; Miller, B.; Clark, C.; Green, R., et al. Reduction of beta-amyloid peptide 42 in the cerebrospinal fluid of patients with Alzheimer's disease. Ann. Neurol. 38:643–648; 1995.
7. Tamaoka, A.; Sawamura, N.; Fukushima, T.; Shoji, S.; Matsubara. E.; Shoji. M.; Hirai, S.; Furiya, Y.; Endoh, R.; Mori, H. Amyloid b-protein 42 (43) in cerebrospinal fluid of patients with Alzheimer's disease. J. Neurol. Sci. 148:41–45; 1997.
8. Scheuner, D.; Eckman, C.; Jensen, M.; Song, X.; Citron, M.; Suzuki, N.; Bird, T. D.;

Hardy, J.; Hutton, M.; Kukull, W.; Larson, E.; Levy-Lahad, E.; Viitanen, M.; Peskind, E.; Poorkaj, P.; Schellenberg, G.; Tanzi, R. E.; Wasco, W.; Lannfelt, L.; Selkoe, D.; Younkin, S. Aβ42(43) is increased in vivo by the PS1/2 and APP mutations linked to familial Alzheimer's disease. Nature Medicine 2:864–870; 1996.

Tau

 9. Arai, H.; Nakagawa, T.; Kosaka, Y.; Higuchi, M.; Matsui, T.; Okamura, N.; Sasaki, H. Elevated cerebrospinal fluid tau protein level as a predictor of dementia in memory-impaired individuals. Alzheimer's Res. 3:211–213; 1997.
10. Clark, C. M.; Ewbank, D.; Lee, V.; Trojanowski, J. Q. Molecular pathology of Alzheimer's disease: Neuronal cytoskeletal abnormalities. In: Growdon, J. H.; Rossor, M., eds., The Dementias. Newton, MA: Butterworth Heinemann; (in press).
11. Trojanowski, J. Q.; Clark, C. M.; Arai, H.; Lee, V. Elevated levels of tau in cerebrospinal fluid: Implications for the antemortem diagnosis of Alzheimer's disease. Alzheimer's Disease Review 1:77–83; 1996.

Neuronal Thread Protein

12. de la Monte, S. M.; Ghanbari, K.; Frey, W. H.; Beheshti, l.; Averback, P.; Hauser, S. A.; Ghanbari, H. A.; Wands, J. R. Characterization of the AD7C-NTP cDNA expression in Alzbeimer's disease and measurement of a 41-kD protein in cerebrospinal fluid. J. Clin. Invest. 100:3093–3104; 1997.
13. de la Monte, S. M.; Volicer, L.; Heuser, S. L.; Wands, J. R. Increased levels of neuronal thread protein in cerebrospinal fluid of patients with Alzheimer's disease. Ann. Neurol. 32:733–742, 1992.
14. de la Monte, S. M.; Wands, J. R. Neuronal thread protein overexpression in brains with Alzheimer's disease lesions. J. Neurol. Sci. 113:152–164; 1992.

Neurotransmitter

15. Beal, M. F.; Growdon, J. H. CSF neurotransmitter markers in Alzheimer's disease. Prog. Neuro-psycholpharmacol. & Biol. Psychiat. 10:259–270; 1986.
16. Beal, M. F.; Growdon, J. H.; Mazurek, M. F.; Martin, J. B. CSF somatostatin-like immunoreactivity in dementia. Neurology 36:294–297; 1986.
17. Terry, R. D.; Davies, P. Dementia of the Alzheimer type. Ann. Rev. Neurosci. 3:77–95; 1980.

Systemic

18. Davis, R. E.; Miller, S.; Hernstadt, C.; Ghosh, S. S.; Fahy, E.; Parker, W. D. Jr. Mutations in mitochondrial cytochrome C oxidase genes segregate with late-onset Alzheimer disease. Proc. Natl. Acad. Sci. USA 94:4526–31; 1997.
19. Etcheberrigaray, R.; Ito, E.; Oka, K.; Tofel-Grehl, B.; Gibson, G. E.; Alkon, D. L. Potassium channel dysfunction in fibroblasts identifies patients with Alzheimer disease. Proc. Natl. Acad. Sci. USA 90:8209–13; 1993.
20. Gasparini, L.; Benussi, L.; Curti, D.; Racchi, M.; Govoni, S.; Bianchetti, A.; Trabucchi, M.; Ginetti, G. Inhibition of energy metabolism alters APP secretion in Alzheimer's disease fibroblasts. Soc. Neurosci. Abs. 23:332–3; 1997.
21. Govonl, S.; Bergamaschi, S.; Racchi, M.; Battaini, F.; Binetti, G.; Bianchetti, A.; Trabucchi, M. Cytosol protein kinase C down regulation in fibroblasts from Alzheimer's disease patients. Neurology 43:2581–86; 1993.

22. Growdon, J. H.; Graefe, K.; Tennis, M.; Hayden, D.; Schoenteld, D.; Wray, S. H. Pupil dilation to tropicamide is not specific for Alzheimer disease. Arch. Neurol. 54:841–44; 1997.

23. Hirashima, N.; Etchabarrigaray, R.; Bergamaschi, S.; Racchi., M.; Battaini, F.; Binctti, G.; Govoni, S.; Alkon, D. L. Calcium responses in human fibroblasts: A diagnostic Molecular profile for Alzhchner's disease. Neurobiol. Aging 17:549–55; 1996.

24. Joachim, C. T.; Mori, H.; Selkoe, D. L. Amyloid β-protein deposition in tissues other than brain in Alzheimer's disease. Nature 341 :226–30; 1989.

25. Kennard, M. L.; Feldman, H.; Yamada, T.; Jeffries, W. A. Serum levels of the iron binding protein p97 are elevated in Alzheimer's disease. Nature Med. 2:1230–35; 1996.

26. Kish, S. J.; Bergeron, C.; Rojput, A.; Dozic, 9.; Mastrogiacomo, F.; Chang, L.-J.; Wilson, J. M. Brain cytochrome oxidase in Alzheimer's disease. J. Neurochem. 59:776–9; 1992.

27. Parker, W. D. Jr.; Filley, C. M.; Parks, J. K. Cytochrome oxidase deficiency in Alzheimer's disease. Neurology 40:1302–3; 1990.

28. Scinto, L. F.; Daftner, K. R.; Dressler, D., et al. A potential noninvasive neurobiological test for Alzheimer's disease. Science 266:1051–54; 1994.

29. Talamo, B.; Feng, W.-H.; Perez-Cruet, L.; Adelmen, L.; Kosik., K.; Lee, V.M.-Y.; Cork, L. C.; Kauer, J. S. Pathologic changes in olfactory neurons of Alzheimer's disease. Ann. N. Y. Acad. Sci. 640: 1–7; 1991.

30. Wallace, D. C.; Stugard, C.; Murdock, D.; Schurn, T.; Brown, M. D. Ancient mtDNA sequence in the human nuclear genome: A potential source of errors in identifying pathogenic mutations. Proc. Natl. Acad. Sci. USA 94:14900–14905; 1997.

31. Zubenko, G. S.; Cohen, B. M.; Boller, F.; Malinakova, M. S.; Chojnacki,, B. Platelet membrane abnormality in Alzheimer's disease. Ann. Neurol. 22:237–44; 1987.

32. Zubenko, G. S.; Cohen, R. M.; Growdon, J. H.; Corkin, S. Cell membrane abnormality in Alzheimer's disease. Lancet 2:236; 1984.

33. Zubenko, G. S.; Teply, M. S.; Winwood, E.; Huff, T. J.; Moossy, J.; Sunderland, T.; Martinez, A. J. Prospective study of increased platelet membrane fluidity as a risk factor for Alzheimer's disease: Results at 6 years. Am. J. Psychiatry 153:420–23; 1996.

Appendix

Members of the Working Group submitted position papers. The ideas and the perspectives represented in these papers helped shape the consensus statement and were useful in the preparation of the final report. The Advisory Committee of the Working Group gratefully acknowledges the contribution of these authors. Some of these papers, listed below, are being published in this supplement.

The Working Group Advisory Committee

Peter Davies, Ph.D., Judith and Burton Resnick Professor of Alzheimer's Disease Research, Albert Einstein College of Medicine of Yeshiva University, Bronx, New York.

Sid Gilman, M.D., Chair, Department of Neurology, Michigan Alzheimer's Disease Research Center, University of Michigan, Ann Arbor, Michigan.

John H. Growdon, M.D., Chair, Professor, Department of Neurology, Massachusetts General Hospital, Boston, Massachusetts.

Zaven S. Khachaturian, Ph.D., Director, Ronald and Nancy Reagan Research Institute, Alzheimer's Association, Chicago, Illinois.

Teresa S. Radebaugh, Sc.D., Deputy Director, Ronald and Nancy Reagan Research Institute, Alzheimer's Association, Chicago, Illinois.

Allen D. Roses, M.D., Vice-President and World-Wide Director, Genetics, Glaxo Wellcome Research and Development, Research Triangle Park, North Carolina.

Dennis J. Selkoe, M.D., Director, Center for Neurologic Diseases, Brigham & Women's Hospital, Boston, Massachusetts.

John Q. Trojanowski, M.D., Ph.D., Professor, Pathology & Laboratory Medicine, University of Pennsylvania Medical Center, Philadelphia, Pennsylvania.

The Members of Working Group

John P. Blass (Gary E. Gibson, K.-F. R. Sheu), Burke Medical Research Institute/Cornell University Medical College, White Plains, New York.

Kaj Blennow, Department of Clinical Neuroscience, Unit of Psychiatry and Neurochemistry, University of Goteberg, Sweden, and the Swedish Medical Research Council, Stockholm, Sweden.

Andre Delacourte, Director of Research INSERM, Place de Verdun, Lille, France.

Giovanni B. Frisoni, Geriatric Research Group, Istituto, Sacro Cuore di Gesu, Brescia, Italy.

Wilfred A. Jefferies, The Biotechnology Laboratory and the Departments of Medical Genetics, Microbiology and Immunology, and Zoology, the University of British Columbia, Vancouver, British Columbia, Canada.

Amanda McRae, Department of Anatomy and Cell Biology, University of Goteborg, Goteborg, Sweden.

H. M. Wisniewski (P.D. Mehta, T. Pirttla), New York State Institute for Basic Research in Developmental Disabilities, Staten Island, New York.

Ram Parshad, Department of Pathology, College of Medicine, Howard University, Washington, D.C.

Leonard F. M. Scinto, Laboratory of Higher Cortical Functions, Brigham and Women's Hospital, Boston, Massachusetts.

Philip Scheltens, Department of Neurology, Academisch Ziekenhuis Vrije Universiteit, Amsterdam, The Netherlands.

Paavo J. Riekkinen (Hilkka S. Soininen), Department of Neuroscience and Neurology, Kuopio University, Kuopio, Finland.

Gregory R. J. Swanwick, Mercer's Institute for Research on Ageing, St. James's Hospital, Dublin, Ireland.

Lars-Olof Wahlund, Department of Clinical Neuroscience and Family Medicine, Karolinska Institute, Huddinge University Hospital, Huddinge, Sweden.

John Q. Trojanowski (S. E. Amoltl, Virghlia M.-Y. Lee), Department of Pathology and Laboratory Medicine, University of Pennsylvania, School of Medicine, Philadelphia, Pennsylvania.

Bengt Winblad (Lars-Olof Wahlund), Department of Clinical Neuroscience and Family Medicine, Karolinska Institute, Huddinge University Hospital, Huddinge, Sweden.

Yasuo Ihara (Tsuneo Yamazaki), Department of Neuropathology, Faculty of Medicine, University of Tokyo, Tokyo, Japan.

Position Papers Published in this Volume

Hiroyuki Arai, Christopher M. Clark, Douglas C. Ewbank, Sadao Takase, Susumu Higuchi, Masakazu Mirua, Hisatomo Seki, Makoto Higuchi, Toshifumi Matsui, Virginia M.-Y. Lee, John Q. Trojanowski, Hidetata Sasaki, Department of Geriatric Medicine, Tohoku University School of Medicine, Sendal 980, Japan. "Cerebrospinal Fluid Tau Protein as a Potential Diagnostic Marker in Alzheimer's Disease."

Norman L. Foster, Michigan Alzheimer's Disease Research Center, University of Michigan, Ann Arbor, Michigan. "The Development of Biological Markers for the Diagnosis of Alzheimer's Disease."

Douglas Galasko, Department of Neurosciences, University of California, San Diego, San Diego, California. "CSF Tau and AB42: Logical Biomarkers for Alzheimer's Disease?"

Christoph Hock, Department of Psychiatry, University of Basel, Basel, Switzerland. "Biological Markers of Alzheimer's Disease."

Bradley T. Hyman, Harvard Medical School, Boston, Massachusetts. "Biomarkers in Alzheimer's Disease."

P. H. St. George-Hyslop, Center for Research in Neurodegenerative Diseases, University of Toronto, Toronto, Canada. "Role of Genetics in Tests of Genotype, Status and Disease Progression in Early Onset Alzheimer's Disease."

Takeshi Iwatsubo, Department of Neuropathology and Neuroscience, University of Toyko, Toyko, Japan. "Amyloid B Protein in Plasma as a Diagnostic Marker for Alzheimer's Disease."

Malcolm Kennard, The Biotechnology Laboratory, The University of British Columbia, Vancouver, British Columbia, Canada. "Position Paper Regarding: Diagnostic Markers for Alzheimer's Disease."

William E. Klunk, University of Pittsburgh Medical Center, Laboratory of Neurophysics, Pittsburgh, Pennsylvania. "Biological Markers of Alzheimer's Disease."

Lars Lannfelt, Karolinska Institute, Department of Clinical Neuroscience (Geriatric Medicine, Huddinge Hospital, Huddinge, Sweden. "Biochemical Diagnostic Markers to Detect Early Alzheimer's Disease."

Irene Litvan, Neuroepidemiology Branch, National Institute of Neurological Disorders and Stroke, National Institutes of Health, Bethesda, Maryland. "Methodological and Research Issues in the Evaluation of Biological Diagnostic Markers for Alzheimer's Disease."

Richard Mayeux, Gertrude H. Sergievsky Center, Columbia University, College of Physicians and Surgeons, New York, New York. "Evaluation and Use of Diagnostic Tests in Alzheimer's Disease."

Alfredo Robles, Division of Neurology, Complejo Hospitalario, University of Santiago, Santiago de Compostela, Spain. "Some Remarks on Biological Markers of Alzheimer's Disease."

Note: The following three additional, previously published, papers were submitted, and are noted for information of the reader.

Fabian, V. A.; Jones, T. M.; Wilton, S. D.; Dench, J. E.; Davis, M. R.; Lim, L.; Kakulas, B. A. Alzheimer's Disease and Apolipoprotein E Genotype in Western Australia: an Autopsy-verified Series, MJA 165:77–80; 1996.

Kennard, M. L.; Feldman, H.; Yamada, T.; Jeffries, W. A. Serum Levels of the Iron Binding Protein p97 are Elevated in Alzheimer's Disease, Nature Med. 2:1230–1235; 1996.

Sweet, R. A.; Zubenko, G. S. Peripheral Markers in Alzheimer's Disease, In: Burns, A; Levy, R., eds., Dementia, London: Chapman & Hall; 1994.

Index